Vaccinating Britain

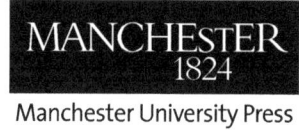
Manchester University Press

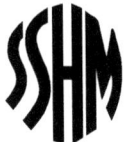

SOCIAL HISTORIES OF MEDICINE

Series editors: *David Cantor* and *Keir Waddington*

Social Histories of Medicine is concerned with all aspects of health, illness and medicine, from prehistory to the present, in every part of the world. The series covers the circumstances that promote health or illness, the ways in which people experience and explain such conditions, and what, practically, they do about them. Practitioners of all approaches to health and healing come within its scope, as do their ideas, beliefs, and practices, and the social, economic and cultural contexts in which they operate. Methodologically, the series welcomes relevant studies in social, economic, cultural, and intellectual history, as well as approaches derived from other disciplines in the arts, sciences, social sciences and humanities. The series is a collaboration between Manchester University Press and the Society for the Social History of Medicine.

Previously published

The metamorphosis of autism: A history of child development in Britain *Bonnie Evans*

Payment and philanthropy in British healthcare, 1918–48 *George Campbell Gosling*

The politics of vaccination: A global history *Edited by Christine Holmberg, Stuart Blume and Paul Greenough*

Leprosy and colonialism: Suriname under Dutch rule, 1750–1950 *Stephen Snelders*

Medical misadventure in an age of professionalization, 1780–1890 *Alannah Tomkins*

Conserving health in early modern culture: Bodies and environments in Italy and England *Edited by Sandra Cavallo and Tessa Storey*

Migrant architects of the NHS: South Asian doctors and the reinvention of British general practice (1940s–1980s) *Julian M. Simpson*

Mediterranean quarantines, 1750–1914: Space, identity and power *Edited by John Chircop and Francisco Javier Martínez*

Sickness, medical welfare and the English poor, 1750–1834 *Steven King*

Medical societies and scientific culture in nineteenth-century Belgium *Joris Vandendriessche*

Managing diabetes, managing medicine: Chronic disease and clinical bureaucracy in post-war Britain *Martin D. Moore*

Vaccinating Britain

Mass vaccination and the public since the Second World War

Gareth Millward

Manchester University Press

Copyright © Gareth Millward 2019

The right of Gareth Millward to be identified as the author of this work has been asserted by him in accordance with the Copyright, Designs and Patents Act 1988.

An electronic version of this book is also available under a Creative Commons (CC-BY-NC-ND) licence, thanks to the support of the Wellcome Trust, which permits non-commercial use, distribution and reproduction provided the author(s) and Manchester University Press are fully cited and no modifications or adaptations are made. Details of the licence can be viewed at https://creativecommons.org/licenses/by-nc-nd/4.0/

Published by Manchester University Press
Altrincham Street, Manchester M1 7JA

www.manchesteruniversitypress.co.uk

British Library Cataloguing-in-Publication Data
A catalogue record for this book is available from the British Library

ISBN   978 1 5261 2675 7   hardback
ISBN   978 1 5261 2676 4   open access

First published 2019

The publisher has no responsibility for the persistence or accuracy of URLs for any external or third-party internet websites referred to in this book, and does not guarantee that any content on such websites is, or will remain, accurate or appropriate.

Typeset
by Toppan Best-set Premedia Limited
Printed in Great Britain
by Lightning Source

Contents

List of figures and tables	page vi
Acknowledgements	vii
Abbreviations	x
Introduction	1
Part I The development and evolution of the vaccination programme	29
1 Diphtheria	31
2 Smallpox	72
3 Poliomyelitis	114
Part II Vaccination crises	147
4 Pertussis	149
5 MMR	180
Conclusion	220
Select bibliography	236
Index	272

Figures and tables

Figures

1.1	England and Wales: diphtheria deaths, 1931–48	page 40
3.1	Poliomyelitis notifications, 1939–69	118
4.1	Pertussis notifications, England and Wales, 1940–2005	154
5.1	Percentage of children receiving first dose of MMR before 24 months in London, rest of England and Scotland, 1999–2000, 2015–16	182
5.2	Mentions of MMR in major daily newspapers, 1996–2016	190
5.3	Notifications of measles in England and Wales, 1940–2015	203

Tables

1.1	Family background and immunisation	51
1.2	Diphtheria notifications and deaths in England and Wales, 1938–60	59
2.1	Importations of smallpox into England and Wales, 1936–70	76–7
2.2	Select vaccination rates as at 31 December 1964	79

Acknowledgements

The research for this book was possible thanks to the generous funding of the Wellcome Trust. It forms part of the Wellcome Investigator Award 'Placing the Public in Public Health: Public Health in Britain, 1948–2010' (grant number WT-100586-Z-12-Z). The work was completed at the Centre for History in Public Health at the London School of Hygiene and Tropical Medicine. I am grateful to the staff at The National Archives, Coventry History Centre at the Herbert Museum and the various digital curators and platform providers for providing access to the material which forms the core of this research. Special thanks are also due to the Wellcome Library for granting permission to reproduce Figure 1.1 from its digitised collection of London Pulse Medical Officer of Health reports. At Manchester University Press, I particularly want to thank Tom Dark for his encouragement and swift replies to garbled emails and Keir Waddington, editor of the Social History of Medicine Series, for his feedback, help and thorough comments.

I owe a huge debt to Alex Mold, the principal investigator on the Wellcome award, my boss and mentor over the three years of my Research Fellowship at the School. She has made sure that I have stayed on course with the research, made my writing more readable and helped guide my career. If this book is useful to anyone it is because of her; and if not, the fault lies with me, the author. I must also thank Martin Moore and Harriet Palfreyman, who have read through countless drafts of this manuscript and offered constructive advice and criticism throughout. They have challenged my assertions and clarified my thinking. I have come to learn that no amount of praise is ever good enough for them. Daisy Payling, Peder Clark and Hannah Elizabeth, my colleagues on

'Placing the Public' have been excellent co-workers, sounding boards and friends over the years. All have helped me to ask new questions of my material, especially Hannah and the work we have done together on the history of emotion within the 1950s polio vaccination programme.

I joined the Centre for History in Public Health as a PhD student in 2009. It has been an uncommonly supportive environment in which to work and study. I must pay particular thanks to my PhD supervisor, Martin Gorsky, who has continued to be a mentor; and the outgoing head of the centre, Virginia Berridge. Ingrid James has been a superb administrator, without whom I am sure I could not have got through the past eight years. Christopher Sirrs and Tim Crocker-Bruque have given useful notes on drafts of work related to this project, for which I am grateful. Thanks too to Stuart Anderson, Hayley Brown, Angela Grainger, Anne Hardy, John Manton, Susanne McGregor, Jane Seymour, Ros Stanwell-Smith, Sue Taylor, Jenny Walke, Mateusz Zatonski and all members past and present for making the Centre a vibrant place to do research.

Claire Frankland, Victoria Cranna, Dolly Padalia and Lisa Heiler were incredibly supportive in the organisation of an exhibition at the School in 2015 which sparked a number of ideas and allowed me to make a number of contacts. So too were Tracy Chantler and Pauline Paterson with a series of symposiums. I am grateful for the time, resources and encouragement of Heidi Larson at the School and Jo Yarwood at Public Health England, whose wealth of experience made the writing of the later chapters much easier and more rewarding. I must also thank Ian Milligan and Niels Brügger for encouraging my work on the Internet Archive and commissioning a book chapter from me which fed directly into the research in Chapter 5. Jane Winters, Richard Deswarte and Peter Webster must also take credit. As I now move on to a new project with the Wellcome Trust, I must also make special mention of Mathew Thomson and Roberta Bivins at the University of Warwick for their encouragement, reading of draft material and sponsoring my application for a post which started in September 2017. It took a lot of stress out of the final months of submitting and revising the manuscript, as did the support of my new colleagues Jenny Crane, Jane Hand, Natalie Jones and Jack Saunders.

I am grateful to the editors and anonymous reviewers at Social History of Medicine and Contemporary British History for accepting my articles on polio and pertussis vaccination controversies. These helped to formulate the arguments in chapters 3 and 4 of this volume. Thanks also to the attendees and organisers of the Modern British Studies conferences in Birmingham (2015 and 2017), the Society for the Social History of Medicine conference in Kent (2016), the European Association for the History of Medicine and Health conferences in Cologne (2015) and Budapest (2017), the Voluntary Action History Society seminar series and the University of Birmingham's medical history seminar series. Baptiste Baylac-Paouly was gracious enough to invite me to speak at the Société française d'histoire des sciences et des techniques conference in Strasbourg in 2017. The feedback on papers given at these has helped enormously.

Finally, I must thank my family. Mom, Dad and Aidan have always encouraged me to pursue this career; and without my wife, Emma, I would not even have been able to start down this path, let alone continue on it. But I must dedicate this book to my uncle Bruce. Although the polio vaccination was available at the time – and even though his older brothers and sister had been given it – Nan decided that Bruce did not need it. Bruce contracted polio. As a result, my parents ensured that I got as many vaccines as they could find. Writing this book has not only given me an insight into the effects of childhood disease long eradicated from Britain, it has made me appreciate how and why people might choose to vaccinate or not. I would like to think it has not just made me understand why my parents were so fearful that they had me vaccinated. It has given me some understanding of why Nan – like a number of parents in Walsall in the 1960s – did not vaccinate uncle Bruce.

Abbreviations

APVDC	Association of Parents of Vaccine Damaged Children
BCG	Bacillus Calmette-Guérin
BMA	British Medical Association
BSE	bovine spongiform-encephalopathy
COI	Central Office of Information
COVER	Cover of Vaccination Evaluated Rapidly
CRS	Congenital Rubella Syndrome
CSM	Committee on the Safety of Medicines
DHSS	Department of Health and Social Security
DT	diphtheria-tetanus vaccine
DTwP	diphtheria-tetanus-whole-cell-pertussis vaccine
HPV	human papillomavirus
IPV	inactivated poliomyelitis vaccine
JABS	Justice Awareness and Basic Support
JCPV	Joint Committee on Poliomyelitis Vaccine
JCVI	Joint Committee on Vaccination and Immunisation
MMR	measles-mumps-rubella vaccine
MOH	Medical Officer of Health
MRC	Medical Research Council
NADBRC	National Association for Deaf/Blind and Rubella Children
NHS	National Health Service
OPV	oral poliomyelitis vaccine
SAGE	Strategic Advisory Group of Experts
SMAC	Standing Medical Advisory Committee
TNA	The National Archives
vCJD	variant Creutzfeldt-Jackob disease
WHO	World Health Organization

Introduction

Why do so many parents vaccinate their children? On a superficial level, this seems like an odd question. In recent years, public health professionals around the world have been much more concerned with parents who do not. A high-profile outbreak of measles in 2015 in Disneyland, California created headlines around the globe, leading the state government to reassess its policy for granting vaccination exemptions.[1] Meanwhile, rising morbidity in Western Europe in 2017 caused many nation-states to increase efforts to vaccinate children against measles, with some even resorting to compulsion.[2] Both in academic and popular media, anti-vaccinationism has been blamed for these trends. In the global North, communities of activists, buoyed by the internet and social media, have caused headaches even in long-established public health systems.[3] Attacks on health workers in the twenty-first-century Global Polio Eradication Initiative showed that resistance to vaccines was still very much a live issue in low-income countries, too.[4] Even where the scientific case has been successfully made that vaccines reduce the burden of infectious disease, moral and ethical concerns can cause much debate. For instance, in the 2010s the human papillomavirus (HPV) vaccine has highlighted trials on human subjects in low-income countries, the potential sexualisation of teenage girls and whether it is acceptable to gender public health responses by excluding boys from routine vaccination programmes.[5]

Despite these anxieties, most citizens and media commentators have appeared to be convinced of the power of vaccination. In February 2016, when the Zika virus was found to cause microcephaly in children born to infected mothers, governments and research institutions around the world clamoured for a vaccine to stem the outbreak.[6] The same was true six months earlier, when the Ebola crisis was declared a Public Health Emergency of International Concern.[7] As for Britain, in 2014–15, 92.3 per cent of children under the age of two years in England received their first dose of measles-mumps-rubella vaccine (MMR) and 94.2 per cent completed their course of vaccines against diphtheria, tetanus, pertussis (whooping cough), polio and Hib (the five-in-one vaccine).[8] Rates in Scotland were even higher.[9] In a 2016 survey conducted by the Vaccine Confidence Project at the London School of Hygiene and Tropical Medicine, 89.6 per cent of British respondents agreed or strongly agreed that vaccines were important; 84 per cent agreed that they were safe; and 86.7 per cent agreed that vaccination was effective.[10] These vaccines have been actively accepted, not just passively tolerated. British parents actively demanded protection for their children. When Faye Burdett, a two-year-old girl from Kent, died of meningitis in February 2016, her parents began a campaign to raise awareness of the existence of the meningitis B vaccine. Ex-England Rugby Union captain Matthew Dawson, whose own son nearly succumbed to the disease, gave added publicity to the cause and it caught national media attention. Over 800,000 people signed a petition demanding that the vaccine be given free to all children, not just those who had been born after 1 July 2015. It was the most-signed online petition since the UK government set up the UK Government and Parliament petitioning system.[11] It appeared that Britain, like the United States, had accepted what Jacob Heller calls "The Vaccine Narrative" – 'We simultaneously understand vaccines as a shield against diseases, a rite of passage for children and parents, and an expression of our science, civilization and morality.'[12]

This book examines how the routine immunisation of children became the status quo in Britain after the Second World War. It tells the story of how vaccination programmes became established in the modern British welfare state, how they expanded and how they were maintained. Successive British governments achieved this by responding to various challenges, including vaccine shortages, public scepticism over safety, scientific controversies and supply logistics. The schedule expanded from just two disease-prevention programmes in 1945 (smallpox and diphtheria) to around twenty routine and optional vaccines in 2018.[13] But this was not simply a government project to improve public health. The British public played a key role in shaping the priorities of the programme, in turn placing expectations on the British state and their fellow citizens. To turn the subtitle of Stuart Blume's latest volume on its head: this is not about "how vaccines became controversial"; it is about how they became ordinary.[14]

It would be obtuse to suggest that vaccines and vaccination are – or have ever been – uncontroversial. There have been countless disputes over the role of the pharmaceutical industry, state power, individual liberty, the diseases from which people require protection, the extent to which science should interfere in "natural" disease patterns and many more besides.[15] We have seen periods in which immunisation rates dropped dramatically as a result of losses in public confidence, most notably the 1970s (whooping cough) and 2000s (MMR). But such drops suggest a relatively robust "normal" from which they could fall. Parents in post-war Britain were much more likely to vaccinate their children than not, and compliance with recommended schedules increased significantly over that time. This volume does not attempt to analyse the individual or social psychologies surrounding decision making about vaccines (topics better addressed by other social science disciplines). Instead, it uses periods of disagreement between various government and public bodies over the post-war period to show how the relationship between the British state and its citizens forged the modern vaccination programme. In the 1940s it was not inevitable that public health and the British public would embrace vaccination in the form that they did. Rather, this emerged from a series of developments in vaccine technology, the expansion of the welfare state and changing expectations on the part of both the government and the public. Moreover, through investigating how vaccination policy changed in post-war Britain we begin to understand the fluid and changing role of the public in the practice of public health.

Vaccination in history

When the story of post-war vaccination is told by public health advocates, it is usually one of progress.[16] This is said to occur on both a scientific basis (the discovery of new techniques leading to the development of new vaccines) and a political one (the development of various administrative and bureaucratic systems for the effective delivery of vaccines to the masses).[17] While vaccines have not been the only factor in reducing morbidity and mortality from once-common diseases, epidemiologists are almost unanimous that improvements in the manufacture, administration and education surrounding vaccination have been vital.[18] Such narratives stress how dangerous infectious diseases were in the past and how their risks have been significantly reduced through the work of public health.[19]

While these Whiggish histories serve a useful political purpose, enhancing the reputation of disciplines and governance structures allied to public health, they do not critically reflect on how the growth in vaccination came about. Where there have been investigations into problematic areas of vaccination, they have focused on crises in confidence, but do so in a way that assumes that the default and rational position of the public is to support vaccination. Declines in vaccination rates or resurgences in once-controlled diseases are thus framed as aberrations caused by outside, irrational factors. Thus, the pertussis vaccine scandal of the 1970s or the MMR controversy of the 1990s and 2000s are studied from the perspective of "what went wrong", in order to prevent or manage such crises in the future.[20] Historians of medicine are wary about "learning lessons".[21] Rather, we tend to investigate the past to understand how people understood health, illness and medical care. These concepts are held to be historically contingent, and meant different things to different peoples at different times. How the public responded to new medical technologies or impositions from governments and health authorities can tell us much about cultures of the past. Existing studies of vaccination, for instance, have exposed Victorian attitudes towards the limits of local and national government,[22] while comparative analyses of poliomyelitis vaccines have shed light on the cold-war geopolitics surrounding the trustworthiness of capitalist or communist epidemiological practice and medical ethics.[23] Crucially for this study, work on diphtheria and tuberculosis immunisations has highlighted how different nation-states' cultural attitudes towards medicine and science produced very different interpretations of the same scientific data.[24] This, in turn, resulted in very different policy choices and outcomes.

Given this history, it is clear that vaccination programmes – like any other political project – are rooted in a wider social context. This book explores this through a series of case studies which highlight the ways in which the public and governments interacted, shaping public health as they went. What was expected of the public and of the government changed over this period; and the debates over vaccination show wider concerns about the relationship between the state, its citizens and the nature of public health governmentality.[25] The book does this by building on existing histories of specific diseases and vaccine crises. This has been a common feature of the historiography of British immunisation policy. Works on the introduction of BCG (Bacillus Calmette-Guérin, an anti-tuberculosis vaccine), diphtheria immunisation, polio vaccine and hepatitis B vaccine have given insight into the scientific, political and cultural context of vaccination and how it was received by the public.[26] Less attention has been paid to the mundane business of established immunisation programmes which did not cause significant controversy. It is generally assumed that health care priorities shifted away from infectious disease control to hospital medicine in the National Health Service (NHS) era, giving an impression that there is nothing of note to study. Where public health is covered, more attention is paid to the management of lifestyles and risk factors.[27] Indeed, Rudolf Klein does not even mention public health in his comprehensive history of the NHS until the HIV/AIDS crisis of the 1980s.[28]

This volume also finds meaning in periods of contestation and in the public attention generated by new vaccines; but by analysing the vaccination programme across the post-war period, we also gain a sense of what made vaccination normal for so many parents. Indeed, the uneventful, mundane administration of vaccination programmes was not peripheral to the history of public health as one might suppose from the literature: it was central to it. The very fact that it has not excited much attention is a testament to how well the concept was established. This book traces how this was done through the early post-war period, and expanded and entrenched during the 1970s and beyond.

This is not to say, however, that notable works on immunisation in general do not exist. James Colgrove's excellent study of vaccination in the twentieth-century United States acts as an instructive contrast to the British story; for instance, there was little fear in the United Kingdom that polio was the harbinger of "socialized medicine", nor did British subjects have problems accessing many vaccines on account of fees charged by private family physicians.[29] Similarly, Bob Reinhardt and Sanjoy Bhattacharya have expertly analysed the smallpox eradication programmes in Africa and Asia with a critical gaze on dominant constructions of global public health and the scientific and administrative procedures which underpinned their success in eliminating the disease in the wild.[30] Most recently, Stuart Blume has detailed the scientific development of vaccination technology and the reasons why vaccination has been controversial across the world.[31] These are still rare exceptions, and until now there has not been such a comprehensive review of the public and vaccination in post-war Britain.

There are also works that have explored the relationship between the public and public health in the United Kingdom. There is a well-established scholarship on such matters in the nineteenth century and on the changing nature of public health governance in the first half of the twentieth century.[32] For the period after 1945, there is growing interest in the meaning of the concept of "the public" within public health, on the part of practitioners themselves and of historians. But while vaccination has been used in part to illuminate this relationship – notably in the work of Roberta Bivins on ethnicity and public health with regard to tuberculosis and smallpox in immigrant populations – none has centred their analysis on the wider context of mass vaccination in post-war Britain.[33]

This is important because Britain's vaccination programmes give new insights into how the relationship between the government and its citizens changed after 1945. It was precisely because infectious disease had become preventable that the public placed greater expectations on the government and fellow citizens.[34] Outbreaks became less common, but were a bigger scandal when they occurred. Governments that were unable to plan and run large-scale immunisation programmes were seen as deficient. This book helps to explain how and why vaccination was a key tool in protecting not just the health of the British people but the reputation of public health and the British state in general. These issues of citizenship were not simply a product of an age of consumerism or individualism that is assumed to have developed during the 1970s and under the New Right governments of the 1980s.[35] During immunisation campaigns in the 1940s questions were raised about the role and responsibility of citizens for their own and their families' health. Similarly, the technologies of managing risk, often attributed to the 1970s and beyond, were present in an earlier period.[36] Many of the facets of a supposed golden age of technocracy existed both before and after the heyday period of the late 1950s to mid-1970s.[37] As these chapters show, targets, statistical monitoring and central direction of regional authorities were employed throughout the post-war period in attempts to immunise the population and reduce the burden of preventable disease.

As with any work of historical scholarship, the researcher must make choices not just about what is included, but also about what must, for reasons of space, time and coherence, be excluded. This book will at no point attempt to assess whether or to what extent vaccines "really" worked, or their relative safety. History does not use the same tools as epidemiology, and these are scientific questions that must be answered using the methods laid out by other disciplines. In any case, these subjects have been tackled in depth both by contemporaries and by those reading back over the extant data.[38] Similarly, deep qualitative analysis of the public's understanding and construction of narratives surrounding vaccination across time are not possible in a volume such as this. Aside from methodological and philosophical issues in determining who the "ordinary" person is, governments have produced far more documentary evidence, and have preserved it in such a way that it is much more accessible to historians.[39] Folklorists are better positioned to explore this terrain, but even here there will be significant issues in accessing the memories of those who are no longer alive to tell their stories.[40] This is not to say that the public is not present in this volume. Members of the public continued to speak back to authorities and each other through letters, public utterances and more diffuse behaviours for which we can find empirical evidence.[41] Instead, this analysis addresses how concepts such as safety and efficacy were expressed by health authorities, politicians, the medical profession, the media, non-governmental organisations and, indeed, members of the public themselves. It is through these that the wider relationship between the public and public health can be grasped.

Not every vaccine used in Britain since the Second World War can be covered in detail. This book focuses on routine childhood immunisation – which necessarily excludes vaccines given to foreign travellers (such as yellow fever), to protect individuals at immediate risk (rabies), to protect subgroups of people considered to be at potential risk (hepatitis B, before 2017) or to protect the military from bioterrorism (anthrax). Even widely used vaccines, such as those against influenza,

HPV or tuberculosis, are not given their own chapters. There were also vaccines for which the public and medical authorities expressed a desire (such as for HIV/AIDS) but which were never developed.[42] Where these diseases and their associated immunisation are relevant to the overall narrative, they will be discussed. However, the chapters that are included here exemplify the broad trends and concepts that are crucial to understanding the relationship between the public and public health authorities during the post-war period.

Finally, any history of Britain needs to engage with the "four nations" question. Political events from devolution in the 1990s to the Scottish and European independence referenda in the 2010s have made British citizens even more aware that "Britain" is not simply "England". The Ministry of Health and its successors had direct jurisdiction over England and Wales, and evidence from these regions is given greater focus than that from elsewhere in the Union. However, it is important to stress that vaccination policy in Britain was *British*. Until 1974, local authorities had responsibility for the implementation of vaccination programmes through Section 26 of both the National Health Service Act 1946 and National Health Service (Scotland) Act 1947. But many of the decisions over immunisation policy at national level were taken cooperatively. As will be shown in Chapters 2 and 3, the "Joint" in Joint Committee on Vaccination and Immunisation refers to the cooperation between the Scottish, Northern Irish and English health authorities on vaccination. Local and national bodies worked with and learned from each other within this framework. Where appropriate, Scottish examples are used to highlight these national issues (such as the 1949 Glasgow smallpox outbreak, or differences in approach between English and Scottish health authorities during the MMR crisis). The focus here is not on particular British cultures of vaccination, but on the British vaccination system. The administrative links between and across regional, national and transnational public health bodies were all important in creating that system.

Vaccination and the public

As indicated in much of the existing literature, the development of vaccination programmes in Europe during the eighteenth and nineteenth centuries was intimately connected with the expansion of central state authority over the public's health, and a widespread political contestation of the precise limits of state authority in relation to the citizen-subject. Vaccination has been associated with state power ever since. Indeed, this contested relationship between individual liberty and collective responsibility with regard to infectious disease control has been central to debates over vaccination and other public health programmes.[43] Who "the public" are within these structures is difficult to define precisely. Where we can discern attempts to define publics (both by contemporaries and by later analysts), we see them mainly through two lenses. There is what we might call a demographic approach, which views publics as populations of people that can be measured according to some set of common criteria. Then there is an identity approach, in which the public as a mass collection of individuals believes itself to have common attributes that allow it to exist as a political force. Thus, publics could be constructed through governance structures as well as construct themselves through voluntary or mutual action.[44] Publics could and did speak and act in myriad ways that disrupted public health policy, and their concerns changed over time. However, this book does not provide a grand unifying vision of who or what the public really was in post-war Britain. Instead, it investigates the ways in which authorities constructed ideas of the public through their vaccination policies. Here, governments identified problems, measured their effects and interpreted the public's behaviour on their terms. But, in doing so, the public spoke back, often complicating authorities' plans and forcing new interpretations of policy. For the government, the voices of individuals and of the public in general were always mediated through these interactions – and the complex ways in which these shone through tell us much about post-war British politics.

Whatever our conception of "the public", public health has maintained a disciplinary function, and much has been written about how governance structures acted upon the public from a medical perspective.[45] Somewhat paradoxically, the imprecision of definitions of "the public" and "public health" have, according to Jane Lewis, been both a strength and a weakness of public health governance and the public health profession.[46] In the supposed heroic age of the nineteenth century, large-scale infrastructure projects, such as water purification and sewerage, had a demonstrable impact upon the health of urban environments following the rapid urbanisation that began in the previous century. Such projects were pushed through by national governments despite objections from local authorities; although it should be noted that local innovation and pressure often had an impact on national policy and the understanding of public health problems.[47] As health systems developed and the power of medical science increased, Medical Officers and local authorities became more heavily involved with the running of municipal hospitals and other Poor Law institutions such as asylums. The looseness of the definition of public health thus allowed Medical Officers to gain significant power during the nineteenth and early twentieth centuries. Yet, as Lewis argues, it also meant that once health systems became increasingly complicated and relied upon ever-centralised power (such as the creation of the NHS), public health became a side-lined profession.[48]

John Welshman and Martin Gorsky have questioned this narrative, arguing that Medical Officers of Health (MOHs) continued to perform important public health functions.[49] It is generally acknowledged, however, that public health transitioned from concerns about infectious disease and epidemic control towards the management of chronic conditions. As hygiene improved, issues such as lung cancer and heart disease proved more pressing. Virginia Berridge tracks this evolution in post-war public health through the lens of smoking.[50] The story of post-war vaccination complicates this picture. MOHs and the British government in general put significant resources into vaccination in the name of controlling infectious disease. This was not in the same vein as the large Victorian sanitation projects, nor were MOHs called into action to contain outbreaks of diseases such as smallpox with the same regularity as in previous decades. But infectious disease did not disappear. Rather, the *risk* of infectious disease became the subject of public health intervention. And, as Berridge also notes of smoking, this did concentrate more closely on individual behaviour, use of the mass media and evidence-based medicine.[51]

Practices of immunisation are woven into this wider history of public health, with the resistance against, and slow uptake of, these technologies haunting government perceptions of the public and vaccination long into the twentieth century. Variolation – the introduction of smallpox into a healthy person to give them a mild form of the disease and confer immunity – was popularised among the British nobility in the early seventeenth century by Lady Mary Montagu.[52] The development and growing acceptability of inoculation techniques, and statistical methods for assessing their efficacy, led some local authorities to use the technique on a wider population as a form of public health protection.[53] Edward Jenner's experiments with cowpox provided a new, safer form of immunisation against smallpox in time for the aforementioned growth in the centralised state public health apparatus.[54] Various Vaccination Acts over the Victorian period placed a duty on local authorities to provide vaccination free of charge, and in 1853 made routine childhood vaccination compulsory.[55] This caused much resentment from a number of constituencies, creating large anti-vaccination societies that objected to the procedure on the grounds of local autonomy, scientific doubt, personal freedom, the intrusion of the state into private matters of child rearing, religious objection, animal rights and resentment at the use of Poor Law institutions to treat the middle classes.[56]

Developments in bacteriology and medical procedures that had given rise to the power of biomedicine and hospital-based medicine in the late nineteenth century also provided new avenues for vaccination.[57] Louis Pasteur's work with anthrax, rabies and fowl cholera showed that attenuated forms of the microbes could perform a similar function to vaccination – and, more crucially, that it was possible to mass produce them.[58] However, these were products of a pre-immunology age; it would not be until the very end of the nineteenth century that such developments in bacteriology were met with reformulations of scientific conceptions of immunity and disease transmission.[59]

The production of diphtheria anti-toxoid and its use in mass immunisation campaigns was, as Esteban Rodríguez-Ocaña has described it, 'the crucial link between public excitement about Pasteur's rabies vaccine and the establishment of national campaigns against tuberculosis, sustaining the development of bacteriology-based public health service'.[60] The growing power of biomedical sciences was thus embodied in these new technologies that borrowed from generally accepted principles of immunity.[61] Through example, mass vaccination programmes showed that science possessed the tools not only to discover new prophylactics, but to use them effectively to prevent disease. The articulation of the concept of "herd immunity" in the 1920s gave further statistical credence to the emerging science of immunology.[62] It also showed science's power to react to contemporary problems. Pasteur's anthrax vaccine, for example, was a direct response to the effects of the disease in cattle on agricultural output.⁶³ Diphtheria had been identified as a distinct and significant epidemic disease only in the wake of mass urbanisation in Europe during the mid-nineteenth century. By the end of the century, an anti-toxoid had been developed.⁶⁴

These advances were embraced by local and national governments as symbols of their own advancement and ability to solve complex problems. Governments employed developments in mass communication to ensure that people took advantage of the new vaccines. In New York City, newspapers, poster advertising, the cinema and the wireless were all employed to proclaim the benefits of diphtheria immunisation. Vaccination was offered as a choice, advertised as one might market an automobile; not imposed by the state as had been common for smallpox.⁶⁵ When Britain initiated its diphtheria programme in 1940, it followed New York's lead by focusing on education rather than compulsion. Such tactics had worked in other fields (such as domestic cleanliness), and helped to establish the narrative that liberal British public health worked with its public, rather than imposing an authoritarian state medical police as had been seen in imperial Germany.⁶⁶ British public health authorities openly sought the cooperation of their subjects, rather than compliance alone – though it is instructive that the Ministry of Health continued to refer to its advertising efforts as "propaganda" well after the end of the War. The role of education in constructing and communicating with the public is a key theme of twentieth- and twenty-first-century public health, and will be a recurring theme throughout this book.⁶⁷

While diphtheria immunisation and BCG were embraced by some nations and integrated into their public health programmes in the inter-war years, Britain was more cautious about using these new technologies.⁶⁸ Linda Bryder's and Jane Lewis's work has shown that epidemiological evidence on vaccination could be interpreted in different ways by nation states.⁶⁹ Thus, while one country could justify the use of a particular vaccine, another could see the same immunisation as unsafe or ineffective as compared to existing practices. The British medical establishment considered its anti-tuberculosis measures – including inspection, notification, sanatoria, dispensaries, hospital care and pasteurisation – to be adequate. Rates of infection from tuberculosis and diphtheria also appeared to be lower in Britain than they were in countries that used immunisation, such as France and the Nordic states.⁷⁰

Such a significant change in public health policy was a risk which the British authorities were not willing to take in the 1930s for fear of damaging their reputations. Local governments were given the power to initiate their own campaigns if they so wished but, given that they needed to pay for the vaccines themselves, coverage was inconsistent and often depended on the priorities of the MOH.[71] The continued strength of anti-vaccination and anti-vivisection voluntary societies in the mid-twentieth century also made central government wary of the public backlash from instituting any national mass immunisation programme.[72] High-profile incidents in which people had been injured or killed through improper use of immunisation gave authorities further justification for remaining cautious.[73] This book draws attention to the ways in which national public health programmes framed scientific findings and reached divergent conclusions in the post-war period. The burden of proof required before British authorities would declare a vaccine safe or effective was influenced by politics as much as by science. Once Britain finally did establish a national anti-diphtheria strategy, the success of this campaign softened attitudes. From the 1940s onwards the Medical Research Council (MRC) began to seriously consider other immunisations as potential additions to the public health system.[74]

The success of mass immunisation through the first half of the twentieth century established it as a key tool in public health. This encouraged the development of new vaccines and the willingness of states to consider using them as part of immunisation programmes. During the Second World War, coordination of political aims and scientific research had seen a number of advancements in medicine as a direct contribution to the war effort, including the protection of troops from potential biological warfare and the demands of operating in foreign climates.[75] Contemporary advancements in virology and immunology offered the possibility of controlling – perhaps even eradicating – other infectious diseases, old and new.[76] It is these developments which the chapters of this book discuss in greater detail. The book starts in 1945, in the afterglow of a successful anti-diphtheria campaign by the wartime coalition government. Despite some initial scepticism, immunisation rates grew significantly over the course of the 1940s, and diphtheria morbidity and mortality dropped significantly. With the prospect on the horizon of using new vaccinations against tuberculosis and pertussis (whooping cough), as well as the new state-run NHS, public health and vaccination were both primed for significant administrative and political transformations.

Chapter outline

Given this history, it is clear that vaccination programmes – like any other political project – are rooted in a wider social context. The book explores this through a series of case studies which highlight the ways in which the public and governments interacted, shaping public health as they went. What was expected of the public and of the government changed over this period; and the debates over vaccination show wider concerns about the relationship between the state and its citizens. In explaining how vaccination became ordinary, the volume is split into two parts. Part I shows how the vaccination programme in Britain as we know it today was created and evolved. Part II deals with vaccination crises within an already-established system. The two parts comprise five chapters which explain these trends through five interrelated themes. Each represents a different area of responsibility or expectation on the part of both the public and public health authorities.

Part I begins with *apathy*. Chapter 1 explores this through the diphtheria immunisation programme. Diphtheria immunisation was introduced on a national basis during the Second World War and was initially successful – so much so, that it formed the basis of the voluntary vaccination system that replaced the Victorian Vaccination Acts with the birth of the NHS. In 1949, however, declining vaccination rates concerned the Ministry of Health. The drop was blamed on apathetic parents (particularly mothers), and the Ministry hoped to combat this by reminding parents of young children how dangerous diphtheria still was. When parents did not have their children vaccinated, they could be accused of negligence. However, public health authorities also understood that the reasons for non-vaccination were various and complex. How they used apathy as a rhetorical device in setting local immunisation targets and health education said much about what was considered reasonable behaviour on the part of parents. And, indeed, what reasonable behaviour the public expected of each other.

Chapter 2 examines *nation*. The British vaccination programme was very much a national project. However, it could not function without implementation at the local level and was dependent on international networks of vaccine knowledge. At the same time, the programme exposed the limits of national power and raised questions about who the "British public" were that required protection through public health policy. Elimination of disease within British borders was as vital as preventing the importation of once-eliminated infections from foreign places and peoples. This is examined through debates over the smallpox vaccine from the end of the war in 1945 to the end of routine childhood smallpox vaccination in 1971. Here too, apathy was an important concept. Vaccination rates remained stubbornly low for a disease long since eliminated from British shores. And yet, whenever there was a local outbreak queues would stretch from local Medical Officers' clinics, demanding emergency vaccination to protect local citizens from the disease. The public's view of what protections the government ought to provide – and the form they should take – were not always aligned with the Ministry's.

This leads to the third and final chapter in Part I, which analyses *demand*. While governments were undoubtedly concerned with disciplining parents who did not conform with official advice, members of the public themselves demanded that the state should make immunisation services available to all. In an advanced economy such as Britain's, the expectation that the state would protect citizens from manageable risks became commonplace. Chapter 3 uses the inactivated polio vaccine programme to show the difficult relationship between what the public demanded and what the government was able or willing to provide. The place of the nation was still important here. This was a national programme, but, like all vaccination at this time, it was administered by local authorities who had differing results in terms of uptake. Despite the demand from some quarters, in others the government still had a hard time overcoming what it perceived to be an apathetic public. Similarly, production of the vaccine was made possible only through large-scale cooperation with other nations; and the relationship between British pharmaceutical companies, foreign nations and the British government was key.

Part II begins in the early 1970s. By this time, smallpox vaccination had been removed from the schedule, while polio and diphtheria immunisation were now well established. They were joined by BCG (in schools), pertussis, measles and tetanus. Vaccination had become commonplace, and it was widely accepted that routine childhood immunisation was a useful and important public health tool. However, controversies did rear their heads. The public had consented and cooperated with British public health authorities in developing the vaccination programme. This meant that when confidence in the medical and political establishments became strained, so did faith in vaccination – at least in the case of specific vaccines at specific times. And yet, such crises did not destroy the vaccination or public health systems entirely, and confidence soon recovered.

Thus, Chapter 4 examines *risk* through the 1970s pertussis vaccine crisis. Risk pervaded all aspects of vaccination policy – indeed public health is inherently about the management of disease risks. Attitudes toward which risks were acceptable and which risks were manageable changed considerably during the post-war period, however. Governments had to manage the risks of damage to their reputation from potentially unsafe vaccines versus the benefits of disease control. The public also pushed back against government policy when it felt certain that risks were unacceptable or were being poorly managed. Many other themes can also be identified here. Public health authorities struggled against a form of apathy: the idea that parents no longer feared pertussis because of the success of the vaccination programme. So too did they have to deal with a form of demand. Parents demanded protection for their children, both from the disease and from the vaccine itself. They understood the risks to their children differently from public health authorities, causing greater tension. Once the scientific basis for the vaccine was re-established and an epidemic loomed on the horizon, there was such demand for the vaccine that many local authorities ran short of it. This led to discussions which reflected wider contemporary concerns about the role of the national government and a deeper political crisis in the welfare state.

Finally, Chapter 5 brings these themes together and examines *hesitancy*, a concept that made an entry into global vaccination policy around the year 2010, but that is clearly a product of the lessons that public health has taken from its own history. Recent vaccine crises and narratives that changing approaches to the meaning of "health" in the World Health Organization have led social scientists to focus on individuals' decision-making processes. These start from the premise that uptake of vaccination ought to be universal and that the declines in vaccination rates are not only a sign of wider problems but are also to some extent preventable with adequate communication and monitoring. None of this can be understood without reference to the changing face of apathy, demand, nation and risk in previous decades. This history is explained in Chapter 5 through the changes in government policy during the MMR crisis in the late 1990s and 2000s. Some parents were accused of apathy due to much-reduced measles morbidity since the introduction of measles vaccination in 1961 and of MMR vaccination in 1988. But this does not capture why the majority of parents made the decision to continue to vaccinate, even during the height of the crisis. Nor does it explain why many opponents of MMR vaccination demanded that the government make separate measles, mumps and rubella vaccines available to any parent who asked for them. As with the pertussis crisis, the public's understanding of risk and the reasons for their hesitancy did not always accord with expert opinion. National and devolved authorities used risk-communication techniques and comparisons with other nations to reassert the safety and utility of MMR vaccination when it became clear that the health education tactics of previous decades were not having the desired effect. This shift from education towards analysis of decision making and risk would be a key facet of twenty-first-century public health.

Notes

1 Raya Jalabi, 'California declares Disneyland measles outbreak over as vaccine fight rages on', *Guardian* (17 April 2015) https://www.theguardian.com/society/2015/apr/17/california-declares-disneyland-measles-outbreak-over (accessed 12 January 2018).

2 World Health Organization, 'Measles continues to spread and take lives in Europe' (11 July 2017) www.euro.who.int/en/media-centre/sections/press-releases/2017/measles-continues-to-spread-and-take-lives-in-europe (accessed 12 January 2018); Michael Day, 'Doctor and MPs in Italy are assaulted after vaccination law is passed', *British Medical Journal*, 358 (2017), j3721; Sophie Arie, 'Compulsory vaccination and growing measles threat', *British Medical Journal*, 358 (2017), j3429.

3 David Callender, 'Vaccine hesitancy: More than a movement', *Human Vaccines & Immunotherapeutics*, 12:9 (2016), 2464–8; Eve Dubé, Maryline Vivion and Noni E. MacDonald, 'Vaccine hesitancy, vaccine refusal and the anti-vaccine movement: influence, impact and implications', *Expert*

Review of Vaccines, 14:1 (2015), 99–117; Kenneth Camargo and Roy Grant, 'Public health, science, and policy debate: Being right is not enough', *American Journal Public Health*, 105:2 (2014), 232–5; Ross S. Federman, 'Understanding vaccines: A public imperative', *Yale Journal of Biology and Medicine*, 87:4 (2014), 417–22.
4 WHO, Rotary International, Centers for Disease Control and Prevention and UNICEF, *Global Polio Eradication Initiative Status Report 29 April 2013* (Geneva: Global Polio Eradication Initiative, 2013).
5 The argument against vaccinating only teenage girls has taken two forms: one, that males can carry HPV and therefore ought to be vaccinated to protect females; and two, that since HPV can cause cancer in males, they ought to be offered the same protection. See Aruna Nigam, Pikee Saxena, Anita S. Acharya, Archana Mishra and Swaraj Batra, 'HPV vaccination in India: Critical appraisal', *ISRN Obstetrics and Gynecology* (2014), 1–5; Fouzieyha Towghi, 'The biopolitics of reproductive technologies beyond the clinic: Localizing HPV vaccines in India', *Medical Anthropology*, 32:4 (2013), 325–42; Heidi Larson, 'The world must accept that the HPV vaccine is safe', *Nature*, 528:7580 (2015), 9; Catriona Kennedy, Carol Gray Brunton and Rhona Hogg, '"Just that little bit of doubt": Scottish parents', teenage girls' and health professionals' views of the MMR, H1N1 and HPV vaccines', *International Journal of Behavioral Medicine*, 21:1 (2014), 3–10; Monica J. Casper and Laura M. Carpenter, 'Sex, drugs, and politics: the HPV vaccine for cervical cancer', *Sociology of Health & Illness*, 30:6 (2008), 886–99; Telegraph, 'Boys should get HPV vaccine to protect them from throat cancers, experts say', *Telegraph* (10 July 2016) www.telegraph.co.uk/news/2016/07/09/boys-should-get-hpv-vaccine-to-protect-them-from-throat-cancers/ (accessed 19 August 2016).
6 World Health Organization, 'WHO Director-General summarizes the outcome of the Emergency Committee regarding clusters of microcephaly and Guillain-Barré syndrome' (2016) www.who.int/mediacentre/news/statements/2016/emergency-committee-zika-microcephaly/en/ (accessed 19 August 2016); Siddhartha Mukherjee, 'The race for a Zika vaccine', *New Yorker* (22 August 2016) www.newyorker.com/magazine/2016/08/22/the-race-for-a-zika-vaccine (accessed 19 August 2016); Tulip Mazumdar, 'Zika vaccine possible "within months"', *BBC News* (4 March 2016) www.bbc.co.uk/news/health-35727047 (accessed 19 August 2016); Linda Carroll and Samuel Sarmiento, '"Striking" results from early Zika vaccine trial', *NBC News* (4 August 2016) www.nbcnews.com/storyline/zika-virus-outbreak/striking-results-early-zika-vaccine-trial-n623016 (accessed 19 August 2016).

7 World Health Organization, 'Statement on the 1st meeting of the IHR Emergency Committee on the 2014 Ebola outbreak in West Africa', (2014) www.who.int/mediacentre/news/statements/2014/ebola-20140808/en/ (accessed 19 August 2016); Vauhini Vara, 'The race for an Ebola vaccine', *New Yorker* (25 November 2014) www.newyorker.com/business/currency/race-ebola-vaccine (accessed 19 August 2016); Anne Roemer-Mahler and Stefan Elbe, 'The race for Ebola drugs: Pharmaceuticals, security and global health governance', *Third World Quarterly*, 37:3 (2016), 487–506; Declan Butler, Ewen Callaway and Erika Check Hayden, 'How Ebola-vaccine success could reshape clinical-trial policy', *Nature*, 524:7563 (2015), 13–14.
8 Hib – *Haemophilus influenza* type b – is an infection that can cause meningitis, septicaemia, pneumonia and other complications. See Health and Social Care Information Centre, 'NHS Immunisation Statistics: England, 2014–15' (23 September 2015) http://digital.nhs.uk/catalogue/PUB18472/nhs-immu-stat-eng-2014-15-rep.pdf (accessed 23 August 2017). Acceptance rates fell slightly in the two following years but remain high: 91.6 per cent for MMR and 93.4 per cent for the five-in-one in 2016–17. NHS Digital, 'Childhood vaccination coverage statistics, England, 2016–17' (20 September 2017) https://digital.nhs.uk/catalogue/PUB30085 (accessed 12 January 2018).
9 In 2014–15, 95.4 per cent of children under the age of 2 received MMR, while over 97 per cent received the five-in-one. National Health Services Scotland, 'Childhood Immunisation Statistics Scotland: Quarter and Year Ending 31 December 2015' (22 March 2016) www.isdscotland.org/Health-Topics/Child-Health/Publications/2016-03-22/2016-03-22-Immunisation-Report.pdf (accessed 23 August 2017), p. 5.
10 Heidi J. Larson, Alexandre de Figueiredo, Zhao Xiahong, William S. Schulz, Pierre Verger, Iain G. Johnston, Alex R. Cook and Nick S. Jones, 'The state of vaccine confidence 2016: Global insights through a 67-country survey', *EBioMedicine*, 12 (2016), 295–301.
11 It has been surpassed (as at 15 February 2018) only by the campaign to re-run the 2016 European Union referendum and demands that Donald Trump's 2017 state visit be cancelled. UK Government and Parliament Petitions, 'Petition: Give the meningitis B vaccine to ALL children, not just newborn babies' (15 September 2015) https://petition.parliament.uk/petitions/108072 (accessed 20 August 2016); 'Meningitis B petition becomes UK's most signed', *BBC News* (19 February 2016) www.bbc.co.uk/news/uk-england-kent-35614846 (accessed 20 August 2016); James Cusick, 'Meningitis B: Petition calling for vaccine breaks government

website record', *Independent* (19 February 2016) www.independent.co.uk/life-style/health-and-families/health-news/meningitis-b-petition-calling-for-vaccine-breaks-government-website-record-a6884946.html (accessed 20 August 2016).
12 Jacob Heller, *The Vaccine Narrative* (Nashville, TN: Vanderbilt University Press, 2008), p. 1.
13 National Health Service, 'Childhood vaccines timeline' (16 July 2016) www.nhs.uk/Conditions/Vaccinations/Pages/Childhood-vaccination-schedule.aspx (accessed 12 January 2018).
14 Stuart Blume, *Immunization: How Vaccines Became Controversial* (London: Reaktion, 2017).
15 *Ibid.* See also Paul Greenough, Stuart Blume and Christine Holmberg, 'Introduction', in Christine Holmberg, Stuart Blume and Paul Greenough (eds), *The Politics of Vaccination: A Global History* (Manchester: Manchester University Press, 2017), pp. 1–16.
16 Eugene Straus and Alex Straus, *Medical Marvels: The 100 Greatest Advances in Medicine* (Amherst, NY: Prometheus Books, 2006); Arthur Allen, *Vaccine: The Controversial Story of Medicine's Greatest Lifesaver* (New York: W. W. Norton, 2007), p. 1; Paul A. Offit, *Vaccinated: One Man's Quest to Defeat the World's Deadliest Diseases* (New York: Smithsonian Books, 2007); Gareth Williams and Ray Loadman, *Paralysed with Fear: The Story of Polio* (Basingstoke: Palgrave Macmillan, 2013).
17 Andrew W. Artenstein (ed.), *Vaccines: A Biography* (New York: Springer, 2010).
18 Andrea Kitta, *Vaccinations and Public Concern in History: Legend, Rumor, and Risk Perception* (New York: Routledge, 2012); Artenstein (ed.), *Vaccines*; Paul A. Offit, *The Cutter Incident: How America's First Polio Vaccine led to the Growing Vaccine Crisis* (New Haven, CT: Yale University Press, 2005); Helen Bedford and David Elliman, 'Concerns about immunisation', *British Medical Journal*, 320:7229 (2000), 240–3; H. J. Parish, *A History of Immunization* (Edinburgh: Livingstone, 1965).
19 The debate over the role of medicine and public health on mortality decline since the 1700s has been contested, but this is broadly the consensus among medical professionals. For the debate in historical context see particularly: Thomas McKeown and R. G. Brown, 'Medical evidence related to English population changes in the eighteenth century', *Population Studies*, 9:2 (1955), 119–41; Simon Szreter, 'The importance of social intervention in Britain's mortality decline c.1850–1914: A re-interpretation of the role of public health', *Social History of Medicine*, 1:1 (1988), 1–38; James Colgrove, 'The McKeown thesis: A historical controversy and its enduring influence', *American Journal of Public Health*, 92:5 (2002), 725–9.

20 For examples of medical professionals' interest in the history of anti-vaccination moments in history, see Swansea Research Unity of the Royal College of General Practitioners, 'Effect of a low pertussis vaccination take-up on a large community', *British Medical Journal (Clinical Research Edition)*, 282:6257 (1981), 23–6; Mikio Kimura and Harumi Kuno-Sakai, 'Pertussis vaccines in Japan – a clue toward understanding of Japanese attitude to vaccines', *Journal of Tropical Pediatrics*, 37:1 (1991), 45–7; Robert M. Wolfe and Lisa K. Sharp, 'Anti-vaccinationists past and present', *British Medical Journal*, 325:7361 (2002), 430–2; Richard Horton, *MMR: Science and Fiction – Exploring a Vaccine Crisis* (London: Granta Books, 2004); Tammy Boyce, *Health, Risk and News: The MMR Vaccine and the Media* (New York: Peter Lang, 2007); Paul A. Offit, 'The anti-vaccination epidemic: Whooping cough, mumps and measles are making an alarming comeback, thanks to seriously misguided parents', *Wall Street Journal (Online)* (24 September 2014) www.wsj.com/articles/paul-a-offit-the-anti-vaccination-epidemic-1411598408 (accessed 19 August 2016). Offit's review of the Cutter Incident is more rounded, but explicitly calls for lessons to be learned so that the reputation of vaccination can be defended. Offit, *The Cutter Incident*. Some historical investigations have begun to move away from this narrative as more historical data have become available. See Jeffrey P. Baker, 'The pertussis vaccine controversy in Great Britain, 1974–1986', *Vaccine*, 21:25–26 (2003), 4003–10; Jan Hendriks and Stuart Blume, 'Measles vaccination: Before the measles-mumps-rubella vaccine', *American Journal of Public Health*, 103:8 (2013), 1393–401; Rachel Casiday, 'Risk communication in the British pertussis and MMR vaccine controversies', in Peter Bennett, Kenneth Calman, Sarah Curtis and Denis Fischbacher-Smith (eds), *Risk Communication and Public Health* (Oxford: Oxford University Press, 2010), 129–46; Alison Day, ' "An American tragedy". The Cutter Incident and its implications for the Salk polio vaccine in New Zealand 1955–1960', *Health & History: Journal of the Australian & New Zealand Society for the History of Medicine*, 11:2 (2009), 42–61; Per Axelsson, 'The Cutter Incident and the development of a Swedish polio vaccine, 1952–1957', *Dynamis*, 32:2 (2012), 311–28.
21 Virginia Berridge, 'Using history in policy and practice', in Virginia Berridge, Martin Gorsky and Alex Mold, *Public Health in History* (Maidenhead: Open University Press, 2011), p. 215.
22 Dorothy Porter and Roy Porter, 'The politics of prevention: Anti-vaccinationism and public health in nineteenth-century England', *Medical History*, 32:3 (1988), 231–52; E. P. Hennock, 'Vaccination policy against smallpox, 1835–1914: A comparison of England with Prussia and Imperial

Germany', *Social History of Medicine*, 11:1 (1998), 49–71; Nadja Durbach, *Bodily Matters: The Anti-Vaccination Movement in England, 1853–1907* (Durham, NC: Duke University Press, 2005), p. 1; Stanley Williamson, *The Vaccination Controversy: The Rise, Reign, and Fall of Compulsory Vaccination for Smallpox* (Liverpool: Liverpool University Press, 2007); Michael Bennett, 'Jenner's ladies: Women and vaccination against smallpox in early nineteenth-century Britain', *History*, 93:312 (2008), 497–513.

23 Dora Vargha, 'Between East and West: Polio vaccination across the Iron Curtain in Cold War Hungary', *Bulletin of the History of Medicine*, 88:2 (2014), 319–42; Ulrike Lindner and Stuart S. Blume, 'Vaccine innovation and adoption: Polio vaccines in the UK, the Netherlands and West Germany, 1955–1965', *Medical History*, 50:4 (2006), 425–46.

24 Jane Lewis, 'The prevention of diphtheria in Canada and Britain 1914–1945', *Journal of Social History*, 20:1 (1986), 163–76; Linda Bryder, '"We shall not find salvation in inoculation": BCG vaccination in Scandinavia, Britain and the USA, 1921–1960', *Social Science & Medicine*, 49:9 (1999), 1157–67; Claire Hooker, 'Diphtheria, immunisation and the Bundaberg Tragedy: A study of public health in Australia', *Health and History*, 2:1 (2000), 52–78; Lindner and Blume, 'Vaccine innovation and adoption'; Alison Day, '"The magical formula": Reactions and responses to diphtheria immunisation in New Zealand 1920–1960', *Health & History: Journal of the Australian & New Zealand Society for the History of Medicine*, 15:2 (2013), 53–71.

25 On governmentality and medicine, see Alan R Petersen and Deborah Lupton, *The New Public Health: Health and Self in the Age of Risk* (London: Sage Publications, 2000); Michel Foucault, *The Birth of the Clinic: An Archaeology of Medical Perception* (London: Tavistock, 1973); David Armstrong, *Political Anatomy of the Body: Medical Knowledge in Britain in the Twentieth Century* (Cambridge: Cambridge University Press, 1983).

26 For example, Bryder, 'BCG vaccination'; Lewis, 'The Prevention of diphtheria'; Lindner and Blume, 'Vaccine innovation and adoption'; Jennifer Stanton, 'What shapes vaccine policy? The case of hepatitis B in the UK', *Social History of Medicine*, 7:3 (1994), 427–46.

27 Peterson and Lupton, *The New Public Health*.

28 Rudolf Klein, *The New Politics of the NHS: From Creation to Reinvention*, 7th edn (Oxford: Radcliffe, 2013).

29 James Colgrove, *State of Immunity: The Politics of Vaccination in Twentieth-Century America* (Berkeley: University of California Press, 2006).

30 Sanjoy Bhattacharya, *Expunging Variola: The Control and Eradication of Smallpox in India, 1947–1977* (New Delhi: Orient Longman, 2006); Bob H. Reinhardt, *The End of a Global Pox: America and the Eradication of*

Smallpox in the Cold War Era (Chapel Hill: University of North Carolina Press, 2015).
31 Blume, *Immunization*.
32 On the Victorian era, see Graham Mooney, *Intrusive Interventions: Public Health, Domestic Space, and Infectious Disease Surveillance in England, 1840–1914* (Rochester, NY: University of Rochester Press, 2015); Anne Hanley, *Medicine, Knowledge and Venereal Diseases in England, 1886–1916* (Basingstoke: Palgrave Macmillan, 2016). On the twentieth century, and particularly the inter-war period, see Charles Webster, 'Healthy or hungry thirties?', *History Workshop*, 13 (1982), 110–29; Jane Lewis, *What Price Community Medicine? The Philosophy, Practice, and Politics of Public Health Since 1919* (Brighton: Wheatsheaf, 1986); John Welshman, *Municipal Medicine: Public Health in Twentieth-century Britain* (Bern: Peter Lang, 2000); John Welshman, 'Compulsion, localism, and pragmatism: The micro-politics of tuberculosis screening in the United Kingdom, 1950–1965', *Social History of Medicine*, 19:2 (2006), 295–312; Martin Gorsky, 'Public health in interwar Britain: Did it fail?', *Dynamis*, 28 (2008), 175–98; Jane K. Seymour, Martin Gorsky and Shakoor Hajat, 'Health, wealth and party in inter-war London', *Urban History*, 44:3 (2017), 464–91.
33 Roberta Bivins, '"The people have no more love left for the Commonwealth": Media, migration and identity in the 1961–62 British smallpox outbreak', *Immigrants & Minorities*, 25:3 (2007), 263–89; Roberta E. Bivins, *Contagious Communities: Medicine, Migration, and the NHS in Post-War Britain* (Oxford: Oxford University Press, 2015). See also Petersen and Lupton, *The New Public Health*; Richard Coker, 'Civil liberties and public good: Detention of tuberculous patients and the Public Health Act 1984', *Medical History*, 45:3 (2001), 341–58; Steve Sturdy, 'Introduction: Medicine, health and the public sphere', in Steve Sturdy (ed.), *Medicine, Health and the Public Sphere in Britain: 1600–2000* (London: Routledge, 2002), pp. 1–24; David Cantor, 'Representing "the public": Medicine, charity and the public sphere in twentieth-century Britain', in Steve Sturdy (ed.), *Medicine, Health and the Public Sphere in Britain: 1600–2000* (London: Routledge, 2002), pp. 145–68; Pamela K. Gilbert, 'Producing the public: Public medicine in private spaces', in Steve Sturdy (ed.), *Medicine, Health and the Public Sphere*, 43–59; M. F. Verweij and Angus Dawson, 'The meaning of "public" in "public health"', in M. F. Verweij and Angus Dawson (eds), *Ethics, Prevention, and Public Health* (Oxford: Clarendon Press, 2007), pp. 13–29; John T. MacFarlane and Michael Worboys, 'Showers, sweating and suing: Legionnaires' disease and "new" infections in Britain, 1977–90', *Medical History*, 56:1 (2012), 72–93.

34 Dorothy Porter, *Health Citizenship: Essays in Social Medicine and Biomedical Politics* (Berkeley: University of California Press, 2011), 213–15; Nike Ayo, 'Understanding health promotion in a neoliberal climate and the making of health conscious citizens', *Critical Public Health*, 22:1 (2012), 99–105; Frank Huisman and Harry Oosterhuis, 'The politics of health and citizenship: Historical and contemporary perspectives', in Frank Huisman and Harry Oosterhuis (eds), *Heath and Citizenship: Political Cultures of Health in Modern Europe* (London: Pickering and Chatto 2014), pp. 1–40.

35 On these themes see Petersen and Lupton, *The New Public Health*; Virginia Berridge and Alex Mold, 'Professionalisation, new social movements and voluntary action in the 1960s and 1970s', in Matthew Hilton and James McKay (eds), *The Ages of Voluntarism : How we got to the Big Society* (Oxford: Oxford University Press, 2011), pp. 114–34; Alex Mold, *Making the Patient-consumer: Patient Organisations and Health Consumerism in Britain* (Manchester: Manchester University Press, 2015).

36 On risk, see Chapter 4 and Ulrich Beck, *Risk Society: Towards a New Modernity* (London: Sage, 1992); Mary Douglas and Aaron Wildavsky, *Risk and Culture* (Berkeley: University of California Press, 1983); Jakob Arnoldi, *Risk: An Introduction* (Cambridge: Polity, 2009); Baruch Fischoff and John Kadvany, *Risk: A Very Short Introduction* (Oxford: Oxford University Press, 2011).

37 On technocracy see David Edgerton, 'C. P. Snow as anti-historian of British science: Revisiting the technocratic moment, 1959–1964', *History of Science* 43:2 (2005), 187–208; Mike Savage, 'Affluence and social change in the making of technocratic middle-class identities: Britain, 1939–55', *Contemporary British History*, 22:4 (2008): 457–76.

38 For authors with medical qualifications looking back on the efficacy of vaccines and their worth as public health tools, see Parish, *A History of Immunization*; Kimura and Kuno-Sakai, 'Pertussis vaccines in Japan'; Baker, 'The pertussis vaccine controversy'; David M. Oshinsky, *Polio: An American Story* (Oxford: Oxford University Press, 2005); Offit, *Vaccinated*; Artenstein (ed.), *Vaccines*; Williams and Loadman, *Paralysed with Fear*.

39 Florence Sutcliffe-Braithwaite, 'Discourses of "class" in Britain in "New Times"', *Contemporary British History*, 31:2 (April 2017), 294–317.

40 On the role of folklorists using ethnography to access understandings and meanings of health, see Diane E. Goldstein, *Once Upon a Virus: AIDS Legends and Vernacular Risk Perception* (Logan: Utah State University Press, 2004); Kitta, *Vaccinations and Public Concern in History*.

41 As an example of this, see James Hanley's work on nineteenth-century parliamentary petitions as a way of understanding public reaction to

policy: James G. Hanley, 'The public's reaction to public health: Petitions submitted to parliament, 1847–1848', *Social History of Medicine*, 15:3 (2002), 393–411. See also Daisy Payling on "complaints" to the social survey: Daisy Payling, '"The people who write to us are the people who don't like us": Public responses to the Government Social Survey's Survey of Sickness, 1943–1952', *Journal of British Studies* (forthcoming, 2018).
42 On AIDS, see Jon Cohen, *Shots in the Dark: The Wayward Search for an AIDS Vaccine* (New York: Norton, 2001); Patricia Thomas, *Big Shot: Passion, Politics, and the Struggle for an AIDS Vaccine* (New York: Public Affairs, 2001); Heller, *The Vaccine Narrative*.
43 Colgrove, *State of Immunity*.
44 Sturdy, 'Introduction'; Petersen and Lupton, *The New Public Health*, p. 55.
45 Foucault, *The Birth of the Clinic*; Armstrong, *Political Anatomy of the Body*; Mooney, *Intrusive Interventions*.
46 Lewis, *What Price Community Medicine?*
47 Hanley, *Medicine, Knowledge and Venereal Diseases*; Hanley, 'The public's reaction to public health'; Mooney, *Intrusive Interventions*; Michael Worboys, *Spreading Germs: Disease Theories and Medical Practice in Britain, 1865–1900* (Cambridge: Cambridge University Press, 2000).
48 *Ibid*.
49 John Welshman, 'The Medical Officer of Health in England and Wales, 1900–1974: Watchdog or lapdog?', *Journal of Public Health*, 19:4 (1997), 443–50; Gorsky, 'Public health in interwar Britain'.
50 Virginia Berridge, *Marketing Health* (Oxford: Oxford University Press, 2007).
51 *Ibid*.
52 Diana Barnes, 'The public life of a woman of wit and quality: Lady Mary Wortley Montagu and the vogue for smallpox inoculation', *Feminist Studies*, 38:2 (2012), 330–62; Anne Eriksen, 'Advocating inoculation in the eighteenth century: Exemplarity and quantification', *Science in Context*, 29:2 (2016), 213–39.
53 Anne Eriksen, 'Cure or protection? The meaning of smallpox inoculation, ca 1750–1775', *Medical History*, 57:4 (2013), 516–36.
54 Edward Jenner, *An Inquiry into the Causes and Effects of the Variolæ Vaccinæ a Disease Discovered in Some of the Western Counties of England, Particularly Gloucestershire and Known by the Name of the Cow Pox* (London: Sampson Low, 1789). Benjamin Jesty is often credited as the "inventor" of vaccination, but there were others who had written about cowpox and its potential as a prophylactic against smallpox. See Colin R. Howard, 'The impact on public health of the 19th century anti-vaccination movement', *Microbiology*

Today, 30:1 (February 2003), 22–5; Frank Fenner, Donald A. Henderson, Isao Arita, Jezek Zdenek, Ivan Danilovich Ladnyi and World Health Organization, *Smallpox and Its Eradication* (Geneva: World Health Organization, 1988), p. 258.

55 Vaccination Acts were passed in 1840, 1853, 1867, 1871, 1873, 1898 and 1907. See Deborah Brunton, *The Politics of Vaccination: Practice and Policy in England, Wales, Ireland, and Scotland, 1800–1874* (New York: University Rochester Press, 2008); Hardy, *The Epidemic Streets: Infectious Disease and the Rise of Preventive Medicine, 1856–1900* (Oxford; New York: Clarendon Press ; Oxford University Press, 1993), pp. 110–50.

56 R. E. Spier, 'Perception of risk of vaccine adverse events: a historical perspective', *Vaccine*, 20:Supplement 1 (2001), S78–S84; Colgrove, *State of Immunity*; Nadja Durbach, 'Class, gender, and the conscientious objector to vaccination, 1898–1907', *Journal of British Studies*, 41:1 (2002), 58–83; Durbach, 'Bodily matters'.

57 Foucault, *The Birth of the Clinic*; Armstrong, *Political Anatomy of the Body*; Mooney, *Intrusive Interventions*.

58 As with Jenner and vaccination, there is debate about who was the first to create laboratory-based vaccines, but Pasteur was the first to demonstrate their benefits on a larger scale. Maurice Cassier, 'Producing, controlling, and stabilizing Pasteur's anthrax vaccine: Creating a new industry and a health market', *Science in Context*, 21:2 (2008), 253–78; John D. Grabenstein, 'Toxoid vaccines', in Andrew W. Artenstein (ed.), *Vaccines: A Biography* (New York: Springer, 2010), pp. 105–24.

59 Worboys, *Spreading Germs*; Anne Marie Moulin, 'La metaphore vaccine: de l'inoculation a la vaccinologie', *History & Philosophy of the Life Sciences*, 14:2 (1992), 271–97; Kendall A. Smith, 'Louis Pasteur, the father of immunology?', *Frontier in Immunology*, 3:68 (2012). See also Frank C. Schmalstieg and Armond S. Goldman, 'Birth of the science of immunology', *Journal of Medical Biography*, 18:2 (2010), 88–98; Steven M. Opal, 'A brief history of microbiology and immunology', in Andrew W. Artenstein (ed.), *Vaccines: A Biography* (New York: Springer, 2010), pp. 31–56.

60 Esteban Rodríguez Ocaña, 'The social production of novelty: Diphtheria serotherapy, "herald of the new medicine"', *Dynamis*, 27 (2007), 21–31. See also the special edition of *Dynamis* on diphtheria immunisation, including: Gabriel Gachelin, 'The designing of anti-diphtheria serotherapy at the Institut Pasteur (1888–1900): The role of a supranational network of microbiologists', *Dynamis*, 27 (2007), 45–62; Jonathan Simon, 'The origin of the production of diphtheria antitoxin in France, between philanthropy and commerce', *Dynamis*, 27 (2007), 63–82; Axel C. Hüntelmann,

'Diphtheria serum and serotherapy. Development, production and regulation in "Fin De Siecle" Germany', *Dynamis*, 27 (2007), 107–31.
61 Heller, *The Vaccine Narrative*.
62 W. W. C. Topley and G. S. Wilson, 'The spread of bacterial infection. The problem of herd-immunity', *The Journal of Hygiene*, 21:3 (1923), 243–9.
63 Cassier, 'Producing, controlling, and stabilizing Pasteur's anthrax vaccine'.
64 Ocaña, 'The social production of novelty'.
65 Colgrove, *State of Immunity*.
66 Although, as Patrick Carroll argues, British public health did engage in its own form of policing, and the dichotomy between the British and German systems is more rhetorical than it appears in practice. Patrick E. Carroll, 'Medical police and the history of public health', *Medical History*, 46:4 (2002), 461–94.
67 See Berridge, *Marketing Health*.
68 Bryder, 'BCG vaccination'; Lewis, 'The prevention of diphtheria'.
69 Ibid.
70 Ibid.
71 Lewis, 'The Prevention of diphtheria'; Welshman, 'The Medical Officer of Health in England and Wales, 1900–1974'; Gorsky, 'Public health in interwar Britain'.
72 Lewis, 'The Prevention of diphtheria'. See, for example, the government files detailing correspondence between such groups as the Anti-Vaccination League and the British Union for the Abolition of Vivisection in: The National Archives (hereafter TNA): MH 55/293; MH 55/1720; HO 45/10768/273078; and passim.
73 See Hooker, 'Diphtheria, immunisation and the Bundaberg tragedy'; Peter Hobbins, '"Immunisation is as popular as a death adder": The Bundaberg Tragedy and the politics of medical science in interwar Australia', *Social History of Medicine*, 24:2 (2011), 426–44; Day, '"The magical formula"'; Parish, *A History of Immunization*, pp. 151–3.
74 Trials were published in: Percival Horton-Smith Hartley, *A Study of Diphtheria in Two Areas of Great Britain: With Special Reference to the Antitoxin Concentration of the Serum of Inoculated and Non-inoculated Patients and Other Persons; and the Relation of this to the Incidence, Type and Severity of the Disease* (London: HMSO, 1950); Medical Research Council, 'B.C.G. and vole bacillus caccines in the prevention of tuberculosis in adolescents', *British Medical Journal*, 1:4964 (1956), 413–27; Medical Research Council, 'B.C.G. and vole bacillus vaccines in the prevention of tuberculosis in adolescents', *British Medical Journal*, 2:5149 (1959), 379–96. See also TNA: FD 1/8290; FD 4/272.

75 Kendall Hoyt, *Long Shot: Vaccines for National Defense* (Cambridge, MA: Harvard University Press, 2012); Emma Newlands, *Civilians into Soldiers: War, the Body and British Army Recruits, 1939–45* (Manchester: Manchester University Press, 2014).
76 Nicholas C. Artenstein and Andrew W. Artenstein, 'The discovery of viruses and the evolution of vaccinology', Andrew W. Artenstein (ed.), *Vaccines: A Biography* (New York: Springer, 2010), pp. 141–58.

I
The development and evolution of the vaccination programme

1

Diphtheria

In 1940, diphtheria became the first vaccine of the bacteriological age to be offered free to British children on a national scale. It achieved impressive results in its first years, reducing the case load from over 46,000 in 1940 to just 962 in 1950, and deaths from 2,480 to 49.[1] Medical authorities celebrated this success, but were mindful of the paradox they had created. With diphtheria no longer a common disease, would parents stop immunising their children? And if they did, would a disease that should be eliminated make a deadly return?

These fears appeared to be realised in 1950. After solid progress in immunisation of the child population throughout the 1940s, there was a sudden decline in the number of children being presented for immunisation. While a number of causes were investigated, the main culprit, in the eyes of the Ministry of Health, was apathy. A publicity campaign began and was maintained throughout the 1950s, coordinated through the Ministry of Health and Central Office of Information (COI) and supported through direct interactions with the public by local medical authorities.

This chapter discusses how "apathy" acted as an explanatory model and call to action for health authorities seeking to improve uptake of immunisation services among the population. It played a key role in constructing the public in the minds of policy makers, built out of long-standing paternalistic attitudes towards the working classes, particularly mothers. The Ministry considered apathy a problem because it threatened the successes achieved by public health policy up to this point. Immunisation had reduced the burden of diphtheria on the health services and, it was hoped, could eventually eliminate the disease entirely. The risk was that this apparent progress might stall – or, worse, the disease would return to higher levels. By defining apathy as low uptake of immunisation, the problem could be identified and quantified. In turn, apathy tells us how these authorities viewed the public and their relationship with them. The Ministry of Health focused on encouraging individuals to immunise their children in order to minimise the risk of diphtheria's return. Its campaign ran on the basis that parents no longer feared diphtheria and therefore were unmotivated to present their children for immunisation. Nevertheless, authorities also understood that there were many reasons why parents might not vaccinate. At the local level, medical officers worked with the public and responded to their needs. That is to say, the public was not simply lectured to; rather, policy makers consistently monitored the public through various systems of surveillance for signs that could be interpreted. Apathy actively guided policy in ways that often made immunisation more convenient for parents and children. It was a form of communication; a translation of the diffuse behaviours of the public into a language which administrators and policy makers could understand.

Apathy is an amorphous concept. Indeed, the imprecise nature of the term in itself gives us insight into the motivations and thinking behind local and national policy. This chapter therefore attempts not to deconstruct how the concept was experienced by parents in 1950s Britain but, rather, to explore how it was used – often without precision – by various authorities. Apathy was often invoked to explain public behaviour, and attempts were made to combat it. It was a rhetorical device, one without an objective basis, yet still built into the longer history of British public health practice.

This chapter begins by outlining how the national anti-diphtheria programme came into being during the Second World War. It shows how this continued after 1945, and through the formation of the new NHS. In 1950, however, the Ministry of Health became concerned at declining vaccination rates. The reasons for this are explored, in terms both of changing patterns of behaviour and of the ways in which the statistical indicators available to the Ministry allowed it to "see" (or construct) apathy among parents. The chapter then goes on to explain what national and local government did to combat apathy over the course of the 1950s.

Diphtheria immunisation before 1945

If the decline in immunisation rates suggested that the British people had become complacent about diphtheria, this was not always the case. After some initial difficulties, take-up of diphtheria immunisation was high throughout the later war years and into the late 1940s. Diphtheria immunisation developed out of the work in the emerging science of bacteriology at the turn of the twentieth century.[2] As Claire Hooker and Alison Bashford have argued, 'diphtheria is ideally placed for thinking through the historical connections between bacteriology and applied public health precisely because it was so strongly associated with laboratory medicine and the new capacities to understand and therefore control disease'.[3] The condition itself was discovered to be caused by a bacterium, *Corynebacterium diphtheria*, and tended to attack through the larynx and the tonsils. Complications could include heart disease and paralysis, sometimes leading to death. In Britain during the 1930s, before the introduction of immunisation, an average of 58,000 cases were seen each year, with 2,800 deaths.[4]

However, Britain had not always been so enthusiastic about the procedure. British public health authorities had come to adopt immunisation relatively late, compared to those in other Western nations. Toronto and New York City, for example, had run successful interventions during the inter-war years to significantly reduce morbidity and mortality.[5] Despite this, and although some local authorities had used immunisation prior to the Second World War, Britain was rather conservative with regard to new immunisation technologies. The anti-vaccination and anti-vivisection organisations were still relatively powerful in the 1930s, and the experience of resistance to compulsory smallpox vaccination in the nineteenth century still loomed large.[6] There was also a widespread belief among medical authorities that the well-established public health system in Britain functioned perfectly well without the use of prophylactics. The main example cited was the much lower rates of tuberculosis in Britain as compared to France, despite the latter's use of BCG. Sanatoria and health education were therefore seen by medical authorities as at least as good as BCG, if not better, and so they were not willing to risk introducing a new public health measure that might go wrong.[7] There was no guarantee of vaccine safety, as evidenced by the poisoning of children with contaminated diphtheria toxoid in

Bundaberg, Australia, and contaminated BCG in Lübeck, Germany.[8] While the national government stayed clear of providing the toxoid or centrally funded advertising to promote immunisation, local authorities had been permitted to use it before the war. However, they had to pay for supplies and manpower themselves.[9] Thus, it was embraced with varying levels of enthusiasm and administered with varying levels of competence, resulting in very uneven coverage.[10]

The war provided an impetus to adopt immunisation as a mass public health measure. Mobile populations as a result of evacuation, bomb damage and general dislocation made traditional public health measures more difficult to maintain. Combined with the need to keep the home population healthy for industrial output and morale, diphtheria immunisation was belatedly accepted.[11] From late 1940, a campaign was initiated to immunise all school children. The minimum school leaving age was fourteen, and the school system provided a useful site for vaccination before leavers entered the world of work. The prophylactic was supplied to local authorities free of charge, and the government estimated that around a third of school children up to the age of fourteen had been immunised by September 1941.[12]

After the war

Although in many ways the war-time experience might be seen as atypical, given the number of controls imposed on public life and economic behaviour, immunisation had been shown to be invaluable. Parents thus understood that it was an effective tool and they were keen to have their children protected. If apathy was a problem, authorities were at no great pains to stress it. Indeed, they saw parents' enthusiasm as a sign that modern preventative health care would be seen as a civic duty – states would be obliged to provide services, and good citizens would actively use them.[13] While the British political classes had committed to the social rights of a comprehensive welfare state based on the war-time Beveridge Report, they also came to expect certain behaviours in return.[14] These trends were common in the West during the twentieth century, and accelerated after 1945. Dorothy Porter has argued that it would become increasingly unacceptable for people to be unhealthy and that citizens would be under pressure from the state and from their peers to avoid ill-health.[15] As diseases became "vaccine preventable", not vaccinating became an unacceptable practice. In a speech to the Council for Education and World Citizenship in 1946, Labour Minister of Health Aneurin Bevan cited immunisation as an example of what centrally coordinated health services backed by modern medicine could achieve. Morbidity from diphtheria had effectively halved from its pre-war levels; mortality had been reduced to a third. Bevan further argued 'that in working for a better health service [the Labour Party was] not looking forward to a nation of hypochondriacs, enjoying bad health, but a nation whose members understood and practised the laws of health'. This encompassed a range of health technologies and lifestyle changes, of which immunisation was one. But it would require the 'energetic cooperation of every citizen' to achieve its full effects.[16] Citizens were both the users of services and, through taxation, the funders. Government imposed moral and legal conditions on citizens in return for services, but through democratic channels also could claim to represent citizens. These inherent tensions in health care systems, between individual liberty and collective responsibility, were not new to this period, but they were recast.[17] Indeed, later in the century, as the focus of welfare provision began to shift from a broadly social democratic model to one based more on markets and individual choice within a public-private framework, the relationship between public or preventative health and citizens would change.[18]

This interplay between citizenship and risk management is explored in greater detail in Chapter 4. What is important in the immediate postwar era, however, is that citizens also demanded health protection from the government. The most obvious example of this is the creation of the NHS. T. H. Marshall would describe the coming of the new welfare state as an expression of social rights, a new age in which protection from hardship would be as important as equality under the law and the right to vote in previous decades.[19] If there was a will for greater protection, state planning and modern science appeared to offer a means for its provision. Although much would later be made of the "technocratic age" of the 1950s and 1960s, it was in the 1940s that the British state would begin to take greater control of once-private industries in the name of efficiency and accountability.[20] Indeed, it was through the establishment of monitoring statistics during this time that the

Ministry of Health was able to monitor the apathy that it would see in the 1950s and how it would come to see problems within the rest of the vaccination programme, as described in the later chapters of this book.

Throughout the period discussed in this chapter, the government recommended an initial immunisation of children under the age of twelve months. Young children were at the most risk of death, and early immunisation was considered necessary to increase the efficiency of the programme. This was initial immunisation was "boosted" with a reinforcing dose as the child entered primary school.[21] A combined prophylaxis was also available in some areas, offering protection against both diphtheria and pertussis (whooping cough), which complicated this picture as the 1950s progressed, as authorities could run slightly different programmes to those of their peers. Where the combined vaccine was used the schedule was amended to find a practical and epidemiologically sound compromise between protecting children from pertussis as early as possible and maintaining safety standards. Trials had begun on the pertussis vaccine in 1942, and the combined vaccine was trialled from 1951.[22] By 1957, almost all local authorities had applied for and been granted permission to vaccinate against whooping cough, and many chose the combined immunisation.[23] Because whooping cough was even more dangerous for very young children, this dose was given to children at around six to nine months old. The relationship between the two vaccines – and indeed the two diseases – had implications for the campaign against apathy. The Ministry considered the public much more fearful of whooping cough, and therefore the combined prophylactic was seen as an administratively convenient way of reaching otherwise-apathetic parents. Separate injections may have led parents to "choose" one form of protection over another, further reducing the diphtheria immunisation rate.[24] These are discussions to which this chapter will return.

The use of schools as sites for vaccination was significant for two reasons. First, since attendance was compulsory, schools were historically important as a surveillance tool for health authorities. Height, weight and other measurements were taken in schools to track malnutrition and neglect, primarily to ensure that children grew up healthy enough to work in factories, fight in the army and bear children.[25] Through them, local MOHs could reach almost all children and produce records about their immunisation statuses for routine monitoring and follow-up. Second, this greater efficiency in school-age surveillance meant that there was a significantly higher rate of immunisation among children over the age of five than those of pre-school age.[26] Infants were immunised at clinics held at specific times, usually led by the MOH. This reflected the administrative arrangements for public health at the time, as well as practical considerations with regard to diphtheria toxoid. Immunising from local authority clinics made it easier to store the vaccine, order in bulk and keep track of usage statistics. Clinics could see more patients in a shorter period than general practitioners, who, before 1948, were not contracted to a national health service.[27] Supplying the vaccine to individual surgeries and collating the statistical returns demanded by the Ministry would also add an extra layer of administration. Parents could make arrangements with their own doctor if they wished, with the general practitioner then being compensated by the local authority, but this was less common than attendance at a clinic.[28] This meant that most parents had to make a specific trip to the clinic to get their children immunised, rather than having the procedure done at the same time as a routine visit or check-up at the doctor's surgery.

Through the statistical data available, the Ministry was well aware that uptake among children of different ages varied significantly. This was a cause for concern from the early days of the programme. Pre-schoolers were specifically targeted in 1942, and again after the end of the war, in an attempt to combat the discrepancy.[29] By the birth of the NHS, local authorities were tasked with immunising 75 per cent of children before they reached their first birthday.[30] But uptake rates did not vary just by age. Geography was another major dynamic. Immunisation was managed at the local level under the direction of local MOHs. Local authorities had traditionally enjoyed a good degree of autonomy from central government, meaning that they could often be resistant if the Ministry attempted to interfere too much with regional matters.[31] However, the use of MOHs was administratively convenient – smallpox vaccination had been the responsibility of local authorities before 1948, and this was maintained and formalised by Section 26 of the National Health Service Acts.[32] There was an inherent tension, therefore, between national targets and local circumstances. The attitudes of parents and priorities of MOHs could vary considerably from council to council, and local difficulties could suspend or severely derail efforts to immunise children promptly. For example, in 1946 in London alone the diphtheria immunisation rate of children under five years old ranged from 68 per cent in one borough to just 28 per cent in another; and the figures for five- to fourteen-year-olds ranged from 20 per cent to 86 per cent.[33]

That "convenience" had an effect on immunisation uptake was significant. Indeed, it would be a central part of debates about apathy. For while a parent's unwillingness to surmount inconvenience could be criticised as apathetic behaviour, it could also be seen a reasonable response to failures on the part of public health authorities, in terms of both service provision and education. Regardless, this was something that needed to be tackled. If indeed the problem was one of willingness to act over convenience, the Ministry believed that this could be overcome through education and persuasion. In this sense, apathy was bound to long-held liberal concepts of public health based on individual freedom and the capacity of informed people to make rational (and therefore "correct") choices.[34] Human behaviour was a contributor to the spread of disease, giving moral authority for medical officers to intervene for the good of national productivity and military power.[35] As societies became more reliant on technologies and complex administrative systems, these risks were considered to be manageable. The state's role was therefore to ensure that individuals behaved in ways that did not expose the state or fellow citizens.[36] However, such actions could not unduly interfere with the rights of private citizens. Thus, education was seen by English practitioners as a sign of the nation's democratic values, especially when compared to states like Germany that employed a coercive medical police.[37]

During the inter-war years, national and local health authorities expanded education as a preventative strategy.[38] The creation of the COI from the war-time Ministry of Information also showed that such tactics would become even more important in the NHS era.[39] Apathy was therefore seen as something that could be eliminated, much like sewerage and other public health measures had rid the streets of other "nuisances". Educating the public through "propaganda", as it was termed by public health officials at the time (without the modern negative connotations), was a key tool in the MOH's arsenal.[40] And yet, this also gave rise to the possibility of "victim blaming". Once education and information were put out to the public, only the stupid, obstinate or wilfully neglectful would not follow the "rational" path set out by public health campaigners.[41] The experience of the 1950s shows that this was not always the way apathy was used as a rhetorical tool. Many people who had been exposed to "education" and were still non-compliant could still be depicted as "apathetic". Similarly, the Ministry accepted that lower immunisation rates were a predictable and rational response to the decline of the disease. Moreover, interactions between authorities and the public showed that there were other costs and risks associated with immunisation that informed parents' decisions about their children's health.

Despite this subjective and vague notion of apathy, the Ministry of Health felt that it would undermine the immunisation programme and see the return of thousands of cases of a deadly illness.[42] This attitude reflected a belief that citizens had a duty to be engaged in their own health care – to avoid illness and so not put strain on health resources or harm national productivity. The immediate post-war era was one in which citizens demanded health care as a right from their governments; but it was also one in which governments and fellow citizens demanded mindfulness of those who used those services.[43] As a result, the government identified apathy as a problem and sought to "measure" it, primarily through tracking immunisation rates and commissioning studies from the Social Survey (both of which will be explored in this chapter). Yet as we will also see, publics responded in other ways which showed that they were not as disengaged as headline figures and official thinking might have suggested. This, in turn, affected the ways in which local and national authorities sought to engage the public. It had a major impact in the way in which the 1950s anti-diphtheria campaign would be run.

The 1950s campaign

All the evidence suggested that the immunisation campaign since 1940 had been a public health success story. Local authorities were required to return statistics on the number of immunisations performed, and diphtheria was a notifiable disease. Case load and death rates dropped significantly over the period up to 1950. To celebrate ten years of the NHS, London County Council's Annual Report for 1957 showed the significant decline in mortality in different age groups in an informative chart (Figure 1.1). A trend line was plotted to show just how successful

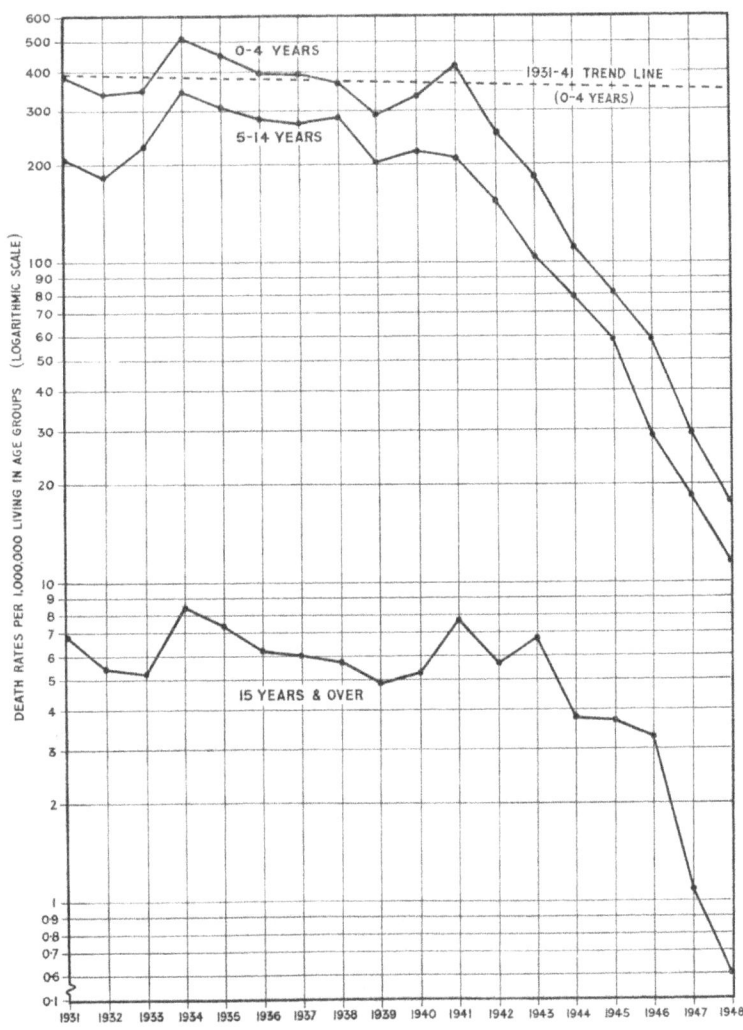

Figure 1.1 England and Wales: diphtheria deaths, 1931–48.
Source: J. A. Scott, *MOH Report, 1957*, p. 65. Reproduced from the digitised Medical Officer of Health Reports by the Wellcome Trust under Creative Commons licence (CC-BY 4.0).

public health provisions had been in the 1940s by comparing actual death rates to a projection based on data from the 1930s.[44] Other graphs produced in MOH reports in the 1950s also included a line plotting 'percentage of population (5–14) not immunised', which further demonstrated the correlation between immunisation rates and declining notifications in London County.[45] Further proof of the impact of immunisation came from official statistics. Those who had been immunised were four times less likely to develop the disease, and if they did, they were twenty times less likely to die of it.[46]

However, the Ministry became concerned at the sudden drop in the number of young children being immunised. In 1949, the government had achieved its target of 75 per cent uptake. Yet, preliminary figures for 1950 suggested a significant decrease, and in 1951 fewer than 30 per cent of children less than a year old were immunised.[47] It was clear that the Ministry had a problem. The question was, what had caused it and what could be done? Very quickly, "apathy" among parents was identified as the main culprit.

The choice to focus on apathy seems at first glance to be a strange one. The decrease in the number of vaccinations was caused primarily by a lack of opportunity. Owing to a national epidemic of poliomyelitis, the campaign had been suspended in areas of particularly high prevalence.[48] This meant that parents' appointments were cancelled, and local authorities could not follow up on young children who had not been immunised.[49] The reason for the suspension was that medical authorities had received some evidence that immunisation (against any disease) might exacerbate the onset of paralysis in the limb in which a person was injected during a poliomyelitis outbreak. Some medical professionals and commentators argued that the act of injection may actually cause polio, reflecting the gaps in knowledge about the disease at the time.[50] A. Bradford Hill and J. Knowelden at the London School of Hygiene and Tropical Medicine performed an analysis on government data and case reports from J. K. Martin,[51] B. P. McCloskey[52] and D. H. Geffen.[53] They concluded that people who developed poliomyelitis within one month of being immunised were much more likely to experience paralysis in the limb in which they were injected. Despite this, it was found that the risks of a recently immunised person developing paralytic symptoms were no greater than those of an unimmunised person – i.e., immunisation did not *cause* paralytic polio.[54] In subsequent years, this allowed the national immunisation campaign to continue, with suspension occurring only in local areas with significant polio outbreaks. National propaganda was, however, suspended during the summer months, the "polio season" in which most cases developed.[55] Despite the clear decline in the percentage of children being immunised, the second biggest reason for the decrease in absolute numbers of immunisations was the lower birth rate of 1949 as compared to the following year of 1950.[56] If the polio season and declining birth rates explained most of the drop-off, then why was the Ministry of Health so concerned with apathy?

Part of the answer lies in how public health authorities monitored and identified public health problems. They concentrated on the areas of low uptake that they could combat directly – that is, the risks that could be managed. Convinced that rates were low even when one made allowances for polio and the birth rate, the Ministry surveyed parents to ascertain their attitudes towards immunisation. It hypothesised that apathy could be a problem; and sought to find it through its new research department, the Social Survey.

The Social Survey had emerged out of the war years and was the successor to the Wartime Social Survey, which was established by the Coalition government as a way of monitoring public attitudes and experiences of government departments so that policies could be more efficiently tailored to the conditions of war-time Britain.[57] Building on sociological and survey methods developed in the earlier period by social research pioneers such as Charles Booth and Joseph Rowntree, and mass participation projects such as Mass Observation, it represented a shift towards technocratic solutions to social problems and an increasing faith in the state to be able to provide rational responses.[58] As Lord Moran showed in 1952, surveys were seen by many in the medical establishment as an excellent tool for judging the public's mood and, in Moran's words, 'persuading them to fall into line' by developing 'new methods of interesting and educating the public' against 'prejudices and old wives' fears'.[59] The Ministry had used the Wartime Social Survey and its successor to assess the impact of its original propaganda campaign during and immediately after the war, interviewing mothers about their knowledge about diphtheria and where they had heard about it.[60] In combination, they suggested that by 1945 most mothers knew about immunisation and almost all had adequate access to clinics. Rates of immunisation were much higher than they had been in earlier years, and apathy is mentioned only as a side concern. By taking those parents who said that they 'have not bothered, not had time yet' and those who had incorrectly believed their children were too young, it estimated 'about 12% of mothers have not had their children immunised owing to ignorance or apathy'.[61] Nine per cent were considered to 'have a positive resistance' through not believing in the procedure, spousal objection or fears the child would be hurt or frightened.[62]

While the 1942 and 1945 surveys had specifically investigated the level of knowledge and effects of propaganda on parents, the 1951 report focused more heavily on the reasons for declining uptake. Many of the questions were similar, to allow comparison across time, but the final report spent much more time analysing the reasons for non-immunisation from mothers of young children. The Ministry hoped to find the extent of apathy and the deeper reasons for parents' reluctance to immunise. Yet, it did not appear that – statistically – apathy could be considered a much larger problem than it had been six years previously. Indeed, direct resistance to immunisation appeared to be much lower than in 1945, with only 3 per cent of mothers considered to be opposed to the procedure.[63] Thirty-five per cent of children who had not been immunised were 'accounted for by apathy and ignorance on the part of the mother'. This, the report concluded, was a similar overall proportion to that identified in 1945.[64] Even the new problem of poliomyelitis did not appear to have had much material effect. The Chief Medical Officer had claimed that the suspension of the programme in some areas had 'naturally aroused apprehension among parents'.[65] But while this was the greatest cause of the lower immunisation rates in 1950, there was little evidence that it had affected parents' decisions about whether to present their children. Very few mothers who had not immunised their children gave the fear of polio as a reason. The debate had received some coverage in the *Manchester Guardian* and *Daily Express*,[66] but despite 'a whole series of questions enabling them to reveal their knowledge on the subject … only 4% of mothers were even aware of the possible association'.[67]

Identifying apathy was not solely an exercise in statistical and sociological methodology. Even if the Social Survey suggested that apathy had not increased, some MOHs and commentators at local and national levels continued to report that they had seen or felt its effects within their communities. Apathy was not, necessarily, something the Social Survey could adequately and objectively capture. It was emotional, identified as a lack of fear among parents. While less tangible than objective survey results, it was no less real to medical officers at the national and local levels. Professional experience and intuition told them that apathy was a bigger problem than it had been in the past; and this perception guided action as much as any material reality. For the Ministry, this was confirmed by their interpretation of uptake statistics. For MOHs, interactions with local citizens confirmed their suspicions. The decline both of parental fear and of the efficacy of public health's ability to communicate risk was reported in multiple forums. The COI had received a lot of praise for the cost-efficiency and positive effects of its campaigning in the 1940s,[68] but the feeling was that the tactics that had been used in previous years were no longer sufficient. The Chief Medical Officer argued that it had become 'less easy to bring home to parents the vital importance of protecting their children than it used to be when most of them had first-hand knowledge of this disease among their own and their neighbours' children.'[69] Others in the press and medical establishment agreed. The Times' medical correspondent wrote of 'a sense of false security' that had tended to 'spread throughout the community'.[70] The London County Council MOH added that 'the low incidence of diphtheria … whilst itself resulting from the successful measures of immunisation, tends to produce apathy in parents to whom the old days of diphtheria scourge were unknown.'[71] Newspaper editorials also reflected concerns after the war that apathy with regard to health care extended beyond diphtheria. 'All the efforts which are being made to improve the health of the nation will come to nothing if people, ignorantly or selfishly, neglect the precautions that are offered them free,' argued the *Daily Mirror*.[72] The *Manchester Guardian* was particularly scathing. The uptake of free orange juice and cod liver oil in schools was at less than half of official targets. Child dentistry, too, was often neglected, despite its availability on the NHS. The public, it argued in an editorial, were apathetic about prophylaxis in general, and neglecting their civic duties.

> We are being kept alive longer, we are surrounded by expensive welfare systems, and yet many of us are too lazy or ignorant to give our children

the safeguards to a healthy life that the State is ready to provide, and too dirty or slovenly in our personal habits to escape outbreaks of food poisoning that should never occur at all. ...

We should be a far healthier nation if we turned as readily to free preventative medical services as we clamour for free aspirin and barbiturates. ... It is a sad indictment of our society that we let free health go begging and then demand money in hundreds of millions to spend on "free" medicine.[73]

These observations, even if they were not borne out by the statistics, dominated the official narrative. They reflected contemporary concerns about good health citizenship in the post-war era, and (at least in the case of the *Manchester Guardian* editorial) appeared to project wider anxieties about other welfare programmes onto vaccination. While good health had come to be seen as a right across economically developed countries after the Second World War, there was also a sense that citizens had a duty to behave in way that did not put their health at risk.[74] Good health meant fewer hospital visits, meaning lower direct health care costs and better productivity owing to fewer work days lost to sickness and disability.[75] This meant citizens making use of welfare schemes that were provided for their own good. Parents ought to want immunisation, and they ought to present their children. If they did not do so, this apathy needed to be eliminated. The national government continued to remind the public of its obligations, but also appealed directly to parents about their own children's health and wellbeing. It stuck to its original premise of attempting to educate parents about the dangers of diphtheria and the benefits of immunisation, in the hope of increasing immunisation rates so that the disease could continue its decline throughout the country. If such tactics had worked in the past, reframing them in the wake of declining fear of diphtheria ought to work again.

The national campaign

The campaign that followed borrowed heavily from posters and tactics that had been used to establish the diphtheria programme during the war. However, the emphasis turned away from simply extolling the virtues of immunisation and towards a concerted effort to explain to parents just why they should still fear the disease, in an effort to combat apathy. The Ministry aimed 'To persuade parents to have their children immunised against Diphtheria *before* they reach the age of twelve months', and 'To raise the level of children immunised to 75% thereby eliminating Diphtheria as an epidemic disease'.[76]

The justification was three-fold. First, the Ministry warned that while morbidity had continued to decline in 1951, so had the immunisation rate. Second, preliminary figures showed the 1952 was on course to be the first year since immunisation began in which mortality had not decreased. Third, the impending introduction of nationwide whooping cough vaccination led the Ministry to worry that parents would choose to ignore diphtheria altogether unless they were made aware of the risks of the disease.[77]

At the national level, the Ministry of Health prescribed propaganda to treat the ailment. It hired billboards for large sixteen-sheet posters, as well as initiating a targeted press campaign. The message throughout the 1950s was that 'diphtheria still kills' and 'diphtheria is deadly'.[78] However, resource constraints limited what the Ministry could do. For 1953 it had wanted to run a nationwide poster campaign costing £21,700. This was denied by the Treasury, who instead allowed a budget of £10,000.[79] The Ministry 'fully agreed that [this] amount ... was insufficient to counteract existing apathy, make parents fully aware of the dangers of diphtheria, and emphasise that the elimination of the disease is conditional upon the maintenance of an adequate level of immunisation'.[80] But what could be done? The Churchill government had placed limits on expenditure – referred to by the Ministry as the 'Salisbury ceiling' – and this was a time of austerity for a number of departments.[81] To make best use of resources, the national campaign was targeted at those areas where the total immunisation coverage in children under five years old had dropped below 50 per cent.[82]

The Ministry of Health acknowledged that such efforts would be in vain without the cooperation of local authorities, showing that the diphtheria programme was not entirely "top down". The Chief Medical Officer explicitly praised MOHs for their work, explaining that the national publicity operation could only help, not replace, the tried and tested campaigning techniques at the local level. This included further targeted advertising, but was also dependent upon the aid of voluntary organisations and efficient use of face-to-face contact between local authority medical staff and parents during the first years of their babies' lives. Thus 'the health visitor, midwife and clinic doctor constitute[d] the joint spearhead of the attack on smallpox and diphtheria'.[83] The campaign was aimed at 'those mothers who have been lulled into a false sense of security', but would 'depend, more than ever, on local initiative'. '*If* local authorities make effective use' of the materials provided, 'there will be fewer mothers saying "if only…" this year – and perhaps in future years too.'[84]

Elements of this campaign were universal in tone, seemingly targeted at all parents. We can see this quite clearly in the centrally produced propaganda materials. The 1951/52 campaign led with a striking and stark poster. It contained no images, but was a simple black typeface on a white background. It read, 'if you had seen a child with diphtheria you would have yours immunised now'. The word 'if' (all in lower case) was larger than the rest of the text, and emphasised by being picked out in red.[85] A later version of the same poster used white text on a black background, but kept the red colour of the opening word.[86] Many leaflets and posters led with (or at least contained) the line 'diphtheria still kills', with emphasis often placed on the word 'still'. Another common line was 'diphtheria costs lives – immunisation costs nothing'.[87] Having been armed with these facts, and being made aware of the real risks of diphtheria, it was argued, parents would make the right choice: 'The wise parent knows … that with the best care in the world any child, and particularly a baby, may fall ill', after all.[88] The only way to insure against this was via immunisation.

Another universal approach was to send postcards to houses where a child was about to reach their first birthday. Decorated like birthday cards, the imagery of celebration helped to present the Ministry's central message. First, it reminded parents of the need to get children immunised before they turned one; and second, it reinforced the idea that immunisation was a gift, and one that both parent and baby would appreciate in time. Local authorities in London found this a particularly helpful tactic, one that was both universal and, by physically entering the homes of potential contacts, in some ways personal. Not everyone could be met by a health visitor, but almost all could be reached through the Royal Mail.[89] It played to the very personal relationship between parents and their young children. 'Only if parents are wise enough to give their babies protection can this deadly disease be held in check,' declared one leaflet.[90] Such rhetoric also emphasised that central tenet of the liberal British public health tradition: immunisation, while clearly desirable and implored by the government, was still a choice.

Despite the universalist overtones, the government was clearly selective in where it targeted its messages. It made very deliberate choices in how and where these messages were sent, telling us much about just whose "apathy" was considered a danger. In doing so, it focused on the group in whom it felt apathy was the most dangerous. As had been made clear from the Social Survey, investigations into parental responses to diphtheria and immunisation had questioned only mothers.[91] Here it had found only a small number of families where immunisation had been refused on the basis of the father's disapproval. These were not further sub-divided in the published statistics, though the report mentioned that about half of those questioned about the father's objection noted bad experience of (smallpox) vaccination in the armed forces and among other parents. All other reasons for non-immunisation were attributed to the mother. Apathy was measured through four categories of response considered to be 'unsatisfactory excuses'. These were 'father does not agree', 'does not believe in it', 'never heard of it' and 'not bothered'. All placed the blame on the mother.[92] This in itself is quite illuminating. 'Never heard of it' would imply a lack of knowledge rather than a lack of care. Yet clearly the authorities were willing to conflate the two. In the midst of a long-running national and local campaign, ignorance was not an excuse. Similarly, 'does not believe in it' and 'father does not agree' would imply positive objection rather than apathy. At face value, only 'not bothered' would constitute indifference. In all of these cases, however, the assumption on the part of health authorities would be that these issues could be cured through education and persuasion. If, in the British liberal tradition of public health, apathy were overcome through giving rational actors the correct facts about health care, then, once mothers (and, in some cases, fathers) were properly educated, these problems would cease. For the Ministry of Health, apathy could cover a range of public responses, so long as they were surmountable through good education.

The focus on mothers can in large part be attributed to mid-century visions of the role of mothers within the family, with women traditionally being seen as the primary – and, at times, only – caregivers.[93] This had been a common theme in public health from the late nineteenth century, the point at which 'motherhood' became an ideological and political state rather than simply a descriptive term for being a mother.[94] But it was not inevitable that fathers would be side-lined. During the interwar years, the role of fathers in the care and raising of children began to gain importance.[95] An agony-aunt column in the *Daily Mirror* clearly felt that fathers had a role, with Sister Clare telling dads to 'put [their] foot down firmly here and insist' that the mother agree to immunisation.[96] The original survey in 1942 did investigate whether 'husbands' were consulted in the decision to immunise the child. Fifty-four per cent of mothers said that they did consult their husband, with 40 per cent declaring that it was their 'own decision'. Husbands from more affluent backgrounds were more likely to be involved, but even in the 'D' social classes, there was an equal split of 'own decision' and 'consulted husband' from those who gave a positive response to the question.[97] The Social Survey did not follow up on this in 1945 or 1951. Since husbands did not appear to be a barrier to immunisation, and wives had shown their capacity to immunise unilaterally, it seems resources were moved to mothers, where they might achieve more immediate results. Apathy among fathers was hence viewed as largely irrelevant; and indeed, their place within this decision-making process was discussed only in relation to their refusal to immunise.

Only one press advertisement in the COI file on the diphtheria campaigns specifically spoke to 'father'; and this had effectively the same content as a contemporary advert showing a picture of a mother with her child.[98] This was a long-running theme. Of the thirty-one magazines listed in the 1942 campaign information brochure, nineteen contained words related to women readers, with none aimed at men.[99] Other actors within this process expressed similarly gender-imbalanced views. The press and local authorities both focused on the sensibilities of the mother. One secretary at a north London town hall objected to the 'ghastly' 'if' posters, sending them straight back to the Ministry. She noted that the mothers in her area would be disturbed by the messages and the imagery, and made a request for the 'pretty' baby posters of previous years.[100] In this specific case, at least, it was felt that apathy could be overcome through a more overtly feminine message rather than through fear. Immunisation messages could also be integrated into pre-existing public health schemes. For example, some local authorities had special film screenings for women, which included other "mothercraft" messages such as disseminating techniques for teaching young children how to walk.[101] Patricia Hornby-Smith, the Minister for Health, gave a speech warning against apathy at press events organised at a new maternal welfare clinic.[102] As for the press, *The Star*, a London-based, populist newspaper, ran a number of stories during 1955 in favour of the immunisation scheme.[103] It was far more explicit about the role of women than the official national propaganda. And far more judgemental. An editorial written by the paper's own 'Harley-st Doctor' put the blame for low immunisation rates on 'Silly Mothers' who 'after all the proofs of its value ... raise silly objections.'[104] Even those with less judgemental tones highlighted the example of the ignorant mother. The Bristol MOH was quoted in a *Bristol Evening World* article recounting a conversation with 'a young mother at a Bristol clinic' after seeing a 'Diphtheria Still Kills' poster: ' "But," she said to the Sister, "I thought it meant only a few spots and Johnny would be over it in a few days. I didn't know it was so dangerous." '[105] If apathy was a problem with parents in general, it was clearly the responsibility of mothers to overcome it.

The 1951 Social Survey indicated some class divide in the uptake of immunisation, as shown in Table 1.1. Sixty per cent of children (of all ages) whose mothers had left school before they turned fourteen were immunised, versus 85 per cent of those whose mothers had been educated beyond the age of fifteen. Similarly, 61 per cent were immunised in households where the main wage earner took home less than £5 per week, as compared to 80 per cent in households where the main weekly wage was more than £10. There was little variation among those outside of the poorest families. The core of the campaign, however, was focused on increasing the immunisation rate in children younger than one year – and here, rates were more even. Fifty-six per cent of children were immunised before twelve months in the lowest earnings bracket, with between 61 and 63 per cent for the higher incomes.[106] Using the 'unsatisfactory excuses' noted earlier, apathy was measured at 36 per cent among least-educated parents, versus 28 per cent for the most-educated. There was a bigger divide across income brackets, ranging from 45 per cent among the poorest to 24 per cent among the better-off.[107] As also shown earlier, in 1942 a greater number of higher-income parents had made a joint decision on whether their child would be immunised.[108]

The Ministry acted upon this information with its propaganda campaign. Although this is not made explicit in the literature, advertising

Diphtheria

Table 1.1 Family background and immunisation

	Proportion immunised	Proportion of immunisations before first birthday	Proportion of mothers' reasons taken as 'unsatisfactory'	Proportion vaccinated [against smallpox]
Mother's education				
Left school before 14 years	60%	60%	36%	28%
Left school when 14 years old	73%	59%	31%	37%
Left school when 15 or over	85%	64%	28%	61%
Weekly income of head of household				
Up to £5	61%	56%	45%	39%
Over £5 to £7 10s	73%	61%	31%	39%
Over £7 10s to £10	80%	63%	27%	43%
Over £10	79%	63%	24%	55%
Not ascertained	70%	58%	21%	46%
Number of children in family				
One	78%	68%	29%	50%
Two	79%	60%	30%	43%
Three	74%	56%	32%	40%
Four or more	55%	50%	35%	26%
All children aged 6 months to under 5	74%	60%	31%	42%

Source: Reproduced from Table 11: Family background and immunisation, in Gray and Cartwright, *Diphtheria Immunisation in 1951*, p. 16.

space was bought in papers such as the *Sunday Express*, *News of the World* and *People*, but not in more middle-class papers such as the *Mail on Sunday*, *Sunday Times* or *Observer*.[109] By 1951 the number of national titles targeted had contracted, but there were still two explicitly mentioned categories of publications: 'the more widely read national Sunday and weekly papers and the most suitable women's weekly magazines'.[110] There was a *prima facie* case for using these periodicals. The more "populist" the titles, the larger the audience, and the more people who would see the advertisement. Local authorities also tried to promote immunisation uptake in traditional "black spots", often in more deprived areas. Manchester used a mobile immunisation van in the 1940s and gained press coverage in the *Manchester Guardian* for it.[111] 'Division 3' in London (covering the boroughs of Finsbury, Holborn and Islington) used a similar vehicle that toured busy shopping centres, hoping to reach children who had not yet been immunised.[112]

Class was not as explicit in the national campaign as gender was. The government had targeted specific locations for increased advertising or epidemiological intervention, but these areas were identified based on their aggregate immunisation rates and not specifically the class composition of local authorities. Partially, this reflected the mass nature of propaganda campaigns. The national government's concern was to tackle apathy by generally raising awareness of diphtheria and the associated risks through a coordinated use of media that would reach the most number of people with the greatest impact. By definition, this would have to be broad and largely "populist". It was the job of local authorities, with their knowledge of the peculiarities of their unique circumstances and demographics to further target the specific populations and families that were non-compliant.[113]

In the press and in the justification for national campaigns against diphtheria, apathy made sense as a central narrative. On the ground, medical authorities presented a different picture of the reasons for non-immunisation and ways of tackling it. A more complex interaction between the public and the immunisation programme emerges, in which the government adapted to parents' concerns. To begin with, the rhetoric of apathy did not necessarily make sense with the data coming back to public health authorities. This was evident even from the way in which the Ministry of Health targeted those local authorities with lower immunisation rates. The Ministry was limited in the direct action it could take, as each authority ran its own public health schemes through its MOH. While the MOHs were empowered or compelled to act in certain ways, prioritisation was a local matter. One direct intervention the Ministry could make was advertising. Originally the plan had been to treat all areas equally, but expenditure limits forced greater selectivity. Instead, the government paid for advertising only in the counties and county boroughs with the lowest immunisation rates.[114] The use of advertising as a public health measure relied on the assumption that lower rates in those areas were due to a lack of knowledge or apathy (in comparison to the better-performing authorities) rather than to any other local peculiarities.[115] Even so, the *Manchester Guardian* noted that the results of the 1945 Social Survey suggested that parents in the northern region knew more about the nature of diphtheria and facts about immunisation, and yet had a lower immunisation rate than the national average.[116] Of the 26 areas targeted due to low immunisation rates in 1952, only 7 were outside the industrial Midlands or the North.[117] Education did not appear to be the problem; the issue was persuasion. As with the 'unsatisfactory excuses', the Ministry's conception of apathy appeared to conflate the issues of ignorance, indifference and disbelief. Despite this contradictory feedback, the government continued to centre its actions on parental apathy.

An outbreak in Coseley, in the Black Country, appeared to justify this approach and confirm judgements about apathy in mothers from certain areas and from certain backgrounds.[118] At the same time, it exposed failures in the logic that education and fear of the disease would be enough to make parents comply with official advice. The town had gone through a diphtheria epidemic in 1951, with 66 cases. Despite an intensive immunisation campaign, there were a further 20 cases in 1952 and 38 in 1953. In 1953, Coseley accounted for almost a third of all cases in England for the year.[119] The intensified immunisation efforts by the local medical authorities succeeded in immunising 78.5 per cent of school children in the district. However, 60 per cent of pre-schoolers remained unimmunised, despite the clear evidence that diphtheria was endemic.[120] According to the Chief Medical Officer's report for 1953:

> In Coseley, as elsewhere in the country, it was found in most instances the parents of unimmunised young children had no objection to the procedure. They were merely indolent and quite apathetic concerning the matter … Later, when the child could be immunised at school,

without any inconvenience, they readily consented. Nevertheless, there was the odd instance of the obdurate parent who could not be persuaded to have his children protected, even though other members of the household had contracted the disease. In several instances in recent years, in Coseley and elsewhere, this refusal has brought tragic consequences – the child not only contracting the disease but succumbing to it.[121]

One of the striking things about this passage is how the Chief Medical Officer repeatedly draws parallels between Coseley and the rest of the country. What happened in Staffordshire could happen anywhere. The tone, however, is far less sympathetic than the content of the national propaganda campaigns. The parents in Coseley were wilfully choosing not to immunise their children. Parents knew that diphtheria was still a menace, yet they were unwilling to make the effort to present their children to medical authorities until the medical authorities came to them. Even then, it could be a struggle. An official from the Staffordshire Health Department despaired, 'we send them forms and tell them of the dangers ... but they don't bother to return the forms.'[122] This interpretation relied on a contradictory definition of apathy. Much like the 'unsatisfactory excuses' in the 1951 Social Survey, the unwillingness or inability to assimilate official advice and make the "correct" decision about immunisation could at once be attributed to wilful resistance *and* apathy. And yet, the education campaign continued. Local Alderman George Newham's response to parents who had fears about immunisation was thus: 'They haven't been educated ... We are still having to teach them.'[123]

Coseley further showed the way in which a number of phenomena could be attributed to apathy. It also highlighted the difficulty of effectively monitoring and intervening in the lives of children without the full cooperation of parents, especially in pre-schoolers. Apathy could therefore also apply to parents who were unwilling to make sacrifices to the greater good. This could include: consent to the procedure in principle; taking the child to the clinic; waiting for the doctor; and having to deal with any potential consequences of the procedure, from irritability to other more serious side-effects. With all these costs and risks, the government was asking a lot of mothers – and it was almost always mothers – with young children. For some, this was part of civic duty, echoing Bevan's words about the 'energetic cooperation of every citizen.'[124] As early as 1946, a coroner in Stoke-on-Trent accused the parents of a child who died of the disease of 'grossly selfish humbug' because 'they had not bothered to have their child Theresa ... immunised'.[125]

Most authorities, however, were much more restrained. For example, the MOH for Camberwell reacted to an outbreak of diphtheria in his borough in 1959 by imploring parents to 'do the right thing' by the country. 'Public apathy and complacency have grown concomitantly with the diminution of a disease, the ravages of which are unknown to the young parents of today,' Chalke wrote.[126] The outbreak served 'as a dramatic reminder ... of the damage that can follow unbelief in the efficacy of immunisation'. Aside from the school absences and risks to the individuals, it was a drain on the time and resources of health workers and hospitals.[127] Despite the moralising tone, there is no evidence in his report that parents were being actively blamed for wanton ignorance or refusal to submit to reason. But there was a sense that some parents were 'lacking a communal health consciousness'.[128] Immunisation was not simply an act for personal protection. It was part of a wider citizenship, both for protecting the "herd" against disease and ensuring that medical resources were not spent fighting a disease that should, but for apathy, be eliminated from British cities. Once again, health care was not only a right of the new, technocratic welfare state; it was the duty of citizens to help themselves and others by availing themselves of these facilities.[129]

Apathy could exist as a general narrative, but this did not have to dictate the specific courses of action taken by health authorities to improve immunisation rates in their local areas. As Jane Seymour and Luke Blaxill's work on the London MOH reports shows, local officers had become less judgemental of citizens as the inter-war years progressed, instead focusing on service provision and understanding of local structural factors to improve health outcomes.[130] London's immunisation rates for children under the age of five remained poor. Only 55.4 per cent of children aged 0–4 had been immunised in 1950. That figure rose to 67 per cent when children under one year of age were discounted.[131] Despite this, apathy was rarely blamed when the disease hit. An outbreak of diphtheria in West Ham had led to an intensified immunisation campaign.[132] Fourteen cases were reported in 1955, and a further two in early 1956. This was the first time since 1948 that the borough had experienced more than five cases in a single year.[133] From

1955 to 1956, the number of children of school age being fully immunised rose from 52 per cent to 87 per cent. Yet the number of pre-school children being immunised remained lower – rising from 56 per cent to 76 per cent.[134] The West Ham MOH reports made no mention of apathy, nor any judgements on the behaviour of parents during this period. The only hint we can find is in the 1956 report, when the Officer makes reference to the number of parents who fail to keep their appointments for the new polio vaccination. He assumed that with this specific vaccine parents 'still had doubts about [its] safety'.[135] A similar picture was found in Finsbury. Blyth Brook, the borough's MOH, mentioned nothing about the behaviour of parents and described a 1959 outbreak as having little more than 'nuisance value'.[136] This may well have been a case of public relations management, downplaying the significance of an infectious disease so as not to stir panic. It was the first time that there had been so many cases of the disease in the borough since 1941, and the first time since 1945 that more than six diphtheria notifications had been made. However, there is no evidence of resistance to this line of reasoning, and no major panic. Blyth Brook's report focused instead on the specific steps that his inspectors and immunisers made in bringing the disease under control. The blame lay in the diphtheria bacillus itself, and was dealt with like any other public health 'nuisance'.

The national government had focused on a publicity campaign partly because this was an area of activity over which it had some control. Local authorities, however, had the advantage of being able to reflect on micro-level issues such as practical access to services. They could, and would, act independently of the Ministry in order to meet their own public health goals. The government acknowledged this in its campaign materials, encouraging MOHs to use their local knowledge, social workers and voluntary organisations to help spread the message about immunisation and raise acceptance rates.[137] Rather than solely blame parental apathy, MOHs did what they could to target black spots and bring immunisation services to parents, rather than waiting for children to come to them. The immunisation vans in Manchester and northern London show this most clearly.[138] Education could also be better targeted according to local custom. R. J. Donaldson (Rotherham's MOH) wrote to the Ministry in 1955 asking for help with locating a film van that he could take around the town. 'I do feel many people fail to read … advertisements,' he lamented.[139] On top of this, traditional services were strengthened. New clinics were set up, and hours extended. Immunisers went to day nurseries and infant welfare sessions to meet parents directly. In one borough, the medical authorities organised an exhibition in which the immunisation session was open to the public to see just how efficient and desirable protection against diphtheria could be.[140] Health visitors were another key tool. These had been used first by voluntary and then by statutory organisations in the field of infant welfare since the late nineteenth century.[141] Their role had become more formalised and professionalised over the twentieth century, and in the post-war years was more akin to that of the social worker as we now know it.[142] From the beginning of the anti-apathy campaign, the direct contact that they enabled with families was considered vital.[143] London County Council considered health visitors along with clinic staff and doctors as the reason why their immunisation programme had been a success.[144] Midwives and health visitors were made aware of every birth in the county and, as part of their other tasks, would press upon parents the need for immunisation.[145] It was always known, then, that propaganda (in the form of posters, press advertisements and film) would not be enough on its own to combat apathy. The government, through its local administrative machinery, had to go to parents and ensure that immunisation fitted in with their lives. As the 1951 Social Survey had found, children in larger families and with poorer parents were less likely to be immunised (see Table 1.1). Better provision of services and direct communication were needed to make parents believe that immunisation was a high-enough priority for them to seek it out. Apathy did not just require a change in parents' attitude, it also needed compromise and cooperation from health authorities.

Indeed, there was an inherent acknowledgement in the 1950s campaign, even in central government, that parents' responses to declining diphtheria rates were rational. While the 'false sense of security' was worrisome,[146] it was 'understandable'.[147] The immediate risk of diphtheria was less obvious to parents, and therefore managing that risk at the individual level was less of a priority.[148] Clearly, parents had concerns over other diseases that felt more immediately threatening – even MOHs themselves had to deal more with outbreaks of poliomyelitis and whooping cough.[149] In another attempt to meet parents' concerns and leverage these to increase diphtheria immunisation, local and national authorities began to use the newly available pertussis vaccine as a way to entice parents to the immunisation clinic and, proverbially, kill two birds with one stone. The 1951 Social Survey had found that parents still found diphtheria to be the most dangerous child illness by some margin, followed by whooping cough.[150] Yet MOHs continued to assert as the decade progressed that they found it easier to convince parents to present their children for pertussis immunisation.[151] In 1953, the Ministry had feared that this would leave diphtheria underappreciated.[152] But widespread use of the combined immunisation just a few years later meant that local MOHs could protect children against both diseases at the same time. Another positive for the Ministry was that whooping cough immunisation was recommended at an earlier age than diphtheria, meaning that there was more time to administer prophylaxis against diphtheria before children turned one year old.[153] In London, protection against diphtheria in children from one to five years old rose from 63.1 per cent in 1953 to 74.1 per cent in 1960 and 94.7 in 1964.[154] The vast majority of these injections came from the combined prophylactic.[155] There were other ways to overcome apathy than education and persuasion. Restructuring of services and response to local circumstance were perhaps more effective in some ways than national propaganda.

Conclusions

The campaign appeared to be a success. As the combined vaccine and other localised public health measures continued, the overall immunisation rate across the country did improve. Immunisation among children under the age of one grew from 28 per cent in 1951 to 44 per cent in 1956.[156] Perhaps more importantly, diphtheria did not make a resurgence. Morbidity and mortality continued to decline, and in 1959 nobody died of the disease (Table 1.2).[157] In the later 1950s, talk of apathy continued in the national press, but at a much lower level than at the beginning of the campaign. This made the occasional outbreak newsworthy rather than a routine occurrence. One major example of this happened in September 1960, when a girl died in Derby. V. N. Leyshon, the city's MOH, sent details of the case to the national press and it gained widespread coverage. It was seen as a warning that parents could not give into complacency – or apathy – and that immunisation against the disease was still necessary. Leyshon reported some days later

Table 1.2 Diphtheria notifications and deaths in England and Wales, 1938–60

	Notifications	Deaths
1938	65,008	2,861
1939	47,343	2,133
1940	46,281	2,480
1941	50,797	2,641
1942	41,404	1,827
1943	34,662	1,371
1944	23,199	934
1945	18,596	722
1946	11,986	472
1947	5,609	244
1948	3,575	156
1949	1,881	84
1950	962	49
1951	664	30
1952	376	23
1953	266	20
1954	173	8
1955	155	12
1956	53	3
1957	37	4
1958	80	8
1959	102	–
1960	49	5

Note: Figures for 1938–43 are not corrected in the same way as those for 1944–60, and are therefore not strictly comparable.
Sources: 1948–50, Ministry of Health, *Report 1950–1951*, p. 25; 1951–1960, Ministry of Health, *Report 1950*, p. 31.

that the publicity had achieved its objective. His clinics had been inundated with requests, and the city's immunisation rate improved dramatically.[158] Even after the relative successes of the 1950s campaign – and despite the experiences of MOHs on the ground over the decade – apathy could still be invoked as a criticism of and warning to parents across the nation.

The anti-apathy campaign had started from the premise that the main issue stopping parents from presenting their children for immunisation was declining fear of diphtheria. In the British public health tradition, the Ministry of Health trusted the power of propaganda, education and persuasion to convince rational citizens to make the right decision for their own and the nation's benefit. In practice, "apathy" served other purposes. It was a convenient scapegoat for local and national authorities attempting to explain their inability to maintain high levels of protection among the public. Local MOHs had to justify their progress (or lack thereof) in their annual reports. The government, too, had clearly assumed responsibility for the health of its subjects and needed to explain how and why outbreaks of a preventable disease had been allowed to happen. Apathy allowed the medical establishment to outline the need for personal responsibility and good health citizenship. It was also clearly a concept that could incorporate a number of different public behaviours and still maintain enough coherence to persuade the Ministry, local authorities and the press that it was a clear danger to public health. Ignorance, indifference, disbelief and unwillingness to perform civic duties were all used in various ways to justify the central narrative of the campaign.

Apathy was also an appealing explanation because the Ministry already had multiple tools and administrative structures with which to combat it. It was a manageable risk. If indeed the issue was one of education and persuasion, the Ministry was in a position to utilise the COI and could build upon a long history of local public health campaigning with voluntary organisations, press cooperation and medical clinics. Citizens could be reminded of their obligations and the Ministry could appeal to parents' self-interest. While this was the main thrust of the campaign, however, in practice national and local authorities realised that "propaganda" alone would not tackle root problems. The government adapted its own tactics in response to the various ways in which parents' apathy spoke to the medical establishment. Through the Social Survey, statistical analyses and contact with parents on a number of levels, health authorities were able to modify their administrative and medical arrangements so that they were better attuned to the public's needs and concerns. It allowed MOHs to see both what was attractive and unappealing about diphtheria immunisation. Longer clinic hours, health visitors, mobile immunisation vans and the use of combined prophylactics were combined with existing propaganda arrangements to make immunisation against diphtheria a more attractive proposition. In other words, to rectify a national public health problem, local service provision had to be improved.

Apathy was a construct, then, that was created by local and national public health bodies as a form of communication: a translation of the diffuse behaviours of the public into a language which administrators and policy makers could understand. It was a framing device that could incorporate elements of public behaviour that were not precisely quantifiable or identifiable. As such, it kept many of the paternalistic elements of 1950s society and attitudes toward women and "the masses". It could simultaneously see resistance, disbelief and indifference as part of the same phenomenon, because all indicated that the public had not yet realised the "facts" on immunisation. But it was not an entirely one-sided conversation. The public could be seen to react and respond to changes in policy through the myriad administrative surveillance tools developed over previous years. In the end, apathy was the overall concept employed by government to justify its propaganda campaign; it was the more nuanced local interactions with the public, though, that made it a qualified success.

Notes

1 Ministry of Health, *Report of the Ministry of Health Covering the Period from 1st April, 1950 to 31st December, 1951. Part II on the State of the Public Health, Being the Annual Report of the Chief Medical Officer for the Year 1950* (Cmd 8582) (London: HMSO, 1952).
2 Steven M. Opal, 'A brief history of microbiology and immunology', in Andrew W. Artenstein (ed.), *Vaccines: A Biography* (New York: Springer, 2010), pp. 31–56; Esteban Rodríguez Ocaña, 'The social production of novelty: diphtheria serotherapy, "herald of the new medicine"', *Dynamis*, 27 (2007), 21–31.
3 Claire Hooker and Alison Bashford, 'Diphtheria and Australian public health: Bacteriology and its complex applications, c. 1890–1930', *Medical History*, 46:1 (2002), 41–64, esp. p. 42.
4 Or a death rate of 4.8%. The National Archives (hereafter TNA): BN 10/229, Ministry of Health, Immunisation against diphtheria, 1957–58.
5 Claire Hooker, 'Diphtheria, immunisation and the Bundaberg Tragedy: A study of public health in Australia', *Health and History*, 2:1 (2000),

52–78; Alison Day, '"The magical formula": Reactions and responses to diphtheria immunisation in New Zealand 1920–1960', *Health & History*, 15:2 (2013), 53–71; Jane Lewis, 'The prevention of diphtheria in Canada and Britain 1914–1945', *Journal of Social History*, 20:1 (1986), 163–76.

6 Lewis, 'The prevention of diphtheria', esp. p. 169.
7 See this argument with reference to tuberculosis in: Linda Bryder, '"We shall not find salvation in inoculation": BCG vaccination in Scandinavia, Britain and the USA, 1921–1960', *Social Science & Medicine*, 49:9 (1999), 1160–1.
8 Hooker, 'Diphtheria, immunisation and the Bundaberg Tragedy'; Bryder, 'BCG vaccination', p. 1158.
9 Lewis, 'The prevention of diphtheria', pp. 166–7.
10 John Welshman, 'The Medical Officer of Health in England and Wales, 1900–1974: Watchdog or lapdog?', *Journal of Public Health*, 19:4 (1997), 443–50, p. 445.
11 Ministry of Health, *Summary Report by the Ministry of Health for the Period from 1st April, 1939 to 31st March 1941* (Cmd 6340) (London: HMSO, 1942), pp. 4–5; Lewis, 'The prevention of diphtheria'.
12 Ministry of Health, *Summary Report, 1939–1941*, pp. 4–5.
13 Dorothy Porter, *Health Citizenship: Essays in Social Medicine and Biomedical Politics* (Berkeley: University of California Press, 2011); Frank Huisman and Harry Oosterhuis, 'The politics of health and citizenship: Historical and contemporary perspectives', in Frank Huisman and Harry Oosterhuis (eds), *Heath and Citizenship: Political Cultures of Health in Modern Europe* (London: Pickering and Chatto, 2014), pp. 1–40.
14 T. H. Marshall, *Citizenship and Social Class, and Other Essays* (Cambridge: Cambridge University Press, 1950); William H. Beveridge, *Social Insurance and Allied Services* (Cmd 6404) (London: HMSO, 1942).
15 Porter, *Health Citizenship*.
16 Bevan quoted in '"Houses in great numbers"', *The Times* (4 January 1946), p. 4.
17 On individual liberty versus collective responsibility specifically in the field of vaccination see James Colgrove, *State of Immunity: The Politics of Vaccination in Twentieth-Century America* (Berkeley: University of California Press, 2006).
18 Candace Johnson Redden, 'Health as citizenship narrative', *Polity*, 34:3 (2002), 355–70.
19 Marshall, *Citizenship and Social Class*.
20 Edgerton, David, 'C. P. Snow as anti-historian of British science: Revisiting the technocratic moment, 1959–1964', *History of Science*, 43:2 (2005), 187–208; Glen O'Hara, 'Towards a new Bradshaw? Economic statistics

and the British state in the 1950s and 1960s', *Economic History Review*, 60:1 (2007), 1–34.
21 See TNA: MH 134/151, Diphtheria Immunisation – Meeting held at the Ministry of Health, 30 March 1949. It was initially envisioned that a further dose would be given at age ten, although in practice this was widely neglected. TNA: MH 134/151, Gordon Lilco [Ministry of Health] to Dr C. B. Crane [MOH, York], 12 August 1954.
22 Anon, 'Prevention of whooping-cough by vaccination', *British Medical Journal*, 1:4721 (1951), 1463–71; Ministry of Health, *Report of the Ministry of Health covering the period from 1st April, 1950 to 31st December, 1951. Part III on the state of the public health* (Cmd 8787) (London: HMSO, 1953), p. 72.
23 Ministry of Health, *Report of the Ministry of Health for the year 1957. Part II on the state of the public health being the annual report of the chief medical officer* (Cmnd 559) (London: HMSO, 1958), p. 44; J. A. Scott, *Report of the County Medical Officer of Health and Principal School Medical Officer for the Year 1957* (London: London County Council, 1958), pp. 66–73.
24 TNA: INF 12/238, Specification Sheet – Campaigns – 14 February 1953.
25 This was a trend across the Western world from the late nineteenth century onwards. See Vibeke Erichsen, 'The health of the school child? An historical comparison of inspection schemes in Britain and Norway', *Dynamis*, 13 (1993), 29–53. In Britain, the Education (Administrative Provisions) Act 1907 had obliged local authorities to monitor the health of elementary school children. See also John Pickstone, 'Production, community and consumption: The political economy of twentieth-century medicine', in Roger Cooter and John Pickstone (eds), *Medicine in the Twentieth Century* (Abingdon: Routledge, 2003), 1–20.
26 MH 55/936, Diphtheria Prophylaxis: Publicity Campaign for Immunisation.
27 Lewis, 'The prevention of diphtheria'.
28 Owing to the local nature of the administration, rates varied. Only one in five immunisations in London was performed by the family doctor in 1957. However, the 1951 Social Survey found that family doctors performed 35 per cent of all immunisations nationwide, and that it was becoming more common. See Scott, *Report, 1957*, p. 68; P. G. Gray and Ann Cartwright, *Diphtheria Immunisation in 1951: An Inquiry Carried out in May 1951 for the Ministry of Health* (London: The Social Survey, 1951), p. 10.
29 MH 55/936, Diphtheria Prophylaxis: Publicity Campaign for Immunisation, attached to letter dated 4 February 1954.

30 *Ibid.* See also TNA: BN 10/229, Ministry of Health and Ministry of Information, Immunisation against Diphtheria Campaign, 1942.
31 Welshman, 'The Medical Officer of Health in England and Wales'.
32 National Health Service Act 1946; National Health Service (Scotland) Act 1947.
33 Scott, *Report, 1957*, p. 64.
34 George Rosen, *A History of Public Health* (New York: MD Publications, 1958), pp. 132–5; David Armstrong, 'Origins of the problem of health-related behaviours: A genealogical study', *Social Studies of Science*, 39:6 (2009), 909–26; Nathan Manning, 'The relational self and the political engagements of young adults', *Journal of Sociology*, 50:4 (2014), 486–500.
35 David Armstrong, *Political Anatomy of the Body: Medical Knowledge in Britain in the Twentieth Century* (Cambridge: Cambridge University Press, 1983); Ina Zweiniger-Bargielowska, 'Raising a nation of "good animals": The New Health Society and health education campaigns in interwar Britain', *Social History of Medicine*, 20:1 (2007), 73–89.
36 On risk, see Chapter 4 and Ulrich Beck, *Risk Society: Towards a New Modernity* (London: Sage, 1992); Jakob Arnoldi, *Risk: An Introduction* (Cambridge: Polity, 2009).
37 Although this narrative has been challenged by historians, it resonated for much of the twentieth century. For a comprehensive review of the debate, see Patrick E. Carroll, 'Medical police and the history of public health', *Medical History*, 46:4 (2002), 461–94.
38 Sue Bowden and Alex Sadler, 'Getting it right? Lessons from the interwar years on pulmonary tuberculosis control in England and Wales', *Medical History*, 59:1 (2015), 101–35; Joseph Melling and Pamela Dale, 'Medical Officers of Health, gender and government responses to the problem of cancer in Britain, 1900–1940', *Medical History*, 53:4 (2009), 537–60; Amanda Engineer, 'Illustrations from the Wellcome Library: The Society of Medical Officers of Health: Its history and its archive', *Medical History*, 45:1 (2001), 97–114.
39 John Welshman, '"Bringing beauty and brightness to the back streets": health education and public health in England and Wales, 1890–1940', *Health Education Journal*, 56:2 (1997), 199–209; Martin Gorsky, 'Public health in interwar Britain: did it fail?', *Dynamis*, 28 (2008), 194–5. See also Brendan Maartens, 'From propaganda to "information": Reforming government communications in Britain', *Contemporary British History* (2016); Mariel Grant, 'Towards a Central Office of Information: Continuity and change in British government information policy, 1939–51', *Journal of Contemporary History*, 34:1 (1999), 49–67.

40 Engineer, 'Illustrations from the Wellcome Library'; Gorsky, 'Public health in interwar Britain'; Welshman, 'The Medical Officer of Health in England and Wales'.
41 See interwar criticisms of public behaviour despite "propaganda" campaigns against tuberculosis in Bowden and Sadler, 'Getting it right?', esp. pp. 117–18. See also criticisms of workers' attitudes with regard to health and safety in the 1970s in Christopher Sirrs, 'Accidents and apathy: The construction of the "Robens Philosophy" of occupational safety and health regulation in Britain, 1961–1974', *Social History of Medicine*, 29:1 (2016), 66–88.
42 Porter, *Health Citizenship*.
43 Huisman and Oosterhuis, 'The politics of health and citizenship'.
44 Scott, *Report, 1957*, p. 65.
45 Unlike in Figure 1.1, these tracked notification rates rather than deaths. The first example is seen in Allen Daley, *Report of the County Medical Officer of Health and School Medical Officer for the Year 1950* (London: London County Council, 1951), p. 18. Versions of this chart were updated and produced until 1955.
46 Ministry of Health, *Summary report of the Ministry of Health for the year ended 31st March, 1943* (Cmd 6468) (London: HMSO, 1943).
47 TNA: BN 10/229, John A. Charles, Chief Medical Officer, 'A letter to Medical Officers of Health', Immunisation against diphtheria, 1957–58; TNA: INF 12/238, IF Armer to Director-General, COI, 12 January 1953.
48 TNA: BN 10/229, A message from the Chief Medical Officer, December 1950.
49 Gray and Cartwright, *Diphtheria Immunisation in 1951*.
50 Ironically, the speed at which the polio vaccine virtually eliminated the disease from high-income countries meant that research on the disease's aetiology remains patchy. The Bradford Hill and Knowelden review (see below) ruled out a causational relationship between injections and polio, but there is much that medical professionals do not know. For more on polio, see Chapter 2. A similar process was found with smallpox, a disease virtually eliminated before modern biomedical techniques could study the disease both in the laboratory and in the wild. See David M. Oshinsky, *Polio: An American Story* (Oxford: Oxford University Press, 2005); Bob H. Reinhardt, *The End of a Global Pox: America and the Eradication of Smallpox in the Cold War Era* (Chapel Hill: The University of North Carolina Press, 2015).
51 J. K. Martin, 'Local paralysis in children after injections', *Archives of Disease in Childhood*, 25:121 (1950), 1–14.

52 Bertram P. McCloskey, 'The relation of prophylactic inoculations to the onset of poliomyelitis', *The Lancet*, 255:6606 (1950), 659–63.
53 D. H. Geffen, 'The incidence of paralysis occurring in London children within four weeks after immunization', *The Medical Officer*, 83 (1950), 137–40.
54 A. Bradford Hill and J. Knowelden, 'Inoculation and poliomyelitis', *British Medical Journal*, 2:4669 (1950), 1–6.
55 TNA: INF 12/238, Note of meeting to discuss the Diphtheria Immunisation Publicity Campaign 1953-4 – 15 October 1952; BN 10/229, Immunisation against diphtheria – National and Local Publicity 1951.
56 Gray and Cartwright, *Diphtheria Immunisation in 1951*.
57 Kathleen Box and Geoffrey Thomas, 'The Wartime Social Survey', *Journal of the Royal Statistical Society*, 107:3/4 (1944), 151–89.
58 Charlotte Greenhalgh, 'The travelling social survey: Social research and its subjects in Britain, Australia and New Zealand, 1930s–1970s', *History Australia*, 13:1 (2016), 124–38; Mike Savage, 'Affluence and social change in the making of technocratic middle-class identities: Britain, 1939–55', *Contemporary British History*, 22:4 (2008), 457–76; Michael Savage, *Identities and Social Change in Britain since 1940: The Politics of Method* (Oxford: Oxford University Press, 2010).
59 'Old Wives' Fears', *Manchester Guardian* (23 April 1952), p. 6.
60 Kathleen Box, *Diphtheria Immunisation: An Inquiry Made by the Social Survey for the Ministry of Health* (London: The Social Survey, October 1945); Anon, 'Social survey of diphtheria immunization', *British Medical Journal*, 2:4461 (1946), 21.
61 Box, *Diphtheria Immunisation*, pp. 32–3.
62 *Ibid.*
63 Gray and Cartwright, *Diphtheria Immunisation in 1951*, pp. 2, 15.
64 *Ibid.*, p. 2.
65 TNA: BN 10/229, A message from the Chief Medical Officer, December 1950.
66 See 'Poliomyelitis', *Manchester Guardian* (12 April 1950), p. 10; 'Poliomyelitis Link', *Manchester Guardian* (5 July 1950), p. 2; Chapman Pincher, 'Injections held up: Paralysis fear', *Daily Express* (10 April 1950), p. 1.
67 Gray and Cartwright, *Diphtheria Immunisation in 1951*, p. 2.
68 The French Report, despite recommending cuts to the COI budget, held up the diphtheria campaign as an example of what information services ought to be doing. See Henry French, *Report of the Committee on the Cost of Home Information Services* (Cmd 7836) (London: HMSO, 1949). See also 'Their £40,000 saves us £1,500,000 a year', *Daily Mirror* (1 December 1948), p. 1; 'Cuts in information services', *Manchester Guardian*

(30 November 1949), p. 8; 'State publicity fails to build an army', *Daily Express* (30 November 1950), p. 5; 'Diphtheria deaths down from 1827 to 85 in eight years', *Daily Mirror* (30 November 1950), p. 5.
69 TNA: BN 10/229, A message from the Chief Medical Officer, December 1950.
70 'Inoculations and child health', *The Times* (9 December 1957), p. 11. See also '"Dramatic drop" in diphtheria cases', *The Times* (11 June 1952), p. 3.
71 J. A. Scott, *Report of the County Medical Officer of Health and School Medical Officer for the Year 1951* (London: London County Council, 1952), p. 68. See also 'County of London population', *The Times* (11 June 1952), p. 3.
72 'Neglectful parents', *Daily Mirror* (20 June 1946), p. 2.
73 'Health goes begging', *Manchester Guardian* (11 December 1953), p. 6.
74 Porter, *Health Citizenship*, esp. pp. 67–9.
75 John Pickstone referred to this as a "productionist" view of medicine. See Pickstone, 'Production, community and consumption'.
76 Emphasis original. TNA: INF 12/238, Specification Sheet – Campaigns – 14 February 1953.
77 *Ibid.*
78 TNA: BN 10/229. See especially Immunisation Against Diphtheria, March 1953; Diphtheria Immunisation 1951. Billboards also made use of the "If" campaign described below.
79 TNA: INF 12/238, J. C. Seldon [Treasury] to O. C. Watson [COI], 29 November 1952.
80 TNA: INF 12/238, Note of meeting to discuss the Diphtheria Immunisation Publicity Campaign 1953–4 – 15 October 1952.
81 *Ibid.* See also the King's Speech in 1951, HC Deb (6 November 1951), vol. 493, cc. 50–3.
82 TNA: INF 12/238, Diphtheria Immunisation, 16-sheet poster campaign 1953, Allen Whitmore to B. Crawter, 17 January 1953.
83 J. A. Scott, *Report of the County Medical Officer of Health and School Medical Officer for the Year 1952* (London: London County Council, 1953), p. 80.
84 Emphasis original. TNA: BN 10/229, Diphtheria immunisation 1952, sent February 1951.
85 TNA: BN 10/229, Poster, May 1952.
86 TNA: BN 10/229, Poster, March 1954.
87 TNA: BN 10/229, Leaflet, 'Protect you child against diphtheria', 1956; newspaper advert, 'Please have me immunised against diphtheria', 1955.
88 TNA: BN 10/229, 'Before the first birthday', November 1950.
89 See e.g.: Scott, *Report*, 1957, p. 68; 'More happy birthdays', *Daily Mirror* (20 December 1949), p. 12.

90 Emphasis mine. TNA: BN 10/229, 'Before the first birthday', November 1950.
91 Wartime Social Survey, *Diphtheria Immunisation Enquiry: A Survey of 2,026 Parents made in July–August 1942, for the Ministry of Health* (London: Wartime Social Survey, 1942); Box, *Diphtheria Immunisation*; Gray and Cartwright, *Diphtheria Immunisation in 1951*.
92 Box, *Diphtheria Immunisation*; Gray and Cartwright, *Diphtheria Immunisation in 1951*.
93 Jane Lewis, *The Politics of Motherhood: Child and Maternal Welfare in England, 1900–1939* (London: Croom Helm, 1980).
94 Ann Daly, *Inventing Motherhood: The Consequences of an Ideal* (New York: Schocken, 1983); Angela Davis, *Modern Motherhood: Women and Family in England, c. 1945–2000* (Manchester: Manchester University Press, 2012).
95 Tim Fisher, 'Fatherhood and the British fathercraft movement, 1919–39', *Gender & History*, 17:2 (2005), 441–62.
96 Sister Clare, 'Remember me? I'm only the father!', *Daily Mirror* (4 October 1949), p. 5.
97 Wartime Social Survey, *Diphtheria Immunisation Enquiry*, p. 17.
98 TNA: BN 10/229, 'FATHER Your child's life is in your hands', May 1951.
99 'Woman', 'wife', 'lady'. See TNA: BN 10/229 Ministry of Health and Ministry of Information, Immunisation against diphtheria campaign, 1942.
100 MH 55/936, S. W. Hivet to B. Crawter, internal memorandum, 7 April 1954.
101 'Films for mothers', *Manchester Guardian* (13 December 1951), p. 8.
102 'Parents warned', *Manchester Guardian* (27 November 1954), p. 3.
103 The Ministry kept a number of these cuttings in TNA: MH 55/2191. *The Star* was a local newspaper that ceased publication in 1960. Not to be confused with the present-day *Daily Star*, a national title which began in the 1970s.
104 TNA: MH 55/2191, Newspaper cutting 'Protect your baby now', *The Star* (25 May 1955). See also TNA: MH 55/936, 'Killer at Bay', *The Star* (13 January 1954).
105 TNA: MH 55/2191, Newspaper cutting 'Diphtheria still a killer', *Bristol Evening World* (4 February 1955).
106 Gray and Cartwright, *Diphtheria Immunisation in 1951*, p. 16.
107 *Ibid*.
108 Wartime Social Survey, *Diphtheria Immunisation Enquiry*, p. 17.
109 TNA: BN 10/229 Ministry of Health and Ministry of Information, Immunisation against diphtheria campaign, 1942.

Diphtheria 69

110 And again, the *Sunday Express*, *Sunday Pictorial* and *Radio Times* are cited, but none of the broadsheets. TNA: BN 10/229, Immunisation against diphtheria, National and local publicity 1951, sent March 1950.
111 'Diphtheria immunisation', *Manchester Guardian* (17 October 1945), p. 8; 'Campaign against diphtheria', *Manchester Guardian* (29 May 1946), p. 3.
112 Allen Daley, *Report of the County Medical Officer of Health and School Medical Officer for the Year 1949* (London: London County Council, 1950), pp. 78–9. See also Scott, *Report, 1951*, p. 81. The van is mentioned in subsequent divisional reports, e.g.: Scott, *Report, 1952*, p. 143; J. A. Scott, *Report of the County Medical Officer of Health and School Medical Officer for the Year 1953* (London: London County Council, 1954), p. 134; J. A. Scott, *Report of the County Medical Officer of Health and School Medical Officer for the Year 1954* (London: London County Council, 1955), p. 132.
113 TNA: BN 10/229, Diphtheria immunisation 1952, sent February 1951.
114 TNA: INF 12/238, Note of meeting to discuss the Diphtheria Immunisation Publicity Campaign 1953–54 – 15 October 1952; *ibid.*, Financial authorities in advance of approval of 1953–54 estimates, O. C. Wilson [COI] to J. C. Seldon [Treasury], 20 November 1952.
115 TNA: BN 10/229, Diphtheria immunisation 1952, sent February 1951.
116 'Immunisation', *Manchester Guardian* (6 June 1946), p. 4; Box, *Diphtheria Immunisation*.
117 TNA: INF 12/238, Diphtheria Immunisation, 16-sheet poster campaign, 1953, Allen Whitmore to B. Crawter, 17 January 1953.
118 Coseley Unitary District was part of Dudley, Staffordshire in the area of the West Midlands known as the Black Country.
119 Ministry of Health, *Report of the Ministry of Health for the year ended 31st December, 1953 part II on the state of the public health* (Cmd 9307) (London: HMSO, 1954), pp. 3, 34.
120 *Ibid.*, p. 34.
121 *Ibid.*
122 TNA: MH 55/936, cutting, ' "Their lives could have been saved" ', *Birmingham Gazette* (12 August 1954).
123 *Ibid.*
124 Bevan quoted in ' "Houses in great numbers" ', *The Times* (4 January 1946), p. 4.
125 'Girl of four died: not immunised', *Daily Mirror* (19 June 1946), p. 3.
126 H. D. Chalke, *Report of the Medical Officer of Health for the Year 1959* (Camberwell: Metropolitan Borough of Camberwell, 1960), pp. 2, 41.
127 *Ibid.*, pp. 2, 42.
128 *Ibid.*

129 Porter, *Health Citizenship*; Huisman and Oosterhuis, 'The politics of health and citizenship'.
130 Luke Blaxill and Jane K. Seymour, 'Adventures in text mining with the London MOH annual reports: towards an alternative history of interwar public health', Conference paper (London Health Histories, Wellcome Trust, London, 26 May 2016).
131 J. A. Scott, *Report of the County Medical Officer of Health and School Medical Officer for the Year 1955* (London: London County Council, 1956), p. 84; J. A. Scott, *Report of the County Medical Officer of Health and School Medical Officer for the Year 1956* (London: London County Council, 1957), p. 75.
132 Around 6 per cent of the child population of the borough was immunised in the final four days of 1955 alone. F. Roy Dennison, *Annual Report on the Health Services for the year 1955* (West Ham: County Borough of West Ham, 1956), pp. 1, 70.
133 *Ibid.*, p. 8.
134 *Ibid.*, p. 70; F. Roy Dennison, *Annual Report on the Health Services for the year 1956* (West Ham: County Borough of West Ham, 1957), p. 68.
135 Dennison, *Report, 1956*, p. 68.
136 C. O. S. Blyth Brooke, *Annual Report on the Public Health of Finsbury for the Year 1959* (Finsbury: The Metropolitan Borough of Finsbury, 1960), p. 3.
137 Scott, *Report, 1952*, p. 80; TNA: BN 10/229, Diphtheria immunisation 1952, sent February 1951
138 'Diphtheria immunisation', *Manchester Guardian* (17 October 1945), p. 8; 'Campaign against diphtheria', *Manchester Guardian* (29 May 1946), p. 3. Daley, *Report, 1949*, pp. 78–9. See also Scott, *Report, 1951*, p. 81.
139 TNA: MH 55/2191, R. J. Donaldson [Rotherham MOH] to S. A. Heald [Ministry of Health], 16 November 1955.
140 Scott, *Report, 1954*, p. 133.
141 Jennifer Smith, 'Illustrations from the Wellcome Institute Library: The archive of the Health Visitors' Association in the Contemporary Medical Archives Centre', *Medical History*, 39:3 (1995), 358–67.
142 Pat Starkey, 'The feckless mother: Women, poverty and social workers in wartime and post-war England', *Women's History Review*, 9:3 (2000), 539–57; John Welshman, 'In search of the "problem family": Public health and social work in England and Wales 1940–70', *Social History of Medicine*, 9:3 (1996), 447–65.
143 TNA: BN 10/229, MH & Min Inf., Immunisation against Diphtheria Campaign, 1942.
144 Daley, *Report, 1950*, p. 1.

145 Scott, *Report, 1952*, p. 80.
146 H. D. B. North, MOH Carlton, Nottinghamshire, quoted in '"False sense of security" on immunisation', *Manchester Guardian* (19 August 1954), p. 5.
147 This phrase was repeated in TNA: BN 10/229 Immunisation against diphtheria, Ministry of Health, 1957–58; *ibid.*, Immunisation against diphtheria, Ministry of Health, 1955–56.
148 On parental decision making see Andrea Kitta, *Vaccinations and Public Concern in History: Legend, Rumor, and Risk Perception* (New York: Routledge, 2012).
149 TNA: BN 10/229 Immunisation against diphtheria, Ministry of Health, 1957–58; *ibid.*, Immunisation against diphtheria, Ministry of Health, 1954–55; *ibid.* Immunisation against diphtheria, Ministry of Health, 1955–56.
150 Gray and Cartwright, *Diphtheria Immunisation in 1951*, p. 18.
151 TNA: MH 55/936, I. G. Davies [MOH, Leeds] to Ministry of Health, 18 March 1954; Scott, *Report, 1957*, p. 70.
152 TNA: INF 12/238, Specification Sheet – Campaigns – 14 February 1953.
153 Scott, *Report, 1957*, p. 70.
154 *Ibid.*, p. 69; A. B. Stewart, *Report of the County Medical Officer of Health and Principal School Medical Officer for the Year 1964* (London: London County Council, 1966), p. 68.
155 Stewart, *Report, 1964*, p. 69.
156 TNA: BN 10/229, Immunisation against diphtheria, Ministry of Health, 1957–58.
157 Ministry of Health, *Report 1950*, p. 25; Ministry of Health, *Report of the Ministry of Health for the year 1960. Part II. On the state of the public health. Being the annual report of the Chief Medical Officer* (Cmnd 1550) (London: HMSO, 1961), p. 31.
158 'Immunization rush in Derby', *The Times* (22 September 1960), p. 3; '"Diph" scare checked – doctor', *Daily Express* (26 September 1960), p. 13; 'Girl diphtheria victim', *Guardian* (21 September 1960), p. 2; 'Parents – don't take a chance', *Daily Mirror* (22 September 1960), p. 2.

2

Smallpox

The supposed apathy shown towards diphtheria by certain sections of the British public was largely overcome by the 1960s – or, at least, immunisation rates had improved to such an extent that the Ministry of Health was no longer concerned about widespread diphtheria epidemics. Yet it did not have the same successes with smallpox vaccination. The problem of low rates of infant vaccination and childhood revaccination among the population remained a continual source of irritation for the Ministry. In the government's favour, the success of international vaccination and public health campaigns was making smallpox an ever-decreasing threat; but taking decisions about when the risk of disease had fallen below the risks posed by the vaccine itself proved to be a political and scientific minefield. Moreover, smallpox may have receded as a quotidian threat to British residents by the post-war period – but in the 1950s and 1960s a series of imported cases from abroad showed that the country was still at risk from foreign contagion.

Smallpox is a unique example of an infant vaccination programme that was shut down in Britain.[1] This chapter explores the slow process of dismantling the British system of routine smallpox vaccination of infants. A procedure that had been made compulsory in England and Wales in 1853 was discontinued in 1971. The chief reason for the end of smallpox vaccination was fairly obvious. The disease had been all but eradicated, and had ceased to be endemic in the United Kingdom since the 1930s.[2] But the timing of this decision was by no means inevitable. Full, worldwide eradication was not declared until 1980, and occasional outbreaks of the disease from foreign travel and laboratory accidents were a not-uncommon problem for post-war MOHs. The way in which these decisions were taken says much about the government's approach to the relative medical, financial and political risks of vaccination and disease. It also showed that the modern British vaccination system was forged by decisions not just about which vaccines to include, but also about which ones should be taken away.

The recurring theme in debates and policy decisions about smallpox was the nation. The discursive relationship between the public and the nation is a long-standing one. This applied to the state's – or the public sector's – provision of public health.[3] Britain was a nation to be protected from foreign diseases.[4] Anxieties were raised whenever an outbreak occurred – a sign of how rare smallpox had become, but also of the dread which it still elicited in the general public. Smallpox represented Britain's vulnerability to outside threats in a world of global mass transport by air and sea. And, as Roberta Bivins has shown, it came to be symbolic of Britain's relationship with her empire as attention shifted away from colonial holdings to a new Commonwealth, post-Suez.[5] The specific politics around smallpox policy help to show how these anxieties manifested in the post-war era. So too do the regional, national and transnational sites of public health control. The state managed the risks to its citizens from smallpox at multiple levels. Local MOHs provided epidemic control on the ground, as well as being responsible for the administration of the routine childhood vaccination programme. The Ministry of Health provided the financial support and national policy impetus for these programmes. The medical civil service headed by the Ministry and the Scottish Office began to centralise immunisation policy further than it had done in previous decades. They did so within a global network of knowledge, coloured by the decline of the British Empire and the United Kingdom's new role in the international community. Britain's national interests therefore extended beyond the immediate medical and public health debates.

Through a series of examples, this chapter explores how concerns over the nation were expressed. First, two outbreaks in England in 1949 and Scotland in 1950 showed how the British public reacted in the face of an epidemic. The effects of smallpox were local. When the disease came to a specific area, its population sought protection via emergency vaccination, even when they had not wholeheartedly embraced routine infant vaccination. While this control worked at a subnational level, it existed to deal with an international threat – and was coordinated by the national government. Smallpox was a foreign disease, particularly prevalent in South Asia, but it was not one that was necessarily brought in by non-whites. Vaccination was therefore seen as a prophylactic that could be used in specific circumstances, such as protecting British people during an outbreak or as a disinfectant of bodies which had been contaminated by infected lands. This leads to the second section, which discusses the 1950s "propaganda" campaign for smallpox vaccination. As with diphtheria in the previous chapter, there was a sense that British parents were apathetic about smallpox, considering it a deadly but highly improbable disease. However, unlike with other forms of immunisation, the Ministry of Health and the COI did not dedicate significant resources to promoting the benefits of routine childhood vaccination. Moreover, deeper cultural and scientific misgivings about the benefits and dangers of smallpox vaccination loomed large. Instead, the Ministry relied on a limited number of materials and the cooperation of enthusiastic voluntary organisations to gently encourage British parents to present their children for the procedure. Again, the material stressed the foreign nature of smallpox. Routine vaccination was presented as something that could protect against imported disease, and as a prophylactic giving children the freedom to visit a world that was being made smaller by the growing accessibility of air travel.

The 1960s brought an end to this general laissez-faire attitude towards routine vaccination. Five cases of importation in 1961 and 1962 coincided with the Commonwealth Immigration Bill and a fierce public debate about Britain's responsibilities towards its old colonies and immigration by "coloured" Commonwealth citizens. The press coverage led to a re-examination of the science on vaccination, which in turn posed serious questions for public health officials on the relative risks of routine vaccination, mass vaccination in times of epidemic and the disease itself. The decision about whom to vaccinate and which groups were most at risk of harming themselves or the wider British population was made more difficult by the fact that vaccination had never undergone the same sorts of trials and generated the type of data that the medical civil service would have required even as early as the 1950s to make acceptable, concrete policy recommendations. In the end, the World Health Organization's (WHO) Smallpox Eradication Programme moved the prophylactic effort away from questions of national immunity and towards direct intervention in infected lands. Transnational networks of diseases surveillance, exchange of medical knowledge and movement of people became increasingly important to British public health over the latter half of the twentieth century.[6] As with other European countries, Britain's position as a declining colonial power changed the dynamics of its relationship with other health ministries across the globe – as did the emergence of the WHO.[7] Thus, while routine vaccination continued until 1971 and ports were monitored for signs of importation, Britain's national protection was to come from international cooperation and a battle fought well away from its own shores.

Before 1946

Smallpox was a deadly infectious disease which came in two forms. *Variola major* had a death rate of around 20 per cent, while the weaker *variola minor* had a death rate of around 1 per cent. All could lead to excessive scarring and complications in survivors.[8] While public health measures (including vaccination) had rid economically developed nations of the disease by the end of the Second World War, it continued to afflict many parts of the world. Outbreaks in Britain were rare, but, due to increased travel by sea and air to, from and through endemic regions, they were not unheard of. Demobilisation of troops and dislocation led to a number of cases of importation directly after the war, with some indigenous cases – that is, secondary infections caught by people in Britain from the imported case. Aside from the smallpox importations in England and Wales detailed in Table 2.1, there were outbreaks in Scotland in 1937, 1942 and 1950.[9]

Britain's public health responses to smallpox were well established, and the medical profession was confident that it could deal with any infection that arrived.[10] Vaccination had been used as a public health tool since the early nineteenth century in three distinct ways. First, routine vaccination of children was seen as the best way to prevent outbreaks from occurring. This led to compulsory childhood vaccination in 1853, causing well-publicised resistance from some quarters. Vaccination rates declined significantly after conscientious objection was permitted from 1907.[11] Still, from 1948 until 1962 official policy was to vaccinate infants (children under the age of 12 months). Revaccination was then encouraged in school children and adults.[12] Second, ring vaccination was used on people likely to have been exposed to the

The development of the vaccination programme

Table 2.1 Importations of smallpox into England and Wales, 1936–70

Year	Air/sea	Country of origin	Imported cases		Indigenous cases	
			Cases	Deaths	Cases	Deaths
1936[a]	?	?	?		4	
1936/37[b]	Sea	?			10	
1937[a]	?	?	?		1	
1937	?	?	?		1	
1938	Sea	India	1	1	5	1
1938	Sea	Portugal	1		2	1
1938[b]	Sea	?			8	
1939	Sea	?	1			
1940	Sea	?	1			
1942			1		6	
1944	Sea	Gibraltar	1		15	3
1945	Sea	Italy	1		3	
1946	Air	India	1		3	
1946	Air	India	1		2	
1946[c]	Sea	India	1			
1946[c]	Sea	India	2		5	1
1946[c]	Sea	India	4	1		
1946[c]	Sea	India	1			
1946[c]	Sea	India	2			
1946[c]	Sea	India	1	1		
1946[c]	Sea	India	1			
1946[c]	Sea	India	1	1		
1947	Air	Pakistan	1		30	6
1947	Sea	France			48	9
1949	Sea	India	12	5	4	
1950	Air	Pakistan	1		28	10
1951	Sea	India	1			
1951/52[a,d]	?	?	?	?	138	
1953[b]	Sea	?	?	?	38	8
1957	Air	Nigeria	1		6	3
1958	Sea	India	1		5	1
1960	Air	Malaysia	1			
1961		Pakistan	1	1	2	
1961		Pakistan	1		1	
1961		Pakistan	1	1	13	6

Table 2.1 Importations of smallpox into England and Wales, 1936–70 (Continued)

Year	Air/sea	Country of origin	Imported cases		Indigenous cases	
			Cases	Deaths	Cases	Deaths
1962		Pakistan	1			
1962		Pakistan	1		46	19
1962	Sea	India	3			
1966ᵉ	?	?	?(1)		?(1)	
1967	Air	Pakistan	2			
1968	Air	Pakistan	1			
Totals			51	11	518	78

Notes:
ᵃ Supposed importation.
ᵇ Supposed infection from imported raw cotton.
ᶜ A further 33 cases (including 10 deaths) occurred in the Southend and Merseyside areas. It is possible that these infections were derived from these importations.
ᵈ *Variola minor*.
ᵉ Suspected importation. Child's mother developed modified smallpox.
Source: Adapted from TNA: MH 154/404, Importations of smallpox into England and Wales 1936–1970.

virus through contact with known cases. This was designed to stop the spread of disease by stopping the chain of transmission. Finally, mass vaccination was used across a large population during times of epidemic when other forms of public health control – such as routine and ring vaccination, quarantine and isolation – had failed.[13] This was never considered necessary in the post-war outbreaks, although many people presented themselves for vaccination when smallpox was detected in their area.

Vaccination, as with other public health reforms in the nineteenth century, reflected the growing power of national government over what had traditionally been local matters, and the imposition of compulsion was resisted in many quarters.[14] Conscientious objection was introduced in 1898 and made easier to obtain in 1907.[15] The Vaccination

Acts were repealed completely by the National Health Service Acts of 1946 and 1947. In many ways, this was an administrative clean-up – conscientious objection had effectively ended compulsion anyway, and with many health services now being pulled together it made sense to unify the legislation. But it was also a response to the success of the diphtheria immunisation programme during the war. Programmes in Britain and elsewhere had deliberately chosen to make diphtheria immunisation optional, as it was felt that education and persuasion would work better with parents.[16] Practice had shown this to work, and the British government hoped that it could rehabilitate the reputation of smallpox vaccination by promoting it alongside diphtheria and the soon-to-be-available whooping cough vaccine.[17] The decision to end compulsion was largely ignored by the press and Parliament and, as this chapter will show, was rarely mentioned even when outbreaks occurred.

This legacy caused some issues for the British government after 1948. Smallpox vaccination was an old technology, a product of a bygone age rather than of the new era of bacteriology and virology. Scientific debates in the 1960s showed that there was no robust statistical evidence that vaccination was the safest way of protecting the general population from smallpox importation. The medical profession and Ministry of Health remained supportive of routine infant vaccination, but had to concede that their main evidence base for this was experience and tradition rather than the modern, randomised-control trials and epidemiological analyses that they demanded for diphtheria immunisation, whooping cough vaccine and BCG.[18] Although still rare, the risk of vaccine injuries was higher for smallpox than for modern, laboratory-developed immunisations. Potential hazards ranged from excessive scarring at the vaccination site up to brain swelling (postvaccinal encephalitis) and death. Given that the annual cases of smallpox could often be counted on the fingers of one hand, the number of vaccine-related injuries often exceeded the number of smallpox cases.[19] Moreover, the smallpox vaccination procedure was less clean and sophisticated than modern vaccines. Instead of a simple hypodermic injection, smallpox vaccination was still performed by making small incisions in the arm. This made it unpleasant for the child and the onlooking parent, and resulted in scarring.[20] Given the unlikelihood of encountering smallpox, the Ministry and local MOHs had difficulty convincing parents to present their children for the procedure. Furthermore, while central government financed the infant vaccination scheme and compelled local authorities to provide the service, MOHs had jurisdiction over how the schemes were run. This meant that local areas had developed their own traditions about how much to prioritise routine childhood vaccination. Some, such as Leicester (where the local population had strongly resisted in the nineteenth and twentieth centuries) saw uptake for infants as low as 1 per cent in 1961.[21] Others regularly outpaced the national average, such as Worcester, which in the same year had uptake of 71 per cent.[22] Even more so than with diphtheria immunisation, local rates varied considerably (Table 2.2).

There were two different types of vaccination: routine vaccination as a preventative measure; and vaccination as a form of epidemic control. The difference in public reactions to these two types showed that the

Table 2.2 Select vaccination rates as at 31 December 1964

	Pertussis[a]	Diphtheria[a]	Polio[a]	Smallpox[b]
England and Wales	70	72	65	32
England	70	72	66	32
Wales	64	68	62	19
Bradford	55	58	49	10
Bristol	66	67	57	10
Cardiff	80	85	69	28
Glamorgan	62	67	60	8
Halifax	32	55	48	13
Huddersfield	63	65	58	25
Leeds	63	64	48	26
Merthyr	69	66	50	6
West Yorkshire	68	73	69	23
Worcester	79	81	74	61

Notes:
[a] Percentage of children born in 1962 who were immunised at any time by 31 December 1964.
[b] Percentage of children under the age of two years vaccinated.
Source: Adapted from TNA: MH 154/61, Immunisation and Vaccination Statistics as at 31st December 1964.

circumstances and administration of smallpox vaccination mattered. Uptake of *routine* vaccination was variable. In times of epidemic, however, the public were quick to present themselves for ring vaccination, whether or not they had been in contact with the disease. As the examples in this chapter show, there was a certain common-sense understanding that in times of epidemic the local authority was supposed to vaccinate the people – a legacy from the days of mass vaccination, and a perception that caused great difficulties for national and local authorities.[23] There was ample evidence to suggest that primary vaccination – that is, the first time one is vaccinated – was more dangerous in adults than it was in young children. One of the reasons for routine vaccination was not simply to develop individual and herd immunity, since the effects of vaccination were known to wear off in about ten years. A secondary function was to make it safer to regularly revaccinate older children and adults to maintain their immunity; and in case of need for travel documentation, joining an at-risk profession (such as the armed forces or nursing) or during a local outbreak.[24] Mass vaccination therefore posed public health risks as much as it offered potential protection. The most vivid example of this was the experience of the 1942 epidemic in Scotland, where four people died as a result of vaccinations gone wrong.[25] The examples given in this chapter show that this paradox – and the relative risks as understood by the lay public – were a continual source of anxiety for the Ministry of Health.

The 1950s

Two examples of importation in the 1950s showed that vaccination was seen mainly as a barrier against foreign infection. Since smallpox was a foreign contagion brought in by travellers to or residents of infected areas, the government and the public showed more concern about the vaccination of at-risk groups, rather than massively expanding routine childhood vaccination. The first example is of a case of smallpox on board the SS *Mooltan*, which arrived in the Port of London from Australia in April 1949. Citizens, politicians and local authorities demanded stricter vaccination and quarantine controls on infected ships and for passengers from certain areas; but there was little discussion of improving Britons' vaccination status. The second example concerns an outbreak in Glasgow in April 1950, brought in by an Indian seaman on board the SS *Chitral*. Here, the majority of victims worked in the city's fever hospital. Although authorities were more concerned with low routine vaccination rates among their population in the Scottish case than in the English case, more attention was paid in Scotland to the vaccination status of hospital staff. Here, anxieties were raised not just about the risk posed to nurses and doctors themselves, but also about the potential for the disease to spread beyond the fever hospital, should staff be inadequately protected.

The SS Mooltan

The secondary cases from the SS *Mooltan* exemplified this. Richard Allen and his wife boarded the SS *Mooltan* at Brisbane, Australia on 8 February 1949. On 10 March the ship docked at Bombay. Mr and Mrs Allen went ashore for a few hours, although it is unclear what they did in the city. Neither one had ever been vaccinated. On 24 March, Mr Allen complained of stomach pains, and the on-board medical staff began to suspect he may have caught chicken-pox. On 25 March the ship docked in Marseilles, but Mr Allen was too sick to disembark. Due to fog, the SS *Mooltan* was delayed in the English Channel, and Mr Allen died at sea on 1 April. The MOH for the City of London asked the ship company's surgeon to go aboard and check the body. He immediately diagnosed the case as smallpox. By this point, Mrs Allen was also showing signs of infection. All the ship's remaining passengers and crew were offered vaccination, but it was too late to stop the spread of the disease. As passengers disembarked and travelled to various parts of the country, the disease was found in London, North Lincolnshire, Aylesbury, Liverpool, Torquay and Cornwall. In all, there would be 16 cases and five deaths, including those of the Allens (see Table 2.1).[26]

Importations through seaports were not unknown. This was, however, the first epidemic in Britain since the formation of the NHS. Criticism of the decision to allow the passengers to travel across the country before the disease's incubation period was over came from many quarters.[27] However, the fact that potential carriers of a dangerous disease could slip through the ports and be thousands of miles away from the place where they had contracted the disease before they showed symptoms showed that port sanitation and quarantine regulations, which had a long history in British public health, were beginning to break down.[28] Local authorities, voluntary organisations and individual citizens wrote in protest to the Minister of Health, Aneurin Bevan, demanding that future cases be subject to quarantine. In Parliament, Jocelyn Lucas (Conservative, Portsmouth South) and Bessie Braddock (Labour, Liverpool Exchange) both spoke about the 'widespread anxiety' and urged the Ministry of Health to tighten its regulations.[29] Braddock in particular called for action to be taken against contacts who refused vaccination.[30] Ernest Bramall (Labour, Bexley) also enquired as to whether the decision to end compulsory vaccination would be reversed.[31] Bevan resisted increasing compulsion for either the general population or smallpox contacts, and argued that the Ministry and port authorities had enough powers to ensure the safety of the population.[32] In response to individual correspondence, the Ministry provided details of the International Sanitary Conventions that restricted its ability to forcibly detain passengers; and further noted that such measures probably would not have done much good.[33] There were only four cases in people who had not been aboard the SS *Mooltan*: all of them in one family living near the isolation hospital in Liskeard, Cornwall.[34]

There was not an extended debate in the national press about the cases arising from the SS *Mooltan*. As the Ministry noted, concerns were raised in local authorities where suspected cases had arisen and from some individuals, but there is little evidence of a great national panic.[35] In the Port of London, the local MOH was relaxed. 'The public have played up very well indeed and there has been very little nervousness,' he wrote in his annual report, 'a fact which I think demonstrates confidence arising from the daily supervision of contact cases.'[36] Discussions among health authorities focused on how to stop importation from outside rather than strengthening British immunity to the disease from within through more widespread vaccination. MOHs publicly demanded that Australian and New Zealand passengers be vaccinated if a ship was due to stop in the Indian sub-continent.[37] The MOH for Lambeth, G. O. Teichmann, noted the double standard of expecting all Indian passengers to be vaccinated, but not requiring the same of 'Australasians' who 'were allowed to wander about the bazaars of Bombay etc. where smallpox is endemic'.[38] The Ministry related these concerns to Peninsular & Oriental, the SS *Mooltan*'s operators, who agreed to actively discourage unvaccinated passengers from going ashore in 'Eastern Ports'.[39]

Thus, foreigners and travellers to foreign lands were seen as a potential threat to British public health. This idea had grown in importance since the end of the First World War. In the nineteenth century, smallpox in India and other parts of the Empire was treated much like it was at home. As the disease ceased to be a major problem in Europe and North America, however, smallpox became viewed as a "tropical" disease, and was treated as a foreign threat.[40] But while some blame for the continued presence of smallpox in the sub-continent was put on the superstitions and habits of Indians, the rhetoric around infection was not necessarily restricted to non-whites: 'Australasians' could themselves become contaminated because of their route through infected places and their lack of vaccination. In the meantime, there was no extended demand for more widespread routine vaccination of infants at home. Other than queues in Liskeard, there was also no great clamour for emergency vaccination. Isolated incidents appeared to grab attention, especially in local areas directly or potentially affected, but this soon died down. Unlike with the outbreaks of 1961 and 1962, the SS *Mooltan* cases did not become a national emergency, nor did they significantly alter attitudes towards smallpox in England and Wales. There was no major political crisis of national identity to refract the news of the outbreak.[41] Instead, criticisms of policy were directed more to the ship being allowed to land than any disquiet over the epidemic controls or Britain's vaccination status.[42] This was despite the ship's ability to remain in the news. A nine year old girl developed suspected smallpox on the Mooltan's return trip to Australia; and later that same year, the ship was quarantined in the Thames due to typhoid.[43]

The SS Chitral

Given the racial element to the 1961/62 outbreak, the SS *Chitral* incident provides an interesting contrast. On 5 March 1950, Lascar seaman Mussa Ali landed at Tilbury on the SS *Chitral* before travelling to Glasgow.[44] His country of origin was smallpox endemic, and he was non-white – unlike the Allens. As a Lascar seaman, it was also unlikely that he or his shipmates had been revaccinated to maintain his immunity, unlike sailors in the Royal Navy.[45] He was admitted to hospital with pneumonia and suspected chicken-pox. This was subsequently found to be smallpox. A doctor who had come into contact with Ali, Janet Fleming, died in the nearby town of Hamilton on 2 April. The outbreak would infect 19 people and kill six.[46] During the epidemic, thousands queued on the streets of Glasgow and Hamilton for vaccination. The incident highlighted some of the differences between the English and Scottish health services' experience of smallpox, but the issue of importation remained central. Here was 'Bombay smallpox',[47] brought in by an Indian seaman and with the potential to affect Scotland's public and economic health. Yet the focus of discussion remained largely on the quality of preventative services at home rather than on concern about immigration.

The Scottish Office had already expressed its concerns with British smallpox policy in 1948. W. M. Ballantine, a Scottish civil servant, noted that 'there is not the same tradition of vaccination in Scotland as in England and the number of vaccinated children is very low'.[48] In an epidemic in 1942, mass vaccination was employed as a form of epidemic control in Edinburgh; but, due to the low rates of primary vaccinations, there were nine cases of encephalitis and four deaths.[49] Ballantine asked if the COI would consider a national (British) smallpox vaccination education campaign. He felt that this would be particularly welcome in Scotland, given that 'the risk of importation of smallpox [was] high' and 'the likelihood of spread [was] greater in Scotland'.[50] The COI declined, as it was more concerned with promoting the new NHS; and when it did return to promoting immunisation, it was more interested in diphtheria and the soon-to-be-available pertussis vaccine. Instead, the COI recommended that local authorities should decide what was needed in their area, and the Central Council for Health Education would provide materials which could be ordered and used.[51]

When the disease broke out in Glasgow and Hamilton during late March and early April 1950, local MOHs offered vaccination to the public. At its peak, a special clinic in Glasgow was reportedly vaccinating 600 people per hour. By 15 April, two days before Glasgow was given the all clear, around 300,000 people had been vaccinated across Lanarkshire and Renfrewshire. The Glasgow MOH, Stuart Laidlaw, was 'very pleased with the public response for vaccination' and thanked the public for having 'acted very wisely'.[52] Indeed, other than demands from politicians on behalf of their constituents for public inquiries due to 'great anxiety in the public mind', the outbreak did not appear to create a massive scandal in the area or in the national press.[53] The *Daily Mail* reported how Ali was cheered out of the hospital when he recovered, and that there 'was no grudge against the man whose illness had cost six lives'.[54] Instead, attention turned to what the Glasgow outbreak said about Scotland's – and Britain's – ability to deal with smallpox and its economic consequences. In this specific incident, all the victims of the disease had been in direct contact with Ali in hospital. However, while the disease had not spread into the wider community, the number of cases and deaths had caused significant harm to Scotland's and Glasgow's tourism industries during the Easter break. The MOHs of Edinburgh and of Corby in Northamptonshire, a town with a sizable Scottish diaspora, advised their residents not to travel to Glasgow, while New York City began to demand more extensive proof of vaccination before allowing travellers from Scotland to land.[55] Due to the damage to the tourism industry, after the epidemic was over Scottish Office ministers called for an extensive advertising campaign to let the world know that 'Scotland was normal again'.[56] This highlighted the transnational character of the epidemic. Not only had it been imported from foreign shores, but its effects on Britain were also global.

There was also some discussion about the victims of the disease. Nine cases came from hospital staff, of whom four nurses and a laundry maid died. The sixth death was a baby; none of the six had been fully vaccinated. While importation of smallpox may have been impossible to prevent in practice, the poor vaccination records of the hospital staff caused disquiet among politicians north and south of the border. The government declined to make vaccination a condition of employment but reiterated 'the need to ensure that vaccination is offered to all persons [working in] fever hospitals and re-vaccination is offered periodically'.[57] It argued that compulsion would be difficult to justify after the repeal of the Vaccination Acts, and would jeopardise recruitment in fever hospitals that were already finding it difficult to hire staff.[58] This response drew criticism in Parliament from both major parties, although the opposition Conservative politicians were most vocal. Lord (John) Llewellin (Conservative) noted that travellers from the United Kingdom were compelled to be vaccinated for their own protection, and so that they did not import smallpox on their return.[59] David Gammans (Conservative, Hornsey) made a similar argument. Given the insistence of 'almost every country in the world' that vaccination be a condition of entry, why were fever hospital staff – the most likely group to come into contact with foreign travellers with the disease – allowed to work without being up to date? He asked the Secretary of State for Scotland, Hector McNeil, 'have we to wait until three women die before we bring in a regulation which every other country in the world insists on?'[60] In this sense, vaccination was a barrier against foreign infection, with fever hospitals acting as a buffer between the public and an infected outside world. Vaccination not only protected British medical staff, but stopped the spread of the disease out into the wider public. The government's counter arguments, however, rested on the idea that staff were themselves members of the public with the same rights to forego vaccination. If vaccination drove even more employees away from fever hospitals, that buffer might not exist at all.

1950s propaganda and education campaign

The outbreaks in 1949 and 1950 did not substantially alter the Ministry's approach to routine vaccination. The Ministry responded to individual enquiries and stressed the need for health visitors to use a 'personal approach' with parents to convince them of the benefits for their child.[61] There was, however, no sustained propaganda campaign. The complications associated with mass vaccination and adult primary vaccination were well known. With growing travel by sea and, increasingly, by air, there was also a potential for the disease to become more common. Experts continued to write to the Ministry expressing concern that vaccination rates were steadily falling among the general public and NHS staff.[62] Yet the Ministry was mindful not to engage in debates with anti-vaccination groups. Although less prominent than in previous decades, the government did continue to receive correspondence from the Anti-Vaccination League and other individuals.[63] In Parliament, Samuel Viant, a Labour MP in Willesden until 1959, asked regular questions about the safety and efficacy of vaccination and the effects of trials on animals.[64] However, these occasional interactions appeared to be rare and sufficiently low level as not to concern the Ministry, highlighting the declining influence of such groups since the end of compulsion and growing confidence in immunisation technologies during the interwar years. Instead, the Ministry preferred to reiterate the benefits of vaccination and argued that since diphtheria and whooping cough immunisation had been such a success parents could possibly be persuaded at the same time to get their children vaccinated against smallpox.[65]

By the middle of the decade, the Ministry began to reassess its approach in light of its wider public health goals. While the government encouraged parents to immunise their children against other diseases – and appeared to be having success in these endeavours – correspondence and vaccination statistics suggested that, regardless of the intention, parents had not been convinced to take up smallpox vaccination as well.[66] An officer from Essex offered some evidence from their area. When asked why mothers might not be presenting their children, home visitors replied that the women they worked with were often told when they arrived that there was not enough vaccination material and they failed to make or complete follow-up appointments. Parents also objected to waiting in a doctor's surgery with a healthy baby among sick patients. In his opinion, 'there is not real apathy among parents but now that compulsion is no longer necessary, effective propaganda and stimulus is essential'.[67] The Chief Medical Officer, John Charles, wrote in his 1954 Annual Report that it was becoming increasingly important that parents should present their children. The older generation, who had been children at the time of compulsory vaccination, were passing away. A new vaccination drive would restore immunity.[68] A circular was sent to all local authorities in 1955 noting Charles's concern 'at the current neglect of vaccination except as an emergency measure during outbreaks of smallpox, and […] the resulting lack of protection for the individual and for the community'.[69] A new poster was designed, and local MOHs were encouraged to give smallpox vaccination greater priority, in the hope of raising infant uptake from a modest 36.4 per cent in 1955 to 75 per cent.[70] The choice of message was revealing. The English and Welsh authorities were inspired by a long-running leaflet in Scotland which had used newspaper headlines from the 1950 outbreak to remind parents of just how dangerous the disease could be. It pulled no punches – the opening paragraph read: 'do you want to take the risk of seeing your child's face pitted by the ugly scars of smallpox?' This type of message was similar to the one used in the diphtheria campaign at the same time, demonstrating a coherent message about vaccination (even if the volume of material and the response to it was not equal across all programmes). Although it did not go so far as to show pictures of diseased children, it used the threat of potential damage through inaction to press home its message. It stressed that vaccination before an outbreak was safer than waiting for one to occur, and ended with the slightly dubious claim that 'vaccination does not upset children, although in adults a first vaccination may be very painful. So have your child vaccinated now! Keep your baby safe!'[71] The resulting English poster tried to emulate the visual impact of the Scottish one, with a bright yellow background and the words 'vaccination' and 'smallpox' in bright red block capitals. The text was less outwardly emotive, simply quoting the Chief Medical Officer: 'VACCINATION of all healthy babies must be our aim if we are to protect the community against a run of SMALLPOX.'[72] The foregrounding of the benefits to the community was in contrast to previous campaign messages which had very deliberately focused on the individual benefits of vaccination to the child and parent.[73] The diphtheria campaign, for example, had foregrounded healthy babies and the protection that parents could gift to their child.

Despite Charles's pronouncement, this would be the extent of the Ministry of Health's propaganda mission. Both the anti-diphtheria and anti-poliomyelitis publicity efforts got far more attention from the Ministry of Health and COI.[74] No major incident in the 1950s forced the government to change tack. There was also evidence to suggest that even some doctors had inferred that the end of compulsion was an admission from the government that it no longer saw routine smallpox vaccination as a priority.[75] As local MOHs and other organisations wrote to the government for advice, the only other promotional offering was a 1951 film called *Surprise Attack*. Film had been used to promote public health messages and inform the public about public health activities for decades.[76] Bermondsey in South London, for example, had established its own film department in the 1920s.[77] At this time, a growing documentary film movement began to be co-opted by government departments that saw it as an effective communication tool, producing a range of materials for the promotion of health and other government activities.[78] *Surprise Attack* starred John le Mesurier as a general practitioner and showed the story of a family whose young girl caught smallpox from a rag doll brought back from 'the east' by her father. In the film's tale of how the MOH tried to keep control of the outbreak, the girl survives with significant scarring. The final few moments have the MOH showing pictures of real smallpox cases to show how gruesome the disease could be – and a call to action for parents to take their children to the clinic to be vaccinated. The film stressed that while parents might think that smallpox was now rare, 'by the time your children are all grown up, air travel will be general'.[79] The dangers of travel – from both foreigners coming to Britain and unprotected Britons bringing disease back – were ever present.[80] However, that *Surprise Attack* had not been updated or replaced by the early 1960s reflected a lack of sustained effort or resource commitment from the authorities.

While the government did not prioritise smallpox vaccination advertising, the public appeared relatively apathetic too. Vaccination rates did recover slightly in the mid-1950s, but not by enough to reach the 75 per cent target set by Charles.[81] However, the government was able to lean on publicity produced by outsiders with an interest in childhood vaccination. This was not a new development. Voluntary organisations had been involved in health care from before the war, from health education to the running of hospitals.[82] The National Baby Welfare Council had expressed considerable concern when it had written to the Ministry asking for a smallpox poster for an exhibition on child health and had been told that there was not one in circulation.[83] The Council sought to fill the gap itself, but when outside bodies created health propaganda they could cause embarrassment for the government. The War Office complained to the Ministry about one poster which presented a returning soldier as a vector of disease and in a dishevelled uniform. Another leaflet contained inaccuracies on vaccination procedure and official government advice.[84] Both pieces did, however, reinforce the "foreign threat" perception of smallpox. The returning soldier was a danger because of where he had been and how quickly he could return home. In the leaflet, a mother is urged to have her daughter 'done', despite the scarring from the vaccination, because 'she may want to be an airhostess' someday. In both pieces, the pain of the adult vaccination was stressed to convince parents that it was best to act now rather than later – deliberately drawing on the experiences of many fathers and husbands who would have been vaccinated for national service during and after the war.[85] Despite the potential embarrassment, the Ministry became increasingly reliant upon these organisations to spread its message. When the Women's Voluntary Service offered to help distribute material in July 1956, the Ministry asked it to contact local MOHs instead.[86] By September, however, it was responding to a national campaign by the Women's Institute by sending hundreds of copies of the yellow poster to branches across the country.[87] Certain sections of the public clearly believed in the importance of routine childhood vaccination; but these were voluntary organisations of a middle-class bent concerned primarily with motherhood.[88] Without central coordination and resources, the campaign never fully developed.

The 1960s – Commonwealth Immigration Bill

The campaign for improved routine smallpox vaccination rates in the 1950s did not see an appreciable increase in uptake. But this did not cause undue anxiety among staff at the Ministry of Health. There were five importations of *variola major* between 1951 and 1960, and all were adequately contained, despite the deaths of twelve people (see Table 2.1). There was also a *variola minor* outbreak in Rochdale in 1951/52, from infected raw cotton, which caused 138 cases but no deaths. It was generally accepted that routine childhood vaccination was desirable, but the Ministry had faith that its existing methods of port control, isolation and vaccination of contacts were enough to protect Britain from external threat.[89] There was some concern about the level of campaigning from the British Medical Association (BMA) at its conference in 1960. Following the conference, the Association wrote to the Ministry to find what publicity material it had available and to urge it to renew the vaccination campaign. The Ministry remarked that it had little of its own material, and that other organisations' efforts were taken into account. More broadly, it had not produced much in recent years because local authorities had shown no demand for materials.[90] This low-level critique from the BMA may not have required much response; however, a major outbreak of smallpox was about to be turned into a national scandal. This saw more attention drawn to smallpox policy, and forced the Ministry to reassess its position.

From 16 December 1961 to 11 January 1962, five separate importations of *variola major* occurred through Britain's airports, all from Pakistani travellers.[91] A smallpox epidemic was raging in Karachi, and planes were able to transport passengers to London in a matter of hours. The volume of passengers had also increased, as immigrants hoped to get to Britain to settle before the Commonwealth Immigrants Act 1962 came into force and restricted movement from Commonwealth countries. From these five, two cases resulted in local outbreaks: one in Bradford and another in Cardiff. A third outbreak then developed near to the isolation hospital in Penrhys, and spread into the Rhondda Valley, South Wales. For anti-immigration politicians, the outbreaks gave legitimacy to their claims for stricter border controls.[92] For the medical profession, this new form of immigration by air raised questions about the ability of existing sanitary regulations to protect the nation from harm.[93] Meanwhile, the British public expressed a range of opinions on smallpox, vaccination, race and government.[94]

Roberta Bivins' work has explored in detail how British attitudes towards the new Commonwealth were manifested during the outbreak. Concerns about the social impact of immigration, particularly from South Asia, were expressed through demands for stricter health checks at ports and proof of vaccination. These were often presented as bureaucratic necessities to protect health, so as to avoid the accusation of direct racism, even though there was little epidemiological merit to the proposals.[95] James Stewart has also collated a rich public history of the outbreak, including contemporary materials and oral histories with survivors.[96] As these demonstrate, routine childhood vaccination was one talking point among many; and certainly not the most important.[97] The outbreak became a scandal because it touched a raw nerve in British politics with regard to Commonwealth immigration, rather than because it was a medical crisis per se. Control of immigration was the main concern. It was therefore as much about protecting Britain's national character as much as its public health. As the public demanded tighter controls on foreigners entering the country, the government was forced to manage a number of risks. Any importation of smallpox at this time was even more politically sensitive than usual. Yet tighter port controls, despite being the apparent "common sense" solution, were likely to be ineffective. There was also the risk that too many draconian regulations could damage international trade, and thus the wider economy.

These issues, especially surrounding race and immigration, have been dealt with effectively by Bivins.[98] However, the wider story of how the Ministry of Health dealt with the situation tells us more specifically about vaccination and the public. Three vaccination strategies emerged: mass vaccination of the indigenous public as a form of epidemic control; selective vaccination of at-risk individuals such as migrants and NHS staff; and routine vaccination of British children as a policy outside of epidemic times or locations. In each, the public and the government had a role to play. The tensions within them were not fully resolved during or in the aftermath of the crisis. Nevertheless, they did lead to a re-evaluation of policy in the years following the end of the epidemic.

The most visible show of support for vaccination came in areas that had confirmed cases of smallpox. Demand for vaccination as protection against a potential epidemic was high, but it caused headaches for national and local health authorities. As there had been in Liskeard and Glasgow in 1949 and 1950, there were queues for vaccination in Bradford, Cardiff and the Rhondda valley. One case had been taken to University College Hospital in the London borough of St Pancras, which also saw lines of concerned members of the public queueing around the block. These images were staples of press and television coverage, much to the chagrin of Chief Medical Officer George Godber. He argued that they reflected panic in epidemic areas, and also fuelled the idea that this was the correct way to behave when smallpox occurred.[99] Mass vaccination was not considered an adequate form of epidemic control, and brought its own problems. Experience in the Scottish epidemic of 1942 had shown that it could lead to complications, aside from the practical undesirability of having thousands of people congregating in one spot in a city with an ongoing epidemic. Enoch Powell, the Minister for Health, declared that 'queues were the evidence of responsibilities neglected' by both the public, who had broken what ought to be 'an almost universal and unquestioned code of behaviour' (i.e. presenting for routine vaccination) and the health authorities, which had not been coordinated or effective enough to ensure that the public understood this.[100]

For Godber, a keen supporter of routine infant vaccination, these queues represented a paradox. As would also be seen with poliomyelitis scares in the 1950s (Chapter 3), mass vaccination enjoyed support in times of crisis that routine vaccination in normal circumstances did not. When reflecting on the 1962 epidemic, Godber remarked:

> Vaccination, of course, played an important part in control ... and in the circumstances of the Rhondda and Bradford the public demand is easily understood. But much vaccination was done as a matter of urgency, where no urgency existed. The population as a whole has, of course, obtained some advantage from this in increased immunity and assurance

of quicker enhancement of that immunity if required in the future. Yet mass demands when smallpox occurred reflect a state of public anxiety attributable in part to the neglect of routine vaccination.[101]

The Ministry was not helped in some areas by its regional lieutenants, who made demands that contradicted central government advice. High demand had led to shortages of vaccine lymph and strict control by central authorities, causing consternation among members of the public as well as MOHs.[102] MOHs in Yorkshire districts near to Bradford demanded more vaccine, and complained when they were not given priority access to limited supplies of lymph. In Halifax especially, the local MOH made the case that because the town had a 'large immigrant population', it required more vaccine to protect its people.[103] This underscored the idea that foreigners were vectors of disease, and foreign lands its source. Queues in other boroughs across the country (and the subsequent shortage of lymph) were also attributed to widespread publicity about the outbreak, and fear of 'coloured' migrants bringing the disease into previously uninfected areas.[104] For other contemporaries, however, the outbreak represented a key tension in public health policy: the fine line between acting to protect the public and *being seen by the public* to act. Even if mass vaccination was not considered medically justified, the MOH for Bradford and his deputy argued that it was a necessary evil to keep the general public calm.[105] Allaying anxieties clearly mattered to local authorities, and, even if people were a little too keen to be vaccinated, MOHs made a point of praising citizens for their cooperation. They had come to expect this after experiences across the country during the post-war period.[106]

While Godber continued to promote the power of routine vaccination, many of the arguments around the 1962 outbreak focused on other forms of prophylaxis. In particular, tighter port controls, vaccination of immigrants and protection of key NHS staff were given far greater coverage in the press, Parliament and medical discourse. Some of this was politically convenient for anti-immigration politicians.[107] For the Ministry, it was another example of common sense being at odds with wider economic and medical wisdom.[108] Despite the panics caused by smallpox in the community, the disease burned out quickly and affected relatively few people. It was considered disproportionate, therefore, to instigate stricter border controls which would adversely affect international travel and trade.[109] Enforcing vaccination or revaccination of travellers from smallpox-endemic countries was resisted, as it might be considered racially motivated, would take up too much time and would have little material effect in preventing importation.[110] Some dissented: one correspondent to the *British Medical Journal* bemoaned that in 'East of Suez there is far too much graft and subterfuge', so that even those with seemingly legitimate vaccination certificates must be considered suspect.[111] However, the two infected individuals who caused the local outbreaks possessed certificates of vaccination and/or showed signs of having been successfully vaccinated in the past. As for the vaccination of at-risk groups – usually taken to mean front-line NHS staff – this was considered administratively impractical. Two-thirds of the indigenous cases were contacted in hospital, affecting staff and patients (a similar pattern to Glasgow in 1950).[112] Staff were prioritised during outbreaks and offered revaccination every three years, but, as in the SS *Mooltan* and SS *Chitral* incidents, it was reiterated that compulsion would have a negative effect on hiring and retention of hospital staff. The Ministry's existing protocols had not been perfect. But it was notable that there were no tertiary outbreaks in Bradford.[113] The disease was promptly kept under control. And while the infectious disease hospitals in some areas were shown to be inadequate, there was never any need to invoke emergency mass vaccination measures.[114] Long-standing public health measures, in line with the International Sanitary Regulations on smallpox, appeared to have worked to keep Britain safe.[115]

However, the level of public disquiet over the 1962 outbreak forced the Ministry to seriously reconsider its routine vaccination policies. The public's faith in vaccination and in their local health authorities during times of epidemic had been demonstrated clearly. But there was a sense in Parliament and the media that local areas had been let down by national government allowing the outbreaks to occur in the first place.[116] There were also criticisms about the lymph shortages and unsatisfactory prioritisation of some areas over others – or, as one correspondent to the *British Medical Journal* put it, 'bureaucratic bumbledom gone bonkers'.[117] Appreciating the failures of vaccination policy, the Ministry of Health re-examined its approach and competing interpretations of the epidemiology. This would eventually lead to the end of routine vaccination in 1971.

The 1960s to 1970s: withdrawal

The Ministry remained confident in its epidemic control policies, but routine vaccination continued to be problematic. The government had consistently fallen well short of its target of 75 per cent childhood vaccination. In analysing its policy, the Ministry collated vaccination statistics, and they made grim reading for proponents of vaccination (Table 2.2). In 1964, the national average for smallpox in England remained at 32 per cent of children under the age of two. Even the most successful local authority, the city of Worcester in the Midlands, achieved only 61 per cent. This was in stark contrast to the relative successes of the pertussis, diphtheria and poliomyelitis immunisation campaigns, which were approaching childhood vaccination rates of 75 per cent, even in areas where smallpox vaccination was unpopular. The figures also suggested that parents saw smallpox vaccination as an epidemic control tool rather than a necessary immunisation for their children. In Bradford, Cardiff and Glamorgan (the epicentres of the 1962 outbreaks), uptake remained below the national average for England and Wales. Indeed, Bradford's rates were equal to the worst in England (Bristol), second only to Merthyr in Wales. The West Yorkshire boroughs which had complained to the Ministry about a lack of lymph during the heat of the crisis also had relatively weak figures. In light of this apathy towards routine vaccination, then, what was to be done? Unlike with diphtheria in the 1950s, it was not sustainable to claim that smallpox was a quotidian threat or that it could ever return as endemic and widespread, regardless of the danger posed in the rare cases of importation. By the same token, it was clear that people were not against vaccination when they felt the threat of smallpox was strong enough. The Ministry embarked on a fact-finding mission to settle these questions of how to protect the nation.

The aftermath of the 1962 outbreak caused debate in the medical press. The dangers of mass vaccination were reiterated, but new concerns were raised about the potential harm of routine vaccination.[118] Three doctors in particular made the argument that routine vaccination ought to be abandoned. The first, George Dick, was Professor of Microbiology at Queen's University Belfast and had worked on oral polio vaccine trials in the early 1950s (see also Chapter 3). His work had shown the risks of cross-contamination, and this had made him very alert to the risks as well as the benefits of vaccination across a large population.[119] The second, Ronald W. Elliott, was the County Medical Officer for West Yorkshire.[120] Both men publicly argued that even if the country could institute 100 per cent uptake of smallpox vaccination, the resulting level of herd immunity would not be enough to prevent occasional outbreaks of smallpox. Moreover, the risk of a smallpox outbreak was low, and getting lower as a result of WHO eradication efforts.[121] By contrast, it was known that between ten and twenty infants died every year from vaccination.[122] In weighing these relative risks and the potential benefits of vaccination, they borrowed from a third doctor, C. W. Dixon. He had calculated that herd immunity from childhood vaccination might not even exceed 10 per cent. Because the effectiveness of the vaccine waned over time, people vaccinated as children would become vulnerable again in young adulthood. Without revaccination, this left a large section of the population vulnerable to infection. This was doubly dangerous because these people might believe themselves to be safe because they had been vaccinated in earlier life and might therefore take risks without knowing it. Dixon concluded that a childhood vaccination programme without a robust adult revaccination programme was worse than useless.[123]

Dick raised his concerns at the BMA's annual meeting in Belfast in July 1962.[124] He was joined by William Edgar, Bradford's Deputy MOH, making a speech to the Royal Society of Health in which he claimed that mass vaccination had not contributed to controlling the outbreak there.[125] The resulting debate was picked up by the popular press, highlighting the strength of feeling on the matter and causing some anxiety on the part of the Ministry of Health. It had hoped to keep the matter relatively private, a discussion between experts in government meeting rooms rather than in a public forum.[126] Correspondents to the *British Medical Journal* were also critical that such a sensitive matter was being aired in a press prone to 'sensationalist' headlines, as evinced by the 'panic' that had followed reports of smallpox during the epidemic.[127] There was a sense, therefore, that the public did not have the knowledge to be able to debate this issue properly and would act emotionally rather than logically.[128] However, the *British Medical Journal* also cautioned its readers that they too held deep emotional positions on smallpox. An editorial quoted the noted epidemiologist Major Greenwood when he said that 'no intelligent person supposes that logic determines practical issues'.[129]

To clarify Dick's comments and the organisation's position on smallpox, the BMA wrote to the Ministry arguing that a new committee should be established to advise the government on vaccination and immunisation policy.[130] That the government agreed to the request shows the power and close relationship that the BMA had with the Ministry at this time.[131] However, when it had requested a more intensive smallpox vaccination campaign some years earlier, this had been treated rather lukewarmly. The formation of a new committee was neither difficult nor out of line with the Ministry's pre-existing plans. The Ministry and Scottish Office's Joint Committee on Poliomyelitis Vaccine (JCPV) which reported to the Standing Medical Advisory Committee (SMAC), was about to expire following the decision to move to oral poliomyelitis vaccine (see Chapter 3).[132] The Ministry had already considered something similar to the BMA's proposal, and therefore established the Joint Committee on Vaccination and Immunisation (JCVI).[133] To respond directly to 'Dick's bombshell', a sub-committee was immediately created within the JCVI to explicitly deal with the questions raised by Dick, Dixon, Elliott and others.[134] Chaired by R. E. Tunbridge, Professor of Medicine at the University of Leeds, the sub-committee's membership included MOHs, general practitioners, researchers and a paediatrician. Elliott himself was co-opted onto the sub-committee. It reported to the main JCVI which in turn reported to the Ministers responsible for health in England, Scotland and Northern Ireland.[135] This reflected the growing influence of expert advice in British health matters in the post-war period.[136]

It also showed that immunisation policy was becoming increasingly standardised. Although the national campaign for diphtheria had begun in 1940, local MOHs were largely responsible for prioritising and administering it at the regional level. The 1950s campaigns had tried to raise uptake in areas of apathy. The JCVI, though, created a dedicated nook of the medical civil service for discussing the issues surrounding vaccination across all diseases and across all the constituent countries of the United Kingdom. Advancing immunisation technology required better planning. Conservative Minister of Health Enoch Powell promised 'a comprehensive and planned programme of immunisation and vaccination in every part of the country'.[137] By focusing on smallpox vaccination, attention had also turned back to indigenous cases – the Ministry acknowledged that importation was impossible to prevent, so it was important to ensure that Britons were best placed to deal with it if or when it arrived.[138] Building on the work of previous organisations such as SMAC and JCPV, this was a national attempt to protect public health. For 'although each outbreak' of infectious disease had 'a focal point of starting ... each focal point [was] of National concern'.[139]

The sub-committee broke down Dick's main critique of vaccination into three areas. First, that 'there is excessive mortality from vaccination'; second that 'smallpox in infancy ... is unlikely to make much contribution to herd immunity'; and third, that 'routine public health control measures would adequately contain epidemic spread'.[140] The first meeting, in April 1963, was a tense affair: the members had strong opinions on vaccination, and were frustrated at the lack of hard evidence to form any concrete advice for the JCVI.[141] A second meeting was called in July to go back over the extant evidence and give Dick, who had been unavailable in April, a chance to present his case more thoroughly.[142] Members seemed to be acutely aware that there was a difference between, as Dick put it, 'paper' and 'de facto' policy.[143] The idea that all members of the public would behave as they were advised – 100 per cent being vaccinated in infancy and then revaccinated regularly throughout childhood and adulthood – was clearly a fantasy. In reality, primary vaccination rates in children were known to be around 40 to 50 per cent (depending on the local authority), and revaccination rates were barely one in ten. C. Kaplan, a member of the sub-committee, wrote in the *British Medical Journal* that this could in fact be worse than nothing, since it might give people (or the country in general) a false sense of security when there was an outbreak.[144] Dick laid down the challenge that the government should either abandon the policy as unworkable, or make genuine attempts to reach the 'paper' policy goal – something it had clearly failed to do during the 1950s.[145] But this too would have de facto problems. Even Elliott, a proponent of ending routine childhood vaccination, argued that 'a not very well-informed public' would see the ending of vaccination as negligent.[146] There had already been a backlash in some quarters when SMAC had shifted the recommendation to vaccinate in the first year of life to vaccination between the ages of one and two years (on the epidemiological evidence that this reduced the risk of complications). H. Josephs, from the Smethwick Local Medical Committee, felt that this would reduce the number of vaccinations in his area, which was dangerous, given the number of 'coloured' immigrants in his borough; W. H. Crichton also argued that mothers preferred to vaccinate at around six months because the children were less mobile and therefore it was easier to deal with the scabs that developed on the arm.[147] Besides, if revaccination was safer than primary vaccination in adults, there were criticisms that Dick's preferred policy of vaccinating only contacts would be unacceptable to the wider public. As the 1962 outbreaks had shown, 'they will come in their hordes and *demand* protection: and no health authority will dare to them say nay'.[148] Most importantly of all, the experts saw their role as one that required firm, unequivocal advice for a public considered unable to make such complex decisions for themselves. The possibility of laying out the risks for parents (and their family doctors) and allowing them to choose was considered absolutely 'unacceptable'.[149]

The paradox of public attitudes to vaccination was again exposed. The public clearly welcomed, even demanded, the protections offered by vaccination in times of epidemic. Doctors working alongside parents and the general public also believed that the removal of routine vaccination would cause considerable disquiet. And yet, primary vaccination rates remained low, with revaccination rates even lower. Even if it could be epidemiologically justified, the removal of what was seen as a necessary protection was problematic. So too was the potential political fallout, should an outbreak occur in the absence of such protection (whether it was a causative factor or not). The hazard of a smallpox outbreak, even a single case, was too much to risk on the incomplete evidence so far accumulated. As the sub-committee noted, there was a general sense that current public health protection methods worked, but there was no reliable experimental evidence to suggest exactly how well they worked, as compared with routine vaccination. There was acceptance that vaccination probably did not prevent many cases, but there was no reliable epidemiological evidence on how few cases it prevented. There may have been little evidence to stop vaccination, but it was also the case that 'smallpox vaccination [was] so much a part of ancient lore that it has not been subjected to the kind of scientific appraisal that other vaccination procedures [had] received'.[150] In these circumstances, the status quo won out, while the sub-committee went in search of the evidence that would allow the JCVI to recommend concrete policy proposals to ministers. Dick's quotation of G. S. Wilson's critique of BCG vaccine was apt: 'It is much easier to introduce a given measure into the public health practice of this country than to remove it once it has become firmly established.'[151]

By the late 1960s, further analyses on the vaccination programme had provided answers to questions about vaccination safety and efficacy. Expert opinion had begun to turn away from the procedure on scientific and practical grounds.[152] More importantly, the smallpox landscape had changed dramatically. The intensification of the WHO Smallpox Eradication Programme from 1967 onwards significantly reduced the areas of the world in which smallpox was endemic.[153] This further increased the risk of vaccine injury relative to the risk posed by the disease itself. While research had been proposed into finding a new, safer immunisation against smallpox, resistance in the WHO, a lack of suitable test populations to assess potency and risk, plus the declining need for it in economically developed nations meant that it never materialised.[154] On the basis of this 'balance of risks', the Secretary of State, Sir Keith Joseph, announced on 28 July 1971 that routine vaccination would end.[155] Both the Department of Health and Social Security (DHSS), which had replaced the Ministry of Health in 1968, and the Scottish Office accepted the JCVI's recommendation that existing public health measures would be enough to control any potential importation. Instead, people in at-risk groups (such as NHS staff, people travelling to smallpox-endemic areas and those requiring vaccination certificates for travel abroad) would be offered vaccination, as would contacts of known smallpox cases.[156]

The decision provoked little debate in the general press. There had not been a confirmed indigenous case of the disease via importation since the 1962 outbreak (see Table 2.1), and there was general confidence in the Eradication Programme. Where one finds isolated voices of dissent, racialised views of the disease were never far away. One concerned resident in Hayes End, Middlesex wrote to her MP that she felt very strongly that 'in our area this is most unwise with considerable numbers of Indians and Pakistanis commuting daily and being employed in local bakeries etc, handling food'.[157] Expert opinion, however, had moved on. Dick gave a summary of the arguments to the

British Medical Journal and was supported by a favourable editorial in the same issue.[158] A few doctors expressed doubts, but it produced far fewer letters than the original 'Dick's bombshell' in the summer of 1962.[159] Much like when compulsory vaccination ended in 1948, the lack of public disquiet showed that the British government had formalised a paper decision that its people had already made de facto. Vaccination and revaccination rates continued to be low, even where uptake for immunisations against other diseases remained relatively robust. The decision also reflected Britain's willingness to act semi-independently from the rest of the world. In the 1960s and 1970s, many other nations, including those in the European Economic Community, continued to make vaccination compulsory for children, or at least heavily promoted it.[160] The United States and Canada had taken similar action to the British government, but these Anglophone countries were outliers. There was a certain privilege to this. Britain and North America had the luxury of weighing up relative risks in a way that, say, India or Somalia could not. The economic and medical maturity of their public health structures allowed their citizens to forego the risks of vaccination at precisely the time that the Eradication Programme was aggressively intervening in the lives of people living in poorer countries.[161] The protection of the British people no longer required its citizens to present themselves for vaccination – indeed, it no longer even required greater controls in Britain's ports. Instead, Britain was to be protected by fighting the sources of smallpox on other continents, rather than by insisting on prophylaxis at home.

Conclusion

Vaccination continued for at-risk groups, and the government maintained stockpiles of freeze-dried and liquid vaccine in case of emergency. This caused some logistical problems, notably the fact that these stores were held by a private company, Listers. Listers had financial troubles in the early 1970s and sold a million doses to Saudi Arabia. This led the government to reassess its storage policies, and highlighted that national British public health resources were not always in public hands.[162] The threat of smallpox faded further during the 1970s, however, and the decision to end routine vaccination was never challenged. Two outbreaks of smallpox resulting from laboratory accidents at the London

School of Hygiene and Tropical Medicine and the University of Birmingham caused scandals that led to the reappraisal of health and safety directives for infectious disease laboratories and the destruction of Britain's remaining *variola* samples.[163] Both incidents were quickly contained to a very few people, and the Birmingham case would turn out to be the world's last smallpox victim. Stores of vaccine thus became largely symbolic. There was a general fear of bioterrorism in the West during the Cold War, and later in the post-9/11 international climate.[164] Yet it was well known that it would be practically impossible to store enough vaccine and distribute it to the entire British population in the case of such an attack.[165] Much like providing mass vaccination in Bradford, calling for tighter port controls and maintaining routine childhood vaccination, being seen to prioritise public health was more important than the relative balance of epidemiological risks.

In the period after 1945, smallpox vaccination had been a tool to defend the British nation from foreign contagion. The nation – Britain – was imagined both as a body to be protected and as a member of an international community. Travellers and medical knowledge moved freely into and out of this nation, creating both opportunities and difficulties. The JCVI smallpox sub-committee noted that vaccination was a 'medical/social/political issue with international aspects and must be resolved in light of all such factors'.[166] Thus, protecting the British public health required a broad view of infectious disease: vaccination was just one tool to achieve this. The British people supported the premise of smallpox vaccination, but saw it as a prophylaxis and form of epidemic control to be used when the local area had become infected. Britain could become a smallpox area – but when it was not, it was difficult to press upon its citizens the need for routine primary vaccination and revaccination. Instead, the government was implored to protect its people by ensuring that ports were properly patrolled, foreign travellers and countries were "disinfected" and, in the rare instances where this failed, to provide vaccination to any Briton who demanded it. The challenge for public health authorities was to placate these demands while stressing that epidemiological evidence might suggest a different weighting of priorities.

Indeed, demand for vaccination would put other stresses on the British government in the 1950s. The next chapter will show how these issues of national protection were stretched by periods of apathy and demand with regard to the new poliomyelitis vaccine. Britain's place within global public health and the international pharmaceutical industry would play a major role in shaping, to borrow from George Dick, 'paper' and 'de facto' policy towards the disease.[167] Unlike with smallpox, the government was able to encourage young adults and parents to have themselves and their children vaccinated – however, it was not an easy process.

Notes

1 The national policy of routine immunisation of school children with BCG against tuberculosis ended in 2005 on the grounds of cost-effectiveness (although some local authorities had made this decision much sooner). This was provided to those between the ages of 10 and 14, whereas primary smallpox vaccination was typically and routinely performed in children in their first or second years of life. See Pat Hagan, 'Routine vaccination for tuberculosis ends in UK', *British Medical Journal*, 331:7509 (2005), 128; Paul Fine, 'Stopping routine vaccination for tuberculosis in schools', *British Medical Journal*, 331:7518 (2005), 647–8.
2 Sarah Rafferty, Matthew R. Smallman-Raynor and Andrew D. Cliff, 'Variola minor in England and Wales: the geographical course of a smallpox epidemic and the impediments to effective disease control, 1920–1935', *Journal of Historical Geography*, 59 (2018), 2–14.
3 Janet Newman and John Clarke, *Publics, Politics and Power: Remaking the Public in Public Services* (London: Sage, 2009), pp. 13–15.
4 David Armstrong, *Political Anatomy of the Body: Medical Knowledge in Britain in the Twentieth Century* (Cambridge: Cambridge University Press, 1983); Dorothy Porter, *Health, Civilization and the State: A History of Public Health from Ancient to Modern Times* (London: Routledge, 1999).
5 Roberta Bivins, '"The people have no more love left for the Commonwealth": Media, migration and identity in the 1961–62 British smallpox outbreak', *Immigrants & Minorities*, 25:3 (2007), 263–89; Roberta Bivins, *Contagious Communities: Medicine, Migration, and the NHS in Post-War Britain* (Oxford: Oxford University Press, 2015).
6 Bivins, '"The people have no more love left"' and Bivins, *Contagious Communities*.
7 On these topics, see Barbara Bush, 'Colonial research and the social sciences at the end of empire: The West Indian Social Survey, 1944–57', *Journal of Imperial & Commonwealth History*, 41:3 (2013), 451–74; Jessica

Pearson, 'French colonialism and the battle against the WHO Regional Office for Africa', *Hygiea Internationalis: An Interdisciplinary Journal for the History of Public Health*, 13:1 (2016), 65–80; James A. Gillespie, 'International organizations and the problem of child health, 1945–1960', *Dynamis*, 23 (2003), 115–42.

8 Frank Fenner, Donald A. Henderson, Isao Arita, Jezek Zdenek, Ivan Danilovich Ladnyi and World Health Organization, *Smallpox and its Eradication* (Geneva: World Health Organization, 1988). When discounting the 138 cases of variola minor in 1952/53, the death rate of indigenous cases in England and Wales was 20.5 per cent. See Table 2.1.

9 There were 1 case in 1937, 101 in 1942 (including 25 deaths) and 19 in 1950 (6 deaths). TNA: MH 55/1836, Ian Sutherland [Department of Health for Scotland] to W. H. Bradley [Ministry of Health], 8 December 1961.

10 G. W. A. Dick, 'Prevention of virus diseases in the community', *British Medical Journal*, 2:5315 (1962), 1275–80; C. W. Dixon, *Smallpox* (London: J. & A. Churchill, 1962); Bivins, '"The people have no more love left for the Commonwealth".'

11 Nadja Durbach, *Bodily Matters: The Anti-Vaccination Movement in England, 1853–1907* (Durham, NC: Duke University Press, 2005); Rafferty, Smallman-Raynor and Cliff, 'Variola minor in England and Wales'.

12 After 1962, evidence on adverse reactions led SMAC to change its recommendation to vaccinate children between the ages of 1 and 2. TNA: MH 154/62, CHSC(VI)(S)(63)2, Note by Ministry of Health – Routine Vaccination, 1963.

13 Fenner et al, *Smallpox and its Eradication*.

14 James G. Hanley, 'The public's reaction to public health: Petitions submitted to Parliament, 1847–1848', *Social History of Medicine*, 15:3 (2002), 393–411.

15 Durbach, *Bodily Matters*.

16 James Colgrove, *State of Immunity: The Politics of Vaccination in Twentieth-century America* (Berkeley: University of California Press, 2006); Jane Lewis, 'The prevention of diphtheria in Canada and Britain 1914–1945', *Journal of Social History*, 20:1 (1986), 163–76.

17 TNA: MH 55/902, Extract from Circular 66/47, 3 April 1947.

18 On the role of scientific evidence in decision making on vaccines see Lewis, 'The prevention of diphtheria'; Linda Bryder, '"We shall not find salvation in inoculation": BCG vaccination in Scandinavia, Britain and the USA, 1921–1960', *Social Science & Medicine*, 49:9 (1999), 1157–67; Jeffrey P. Baker, 'The pertussis vaccine controversy in Great Britain, 1974–1986', *Vaccine*, 21:25–26 (2003), 4003–10; Jennifer Stanton,

'What shapes vaccine policy? The case of hepatitis B in the UK', *Social History of Medicine*, 7:3 (1994), 427–46.
19 Fenner et al, *Smallpox and its Eradication*; Dixon, *Smallpox*; Dick, 'Prevention of virus diseases in the community'.
20 TNA: MH 55/2515, Ministry of Health, Memorandum on Vaccination against Smallpox, 1956; Ministry of Health, Memorandum on Vaccination against Smallpox, 1962.
21 S. M. Fraser, 'Leicester and smallpox: the Leicester Method', *Medical History*, 24:3 (1980), 315–32.
22 Infants were defined as children in their first year of life. TNA: MH 134/156, Immunisation and Vaccination Statistics as at 31 December 1961.
23 See the explanation of people's behaviour in John Douglas and William Edgar, 'Smallpox in Bradford, 1962', *British Medical Journal*, 1:5278 (1962), 612–14. On common sense, see Gareth Millward, '"A matter of commonsense": The Coventry poliomyelitis epidemic 1957 and the British public', *Contemporary British History* 31:3 (2017), 384–406.
24 TNA: MH 154/62, Smallpox Vaccination Group – Routine Smallpox Vaccination, March 1963; MH 55/902, Extract of 'Smallpox Immunisation' by E. T. Conybeare from 'The Practitioner', September 1951.
25 G. Matthew Fyfe and J. B. Fleming, 'Encephalomyelitis after vaccination in Fife', *British Medical Journal*, 2:4325 (1943), 671–4.
26 Richard Allen's wife is only ever referred to as 'Mrs Allen'. TNA: MH 55/1828, Montague Travers Morgan [MOH, Port of London], Smallpox – S.S. 'Mooltan'. Peninsular & Oriental Steam Navigation Co., 20 April 1949; Montagu Travers Morgan, *Annual Report of the Medical Officer of Health to 31st December, 1949* (London: Port of London Health Authority, 1950).
27 TNA: MH 55/1828, P. G. Stock to Melville Mackenzie, Smallpox S.S. Mooltan, 3 May 1949. See also correspondence in TNA: MH 55/1829.
28 Krista Maglen, '"The first line of defence": British quarantine and the port sanitary authorities in the nineteenth century', *Social History of Medicine*, 15:3 (2002), 413–28; Bivins, *Contagious Communities*.
29 HC Deb (5 May 1949), vol. 464, col. 1202.
30 *Ibid.*
31 HC Deb (19 May 1949), vol. 465, col. 608.
32 HC Deb (26 May 1949), vol. 465, cc. 1431–3.
33 See TNA: MH 55/1830, Ministry of Health memorandum, 25 May 1949; TNA: MH 55/1829, N. M. Brilliant to J. A. Marriott, 2 May 1949; N. M. Brilliant to Sandown-Shanklin Urban District Council, 10 May 1949.

34 'Quest for vaccination', *The Times* (10 May 1949), p. 4. It is likely that the disease escaped from the nearby isolation hospital. TNA: MH 55/1829, Unexplained Smallpox in the vicinity of Smallpox Hospitals, May 1949.
35 TNA: MH 55/1828, P. G. Stock to Melville Mackenzie, Smallpox S.S. Mooltan, 3 May 1949.
36 Morgan, *Report, 1949*, p. 17.
37 TNA: MH 55/1829, Stuart Laidlaw to M. T. Morgan, 11 April 1949; 'Smallpox case in train', *Daily Telegraph* (12 April 1949), p. 1; '3 more cases of smallpox from liner', *Daily Telegraph* (20 April 1949), 1.
38 TNA: MH 55/1828, G. O. Teichmann to Dr Thompson, 12 April 1949.
39 TNA: MH 55/1828, Meeting at Ministry of Health on 14 April 1949, to discuss disinfection of ships after smallpox.
40 David Arnold, *Colonizing the Body: State Medicine and Epidemic Disease in Nineteenth-century India* (Berkeley: University of California Press, 1993), esp. pp. 116–58.
41 See discussion of 1961/62 in this chapter. On how events become crises, see Mark Drakeford and Ian Butler, *Scandal, Social Policy and Social Welfare*, 2nd edn (Bristol: Policy Press, 2006).
42 See correspondence in TNA: MH 55/1829.
43 Laboratory tests were subsequently negative for smallpox, but not after the case had made the news. TNA: 55/1829, D. A. Dowling, Chief Medical Officer, Australia House to Ministry of Health, 6 October 1949. On typhoid see Morgan, *Report, 1949*.
44 HC Deb (20 April 1950), vol. 474, cc. 311–12; Anon, 'Epidemiology section', *British Medical Journal*, 1:4658 (1950), 914–15.
45 Tim Carter and Stephen E. Roberts, 'Infectious disease mortality in British merchant seamen and Lascars since 1900: From causes to controls', *International Journal of Maritime History*, 29:4 (2017), 788–815.
46 Anon, 'Epidemiology section'. Nineteen was the revised figure after corrections. MH 55/1836, Ian Sutherland [Department of Health for Scotland] to W. H. Bradley [Ministry of Health], 8 December 1961.
47 'Check on dead doctor's diary to stop smallpox scare', *Daily Mirror*, 3 April 1950, p. 12.
48 TNA: MH 55/902, W. M. Ballantine to Sendall, 15 July 1948.
49 Fyfe and Fleming, 'Encephalomyelitis after vaccination in Fife'.
50 TNA: MH 55/902, W. M. Ballantine to Sendall, 15 July 1948.
51 TNA: MH 55/902, Fife-Clark to W. M. Ballantine, 30 July 1948.
52 'Rush for vaccination', *Scotsman*, 3 April 1950, p. 5.
53 'Fewer vaccinations', *Scotsman*, 14 April 1950, p. 5; 'Smallpox inquiry', *Scotsman*, 25 April 1950, p. 4.

Smallpox 107

54 'Moosa Ali says "sorry about the epidemic"', *Daily Mail*, 20 April 1950, p. 1.
55 'Smallpox city warning', *Daily Express*, 4 April 1950, p. 1; 'New York puts up smallpox barrier as nurse brings death toll to 3', *Daily Mirror*, 8 April 1950, p. 12.
56 'Scotland free from smallpox', *Scotsman*, 28 April 1950, p. 5.
57 HC Deb (20 April 1950), vol. 474, cc. 38–9W. See also MH 55/1836, H.M.(56)79, National Health Service – Hospital Provision for Smallpox, 5 September 1956.
58 HL Deb (19 April 1950) vol. 166, cc. 967–9.
59 *Ibid.*
60 HC Deb (25 April 1950), vol. 474, col. 758.
61 TNA: MH 55/902, Personal approach to Parents on Vaccination and Immunisation, 1953.
62 TNA: MH 55/902, Extract of 'Smallpox Immunisation' by E. T. Conybeare from 'The Practitioner', September 1951; Leonard W. Faulkner [Sheffield Hospital Board] to S. A. Heald, 30 September 1954.
63 See TNA: MH 55/1719; TNA: MH 154/636; TNA: 55/1721; TNA: MH 55/1926; TNA: MH 55/2424.
64 Viant tabled large numbers of written questions on vaccination and immunisation over his career, but some typical examples include: HC Deb (3 May 1950), vol. 474, cc. 206W; HC Deb (7 May 1952), vol. 500, cc. 44–5W; HC Deb (7 July 1955), vol. 543, col. 120W.
65 TNA: MH 55/902, S. A. Heald to Pilditch, 8 July 1953.
66 TNA: MH 55/902, C. B. McArthur [MOH Oswestry] to Ministry of Health, 18 October 1954.
67 TNA: MH 55/902, H. F. Harris, Public Health Nursing Officer, Essex, 6 November 1954.
68 Ministry of Health, *Report of the Ministry of Health for the Year Ended 31st December, 1954. Part II on the State of the Public Health, being the Report of the Chief Medical Officer for the Year 1954* (Cmd 9627) (London: HMSO, 1955), pp. 2–3.
69 TNA: MH 55/902, Circular 6/55 – Vaccination against Smallpox, 6 April 1955.
70 TNA: MH 55/902, Ministry of Health to All Local Health Authorities (England), 9 July 1956.
71 TNA: MH 55/902, Department of Health for Scotland and Scottish Council for Health Education, 'Keep Your Baby Safe', c. 1951.
72 TNA: MH 55/902, Ministry of Health poster, 1955.
73 TNA: MH 55/902, Personal Approach to Parents on Vaccination and Immunisation, undated, almost certainly summer 1953. See also the campaigns against diphtheria in Chapter 1.

74 See Chapters 1 and 3.
75 TNA: MH 55/902, W. M. Ballantine to Ministry of Health, 30 March 1950.
76 Philip Taylor, *The Projection of Britain: British Overseas Publicity and Propaganda 1919–1939* (Cambridge: Cambridge University Press, 2008).
77 Elizabeth LeBas, ' "When every street became a cinema": The film work of Bermondsey Borough Council's Public Health Department, 1923–1953', *History Workshop Journal*, 39 (1995), 42–66. On the use of film as a historical source, see Kelly Loughlin, 'The history of health and medicine in contemporary Britain: Reflections on the role of audio-visual sources', *Social History of Medicine*, 13:1 (2000), 131–45.
78 See Patrick Russell and James Piers Taylor (eds), *Shadows of Progress: Documentary Film in Post-war Britain* (London: British Film Institute, 2010).
79 Ministry of Health, *Surprise Attack* (1951).
80 TNA: MH 55/902, Extract of 'Smallpox Immunisation' by E. T. Conybeare from 'The Practitioner', September 1951.
81 TNA: MH 55/902, Ministry of Health to All Local Health Authorities (England), 9 July 1956.
82 Linda Bryder, 'The King Edward VII Welsh National Memorial Association and its policy towards tuberculosis, 1910–48', *Welsh History Review* 13:2 (1986), 194–216; John Welshman, 'In search of the "problem family": Public health and social work in England and Wales 1940–70', *Social History of Medicine* 9:3 (1996), 447–65; Pat Thane, Melanie Oppenheimer and Nicholas Deakin (eds), *Voluntary Action in Britain since Beveridge* (Manchester: Manchester University Press, 2011).
83 TNA: MH 55/902, B. Crawter to S. A. Heald, 5 October 1954.
84 TNA: MH 55/902, B. Crawter to S. A. Heald, 9 October 1956.
85 TNA: MH 55/902, National Baby Welfare Council poster, c. 1956; Mother What's My Line, National Baby Welfare Council leaflet, c. 1956.
86 TNA: MH 55/902, S. A. Heald to E. Dunbar [Women's Voluntary Service], 25 July 1956.
87 A motion had passed at a recent Women's Institute national meeting. See correspondence in TNA: MH 55/902.
88 Catriona Beaumont, *Housewives and Citizens: Domesticity and the Women's Movement in England, 1928–64* (Manchester: Manchester University Press, 2013).
89 TNA: BD 25/104, Ministry of Health press release, History of Smallpox Outbreak of 1961–62, 24 July 1963.
90 TNA: MH 55/902, S. A. Heald to Assistant Secretary, British Medical Association, 22 February 1960.

91 For medical correspondence on the outbreak, see TNA: 96/1226.
92 Bivins, '"The people have no more love left for the Commonwealth"'; Bivins, *Contagious Communities*.
93 Anon, 'Smallpox in England', *British Medical Journal*, 1:5272 (1962), 164–5.
94 Bivins, *Contagious Communities*.
95 Bivins, '"The people have no more love left for the Commonwealth"'; Bivins, *Contagious Communities*, esp. pp. 115–67.
96 James Stewart, 'Smallpox1962 – an online archive of the outbreaks in Wales and England' (2012) www.smallpox1962.org.uk (accessed 5 April 2017).
97 See, for example, the British Medical Association's insistence on better border checks for foreign visitors. 'BMA criticism on smallpox', *Guardian* (19 January 1962), p. 1; Anon, 'Smallpox in England'.
98 Bivins, '"The people have no more love left for the Commonwealth"'; Bivins, *Contagious Communities*.
99 TNA: BD 25/104, Ministry of Health press release, History of Smallpox Outbreak of 1961–62, 26 July 1963.
100 Anon, 'Immunization ups and downs', *British Medical Journal*, 2:5299 (1962), 250.
101 TNA: BD 25/104, Ministry of Health press release, History of Smallpox Outbreak of 1961–62, 26 July 1963.
102 See R. M. Walters, letter to *The Times* (19 January 1962), p. 11; Alan F. Stewart, letter to *The Times* (20 January 1962), p. 9; 'Smallpox clamour attacked', *Guardian* (18 January 1962), p. 18.
103 Correspondence came from Halifax, Leeds and Huddersfield. TNA: MH 55/2509, Twohig to Dr Bradley, 15 January 1962; Memo to Bradley, 15 January 1962; Tele. Conversation with Leeds CB [County Borough], 16 January 1962.
104 TNA: MH 55/1836, Reprint of Ronald W. Elliott and Joseph Lyons, 'Smallpox 1962 – matters arising', *The Medical Officer*, 107 (1962): 355–61. See also public demand for vaccination in Leeds, Huddersfield, Coventry and other places: 'Rush dries up vaccine', *Daily Mail* (16 January 1962), p. 1; 'Don't panic says Ministry – but a city does panic over smallpox', *Daily Mail* (18 January 1962), p. 1.
105 Douglas and Edgar, 'Smallpox in Bradford, 1962'.
106 Morgan, *Report, 1949*; Bivins, '"The people have no more love left for the Commonwealth"', p. 135; TNA: MH 55/1835, Rochdale County Borough Variola Minor: Comment 8 March 1952; 'Rush for vaccination', *Scotsman* (3 April 1950), p. 5.
107 Bivins, '"The people have no more love left for the Commonwealth"'.

108 See Chapter 3 and the behaviour of certain groups during poliomyelitis epidemics in the 1950s.
109 Bivins, *Contagious Communities*, pp. 148–9.
110 'Unnecessarily exposed', *The Times*, 17 January 1962, p. 11; 'Three irate nurses', Maureen J. Squires, S. Day and A. V. Howell, letter to *The Times*, 20 January 1962, p. 9. M. Schar, 'Vaccination against smallpox', *British Medical Journal*, 1:5275 (February 1962), 403.
111 P. H. Birks, 'Vaccination against smallpox', *British Medical Journal*, 2:5300 (August 1962), 340.
112 TNA: BD 25/104, Ministry of Health press release, History of Smallpox Outbreak of 1961–62, 26 July 1963.
113 That is, no cases resulted from contact with a secondary case. Douglas and Edgar, 'Smallpox in Bradford, 1962'.
114 TNA: BD 25/104, Welsh Board of Health to the Ministry of Health, 24 August 1965. See also HC Deb (24 March 1965), vol. 709, cc. 104–5W.
115 On the role of the International Sanitary Regulations, see Bivins, '"The people have no more love left for the Commonwealth"'.
116 'Unnecessarily exposed', *The Times* (17 January 1962), p. 11; Bivins, *Contagious Communities*, pp. 137–9; Anon, 'Smallpox in England'.
117 Duncan Yuille and Rowland Rogerson, 'Vaccination against smallpox', *British Medical Journal*, 1:5275 (1962), 402.
118 'BMA seeks new smallpox plan', *Guardian* (26 July 1962); Hugh McLeave, 'BMA calls for "jabs" probe', *Daily Mail* (26 July 1962), p. 9.
119 D. S. Dane, G. W. A. Dick, J. H. Connolly, O. D. Fisher, Florence McKeown, Moya Briggs, Robert Nelson and Dermot Wilson, 'Vaccination against poliomyelitis with live virus vaccines', *British Medical Journal*, 1:5010 (1957), 59–74; G. W. A. Dick, 'Epidemiology of poliomyelitis', *British Medical Journal*, 1:5122 (1959), 618–19.
120 MH 55/1836, Ronald Elliott to George Godber, 17 July 1962.
121 Fenner et al, *Smallpox and its Eradication*.
122 Dick, 'Prevention of virus diseases in the community'.
123 Dixon, *Smallpox*, esp. pp. 326–60; C. W. Dixon, 'Vaccination against smallpox', *British Medical Journal*, 1:5287 (1962), 1262–6.
124 Anon, 'Annual meeting, Belfast: Scientific proceedings: Symposium: Virus diseases', *British Medical Journal*, 2:5300 (1962), 318–20. A more detailed precis of his argument was published in November: Dick, 'Prevention of virus diseases in the community'.
125 'B.M.A. await reply on vaccination', *The Times* (26 July 1962), p. 7. See also Douglas and Edgar, 'Smallpox in Bradford, 1962'.
126 TNA: 55/2510, S. A. Heald, Vaccination against smallpox policy, 26 July 1962; 'Smallpox vaccination plan for infants condemned', *Guardian* (25

July 1962), p. 16; 'End routine vaccination of babies for smallpox', *The Times* (25 July 1962), p. 6; Hugh McLeave, 'Stop the jabs!', *Daily Mail* (25 July 1962), p. 6.
127 S. E. Browne, 'Press reports on Belfast', *British Medical Journal*, 2:5300 (1962), 340; Colin Kaplan, 'Vaccination against smallpox', *British Medical Journal*, 2:5298 (1962), 189.
128 See David Cantor, 'Representing "the public": Medicine, charity and the public sphere in twentieth century Britain', in Steve Sturdy (ed.), *Medicine, Health and the Public Sphere in Britain: 1600–2000* (London: Routledge, 2002), pp. 145–68.
129 Major Greenwood, *Epidemics and Crowd Diseases*, quoted in Anon, 'Vaccination against smallpox', *British Medical Journal*, 2:5300 (1962), 311–12.
130 TNA: MH 55/2510, British Medical Association Report of the Infectious Diseases Subcommittee of the Public Health Committee on Certain Matters which had Arisen from the Recent Outbreaks of Smallpox in England and Wales, attached to letter dated 10 July 1962.
131 On professional and voluntary organisations' relationship with policy makers in the postwar period, see Sally Sheard, 'Quacks and clerks: Historical and contemporary perspectives on the structure and function of the British medical civil service', *Social Policy & Administration*, 44:2 (2010), 193–207; Matthew Hilton, Nick Crowson, Jean-François Mouhot and James McKay, *The Politics of Expertise: How NGOs Shaped Modern Britain* (Oxford: Oxford University Press, 2013).
132 TNA: MH 55/2510, Internal Ministry of Health memorandum, 22 August 1962. See also Chapter 3 for context on polio vaccination.
133 TNA: MH 55/2510, Meeting on 21 August to discuss BMA notes and report on recent outbreaks of smallpox.
134 TNA: MH 55/2510, S. A. Heald to Deputy Secretary, Ministry of Health, 26 July 1962.
135 TNA: MH 154/62, CHSC(VI)(S)(63)1, 20 March 1963.
136 Sheard, 'Quacks and clerks'.
137 Anon, 'Immunization ups and downs'.
138 TNA: MH 154/62, CHSC(VI)(S)(63)First Meeting, 9 April 1963.
139 TNA: MH 154/61, Professor J. Knowelden to Professor R. E. Tunbridge, 3 May 1963.
140 TNA: MH 154/61, Professor J. Knowelden to Professor R. E. Tunbridge, 3 May 1963.
141 TNA: MH 154/61, R. E. Tunbridge to W. N. Judd, 7 May 1963.
142 TNA: MH 154/61, CHSC(VI)(S)(63)First Meeting, 9 April 1963; CHSC(VI)(S)(63)Second Meeting, 8 July 1963.

143 MH: MH 154/62, G. W. A. Dick with David Dane, Smallpox Vaccination Policy, discussed at CHSC(VI)(S)(63)First Meeting, 9 April 1963.
144 Kaplan, 'Vaccination against smallpox'.
145 MH: MH 154/62, Dick with Dane, Smallpox Vaccination Policy.
146 TNA: MH 55/1836, Reprint of Ronald W. Elliott and Joseph Lyons, 'Smallpox 1962 – matters arising', *The Medical Officer*, 107 (8 June 1962): 355–61.
147 TNA: MH 154/62, Dr H. Josephs to George Godber, 9 January 1963; Geoffrey Barber to Ministry of Health, 16 August 1963.
148 Emphasis original. E. J. S. Bonnett, 'Vaccination against smallpox', *British Medical Journal*, 2:5305 (1962), 675. See also D. G. Barrowcliffe, 'Vaccination against smallpox', *British Medical Journal*, 2:5306 (1962), 734; R. A. L. Agnew, 'Vaccination against smallpox', *British Medical Journal*, 1:5276 (1962), 482.
149 TNA: MH 154/62, CHSC(VI)(63)9, Note by Secretary.
150 TNA: MH 154/61, J. Knowelden to R. E. Tunbridge, 3 May 1963. See also Ronald W. Elliott to W. N. Judd, 3 September 1963.
151 Dick, 'Prevention of virus diseases in the community'. Quoting G. S. Wilson, 'B.C.G. vaccination in control of tuberculosis', *British Medical Journal*, 2:4534 (1947), 855–9.
152 G. W. A. Dick, 'Routine smallpox vaccination', *British Medical Journal*, 3:5767 (1971), 163–6.
153 Fenner et al, *Smallpox and its Eradication*.
154 Bob H. Reinhardt, *The End of a Global Pox: America and the Eradication of Smallpox in the Cold War Era* (Chapel Hill: University of North Carolina Press, September 2015). See also TNA: MH 154/268, D. G. Evans [Lister] to George Godber, 2 June 1972.
155 MH: 154/268, 'Press release: Halt Called to Routine Vaccination Against Smallpox', 28 July 1971.
156 HC Deb (28 July 1971), vol. 822, col. 126W
157 TNA: MH 154/268, J. R. [name redacted] to Neville Sanderson MP, 5 August 1971.
158 Dick, 'Routine smallpox vaccination.'; Anon, 'For further debate.', *British Medical Journal*, 3:5767 (1971), 129.
159 On doubts, see F. J. G. Lishman, 'Smallpox vaccination', *British Medical Journal*, 3:5773 (1971), 534; Roy G. Condie, 'Smallpox vaccination', *British Medical Journal*, 3:5773 (1971), 534; S. Davies and W. H. Crichton, 'Smallpox vaccination', *British Medical Journal*, 3:5771 (1971), 430–1. On support for the decision, see Guy Bousfield, 'Smallpox vaccination', *British Medical Journal*, 3:5769 (1971), 302.

Smallpox 113

160 TNA: MH 154/268, DHSS to the Council of Europe (UK(72)25PA), 1972; MH 154/62, Vaccination against smallpox in Europe.
161 Reinhardt, *The End of a Global Pox*.
162 TNA: MH 154/268.
163 P. J. Cox, *Report of the Committee of Inquiry into the Smallpox Outbreak in London in March and April 1973* (Cmnd 5626) (London: HMSO, 1974); R. A. Shooter, *Report of the Investigation into the Cause of the 1978 Birmingham Smallpox Occurrence* (HC-668, 1979–80) (London: HMSO, 1980).
164 Reinhardt, *The End of a Global Pox*.
165 See debates in: TNA: MH 148/164; MH 154/270; EF 7/2998.
166 TNA: MH 154/62, CHSC(VI)(63)9, Note by Secretary.
167 MH: MH 154/62, G. W. A. Dick with David Dane, Smallpox Vaccination Policy, discussed at CHSC(VI)(S)(63)First Meeting, 9 April 1963.

3

Poliomyelitis

Indigenous smallpox had been eliminated from Britain in the 1930s, reducing its threat to the day-to-day lives of British people. The public had, however, come to fear a new disease which first reached epidemic proportions in 1947 – poliomyelitis. From that year onwards, regular outbreaks occurred during the "polio season" each summer. No cure was ever found. The only thing authorities could do was provide treatment for acute symptoms and continue research efforts into a preventative vaccine. By the end of the 1960s, the number of annual cases could be counted on one hand, but the vaccination programme that achieved this decline did not eliminate polio overnight; nor was it without significant financial and logistical difficulties.

This chapter focuses on the theme of demand. This was not unique to polio. As has been seen in previous chapters, the British public had come to demand health and other welfare protections from the government, particularly since the 1940s. There was active demand for emergency vaccination during smallpox epidemics. What set polio apart is that we see clear evidence of public demand for a coordinated routine immunisation campaign. In part, this was because of higher levels of anxiety about polio than about other diseases, but it was significant that the specific solution to this problem would be vaccination. The antidiphtheria, pertussis and smallpox programmes offered a template; and new vaccine technology made this possible. Initially this involved the mass polio vaccination of all children and priority groups. Later it would evolve into a programme for all young children as they became old enough to be eligible, and specific campaigns to vaccinate young adults to protect them from the disease.

It is clear from contemporary media coverage and internal government files that the British people wanted protection from polio. As in many Western countries, large charities solicited donations to polio research and care and there was extensive interest in the massive field trials of a new vaccine being developed in the United States in 1954 and 1955.[1] Even when the vaccine became available, many of these charities continued to provide aftercare and support for affected children and adults – and while the majority of publicity for vaccination would come from health authorities, the climate of concern around polio stimulated discussion and demand. Such was this demand that during the period from the introduction of the UK polio vaccine programme in 1956 to the switch to oral poliomyelitis vaccine in 1962, the government faced significant criticism for being unable to provide vaccine to all who wanted it, due to acute and chronic supply shortages. And yet the Ministry of Health also worried that certain sections of the public were too apathetic towards the new technology and needed to be convinced of the benefit both to themselves and to the wider population.

Demand appears in two main contexts throughout this chapter. First, it could be a statistical artefact – a measurement of how many people had requested polio vaccine. Demand could be measured through the registration system established in 1956 as well as the various requests from local health authorities for vaccine supplies when there were surges of requests in any given area. In these cases, demand could be compared with expected or actual supply; and, indeed, demand could be predicted based on past trends, advertising campaigns and the demographics of priority groups under the scheme. Here, demand could be interpreted as an administrative issue. When demand was too high, supplies had to be augmented through more orders for the vaccine from pharmaceutical companies. When demand was too low, either relative to the programme's goals or the amount of available vaccine, it was stimulated through local and national advertising efforts. This administrative balancing act occurred throughout the period, not always successfully, as this chapter will demonstrate. The second context of demand was more subjective. The public in general believed that the government ought to provide polio vaccination to its people. Universal polio vaccination was a symbol of a modern, rational state. Politically, therefore, the vaccination programme was created and expanded not entirely due to administrative or epidemiological measurement, but on what various branches of government believed would be popular with the wider public. Similarly, there was nothing inevitable about the negative political, media and public attention directed towards the various supply crises across the 1950s. Delays in vaccination represented wider concerns, particularly among the public, with governmental administration than simply the immediate benefits to direct beneficiaries.[2]

This chapter begins by outlining the development of the polio vaccine up to the mid-1950s. This was a result of international cooperation and charitable donations, resulting in one of the iconic scientific discoveries of the early Cold War era. However, a high-profile laboratory accident severely dented the reputation of this new technology. Traditionally cautious, British health authorities created their own version of the vaccine. After outlining this British variant and the difficulties it caused, the chapter explores the development of the poliomyelitis vaccine campaign. This was continually affected by supply problems. Partly, this was because of the demands placed on the system by the public. A greater problem was the inability to either produce or source enough vaccine, especially when there were surges in demand. Two incidents in particular are highlighted: an epidemic in Coventry in 1957; and the death of the professional footballer Jeff Hall in 1959. The chapter ends with the introduction of oral poliomyelitis vaccine and the end to these long-running supply issues.

As well as covering demand, the rhetoric around polio vaccine exposes other themes that we have already encountered in the 1950s and 1960s vaccination programmes. The general climate of demand was welcome, but the government was consistently worried about pockets of apathy shown by parents with regard to polio vaccine, and made significant attempts to convince the public to register themselves for the scheme. The public did not act in unison, much to the government's chagrin. Similarly, the nation is an integral part of understanding why the British government chose to prioritise British-made vaccine, even though it was more expensive and difficult to produce than its American equivalent, and even when the resulting supply shortages caused the government significant embarrassment.[3] With the polio vaccine programme finally established, however, the modern post-war vaccination schedule as we know it today had become firmly entrenched in British health care.

Poliomyelitis and the vaccine

While much has been written about polio, it is worth taking some time to explain the context for the new vaccine that became available in the 1950s. In particular, this context explains why parents had come to fear the disease – a subject which has received significant attention from historians.[4] Poliomyelitis is caused by poliovirus, of which there are three types.[5] It is spread through the gut, most commonly through traces of faecal matter entering the mouth. It is asymptomatic in around 70 per cent of infections, but can cause limb weakness or even paralysis in a minority.[6] Despite the higher death rate among infected adult patients, the crippling effects it could have on children gave polio the reputation as a childhood disease. Indeed, it was often called infantile paralysis, although by the post-war period poliomyelitis – or simply polio – became the preferred nomenclature.[7] Given how widespread natural poliovirus was in England and Wales, this led to an average annual case load of acute poliomyelitis of 524 for the five years to 1946, and 5,197 for the five years including and after the first widespread epidemic of 1947 (Figure 3.1). Although there is evidence to suggest that polio has infected humans for millennia, the first full-scale epidemics of the disease were not seen until the late nineteenth century, in American and Scandinavian cities. For this reason, it has been described as a 'virgin soil infection' by J. N. Hayes – one that was shocking to the public because of its apparent novelty and a lack of medical or lay experience with regard to its spread and control.[8] It appeared to affect rich and poor communities with the same force, unlike other infectious diseases such as tuberculosis. A cure has never been found, although a series of therapies were developed across the twentieth century to deal with the acute problems of paralysis and the chronic rehabilitation required to restore some function to affected parts of the body. The most iconic of these was the iron lung, both a symbol of modern medicine's ability to fight against death and a fearful reminder of the severity of the disease. The sight of crutches and callipers on survivors also represented the permanent impairment and disability left in the wake

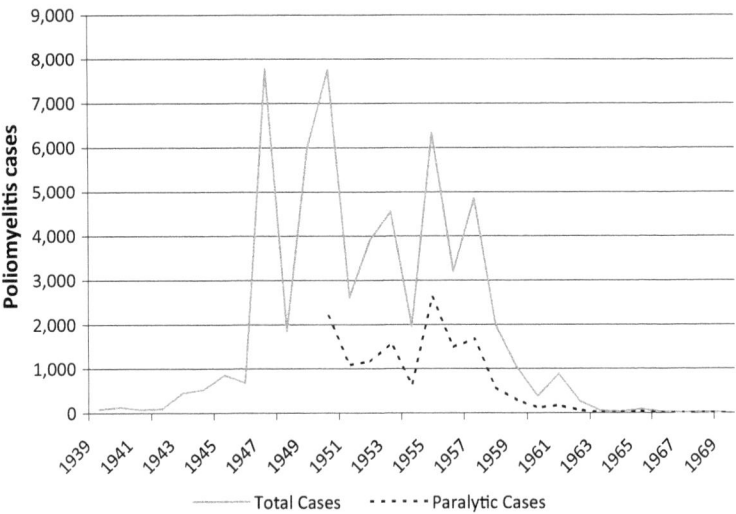

Figure 3.1 Poliomyelitis notifications, 1939–69. Paralytic cases separated from overall notifications from 1950 only.
Source: Public Health England, 'Notifiable diseases: historic annual totals', 28 November 2016. www.gov.uk/government/publications/notifiable-diseases-historic-annual-totals (accessed 5 May 2017).

of an outbreak.[9] The only defence against polio would therefore be prevention of infection, which was, paradoxically, more difficult in more economically developed nations. The prevailing hygiene thesis is that most children in countries with poor sanitation are exposed to poliovirus at an early enough stage that they retain some immunity from their mothers; most therefore develop mild or asymptomatic polio and lifelong immunity. In communities with fully functioning sewerage systems and a culture of handwashing, children and young adults are exposed much more infrequently, and so are more likely to develop a more acute version of the disease later in life. This can explain in part why cases became widespread enough that polio became a notifiable disease in the early twentieth century, although it does not fully account for why Britain was affected by epidemic polio much later than many other nations.[10]

Across the Western world during the early twentieth century a number of organisations were established to raise funds for research into polio and a potential cure. The most high-profile of these was the National Foundation for Infantile Paralysis, also known as the March of Dimes. Established by Franklin Roosevelt in the United States in the 1930s, it received millions of dollars from the American public and helped to fund the research which would produce the first commercially available vaccines. In the United Kingdom, where epidemic polio had begun much later than in the USA, the National Fund for Poliomyelitis Research was established in 1952.[11] When the US team led by Jonas Salk announced at a press conference in 1955 that it had successfully developed an inactivated poliomyelitis vaccine (IPV), the world's press and television attended. The US government licensed it for use within hours.[12] It was an archetypical example of the new, coordinated "big science" of the mid-twentieth century, reliant upon large budgets and teams of scientists and institutions focused on a single problem.[13] The polio vaccine trials were among the biggest medical experiments ever conducted, becoming a model of randomised controlled trials for researchers and pharmaceutical companies around the world.[14]

The Ministry of Health knew that the Salk announcement would stimulate interest in Parliament and in the media. Newspapers had covered the trials as they were being conducted, and regularly reported from international conferences on polio and immunisation.[15] The National Fund for Poliomyelitis Research had contacted all the major news outlets to direct their attention to Salk's results (and to publicise its own work), and the MRC was within a fortnight of being able to release its own data.[16] In the House of Commons, Minister of Health Iain Macleod took a series of questions on the announcement and pledged to move as quickly as possible to bring IPV to the British public, subject to proper testing.[17]

British IPV

Despite this positive publicity, the American IPV programme suffered a major setback almost as soon as it had begun. A batch of the vaccine from the Cutter Laboratories had not been inactivated properly, leading 120,000 children to be injected with live poliovirus.

Subsequently, 260 cases developed, of which ten were fatal.[18] While this caused governments across the world to reassess their commitment to IPV, the British were particularly cautious.[19] Authorities in the United Kingdom had historically been risk averse toward new vaccines, often insisting on a higher burden of proof for their safety than other high-income nations did – most notably in the cases of BCG and anti-diphtheria immunisation.[20] The MRC was keen to ensure that any vaccine used in Britain was as safe and effective as possible. Trials using the Salk vaccine were suspended, and the MRC sent a delegation to the United States to ascertain what had occurred.[21] Through the course of its research and new trials, the MRC recommended that a British vaccine should replace the Mahoney type-I strain of poliovirus in the American vaccine with a less virulent strain; this not only would reduce the risk of another Cutter incident, but would also be more effective in conferring immunity.[22] The MRC was confident that, when combined with the longer and more rigorous testing period demanded by British authorities, the United Kingdom's IPV would be safer and more potent than the American Salk. It advised the government not to use Salk vaccine at all in Britain.[23] The Ministry of Health and the Scottish Office established an advisory body, the Joint Committee on Poliomyelitis Vaccine (JCPV), to guide British health departments on the medical and administrative issues surrounding vaccination.[24] After securing assurances that Glaxo and Burroughs Wellcome would produce the vaccine, on 19 January 1956 Robin Turton (the Minister of Health) announced to a large press conference that children under the age of ten would be eligible for polio vaccination. Parents would register their children, and local authorities would distribute the vaccine as supplies became available.[25] Initially, children were to receive two doses of IPV by injection, but this was extended to three doses in 1958.[26]

The speed at which the scheme was initiated indicated that the Conservative government thought polio vaccination would be a popular move.

> There is something peculiarly distressing about poliomyelitis ... Not only does it kill especially the young, but of those who survive 10 per cent remain severely paralysed and a further 20 per cent retain throughout their lives a degree of paralysis. [Turton] was confident that every father and mother would wish God's speed [sic] to the new plan.[27]

Yet the way in which the scheme was initiated caused a number of problems which had long-standing consequences that would not be fully resolved until the following decade. First, the use of local authorities under Section 26 of the National Health Service Acts meant that administration of the scheme was carried out by councils and MOHs. This caused great variation in the registration and uptake rates for vaccination across the country, as MOHs had different priorities and capacities within their local authorities (as was seen earlier with diphtheria and smallpox immunisation). In two cases, local scepticism even saw local authorities opt out of the scheme altogether. The health committee and MOH of Burton-on-Trent, Staffordshire believed that the national programme was in effect a giant experiment. They also objected to central government guidelines and control. Initially, therefore, the council refused IPV, arguing that more proof was needed that it was safe and effective.[28] By April, Burton had reversed its decision under pressure from pro-vaccine parents. It was considered wrong to deny parents the opportunity to consent to vaccination if they were informed and wanted to take the risk. Moreover, as the Deputy Mayor asked, 'has Burton the right to tell the rest of Britain they do not know what they are doing?'[29] In Wakefield, West Yorkshire the council held out even longer, although by the end of 1957 it had agreed to administer the scheme. Here, the local MOH believed that natural immunity against polio was high in the town, owing to its poor levels of sanitation. Besides, even if polio vaccination could help Wakefield, the MOH argued that the government's approach was inadequate. The council also remained critical, proposing that the scheme should not be implemented until every child could be guaranteed a third dose (as was the norm in the United States).[30] In each of these cases, there was demand for protection from polio. Neither Burton nor Wakefield appeared to be anti-vaccine, or even anti-IPV, in principle. Rather, their concerns stemmed from the administrative arrangements and evidence base around the vaccination programme during the early months of its operation.

The second – and more politically sensitive issue – was that of supply. In changing the formula of the vaccine from American to British IPV, pharmaceutical companies were unable to produce large quantities of the vaccine in time for the beginning of the programme. Burroughs Wellcome had significant delays getting its plant online and so, for long periods of 1956 and 1957 Glaxo was the sole producer.[31] Moreover, in response to the Cutter incident and to maintain public confidence in the safety and potency of British IPV the government had mandated that each batch had to be analysed by the MRC before it could be used on the population. This procedure took around three months. Due to limited laboratory capacity, one batch had to complete the entire testing process before testing could begin on another. Thus, the British IPV supply was released to the public through a narrow "pipeline", with several stages along the process limiting how quickly it could be made available.[32] All this was complicated further by the suspension of vaccination during the polio season.[33] The diphtheria immunisation campaign had also been suspended in the summer months, as there was a suggestion that injections could exacerbate paralysis in the limbs of patients who were subsequently infected with poliovirus.[34] The restriction on vaccinating during summer months was subsequently lifted following re-examination of the medical evidence, but, even so, it was difficult for British firms to produce IPV promptly enough to meet demand.[35]

To manage these stresses, the Ministry initiated a registration scheme. Parents would sign their children onto a register with the local authority, which would then distribute IPV as it became available. This started with two priority groups: children aged 12 months to 4 years; and those aged 5 to 9 years. Initially, the plan had been to vaccinate everyone in this cohort, but the supply problems meant that the government and MRC used this as an opportunity to compare the effectiveness of the vaccine in younger and older children by prioritising children born in specific months.[36] This had been one of Burton's objections – that central government would dictate who received the vaccine rather than allowing local authorities to exercise their discretion. The registration scheme was unlike for other vaccines, where parents could present their children to the clinic and have the procedure done. Nevertheless, it created a framework which could be extended to other cohorts as new vaccine became available and as the backlog of patients was cleared. Each year, children over the age of 6 months were added to the scheme. Further, children up to the age of 14 became eligible in 1957; young adults up to the age of 26 in 1958; and older adults up to the age of 40 in 1960.[37]

The Ministry had warned local authorities that 'disappointment may be inevitable', and the registration system would provide for only a proportion of the children whose parents demanded it in the first year.[38] Before the programme even began senior civil servant Dame Enid Russell-Smith warned that 'there may be a considerable danger that parents may react adversely' or become 'intensely emotional' to 'a method smacking of the village raffle applied to something which might be so important for their children'.[39] Even so, the degree and nature of supply shortages was an embarrassment. Glaxo continued to have production difficulties, caused by the technical nature of vaccine production and a shortage of available monkeys for testing.[40] When a vial of vaccine changed colour in early 1957, possibly because of bacterial contamination caused by improper storage during transit, the entire batch had to be withdrawn, causing significant delays.[41] An editorial in *The Times* summed up the mood:

> The frustrating series of official announcements can give rise to nothing but concern ... What should be made abundantly clear is that these delays are in no way the fault of the MRC or [Glaxo]. ... What seems to have happened is that the Minister took a gamble and announced the probable date on which vaccine might be ready, knowing full well that no one could give any guarantee.[42]

The *British Medical Journal* also admonished the Minister for his press conference in the "American" style, which seemed more about gaining political capital than good public health policy.[43] The Ministry had been advised against the press conference because the media were 'extremely sensitive on the subject of poliomyelitis and have been inclined to treat it sensationally'. The programme should have been 'presented in a sensible and unemotional manner', lest it 'evoke embarrassing reactions from the millions of parents who will be involved'.[44]

Many of these problems were of the government's own making. The choice to use British IPV exclusively placed the programme in a vulnerable position. Production was complex, reliant upon new technologies and expertise that were difficult to procure. Glaxo continued to negotiate with the Ministry of Health on the price and quantity of vaccine which it could supply.[45] Manufacturers were also well aware that the profit-making window for the technology was likely to be small. There was a large market in the short term, as the government planned to vaccinate every child and young adult in the country; but unless suppliers were allowed to export their stock, the demand for vaccine in

Britain would eventually dwindle to the annual birth rate. Manufacturers were therefore reluctant to invest massive amounts of capital into producing the vaccine unless the Treasury was willing to compensate them for inevitable future losses. Of the vaccine that they did produce, the government was also keen to allow British companies to export a proportion of it to other nations. It especially wanted British IPV to be used in the Commonwealth, as it would raise the profile of the pharmaceutical industry and ensure that the economy as a whole remained a global player in these new technologies of the Cold War (and, very shortly, post-Suez) world.[46] If it did not, there was a danger that American companies would gain a monopoly.[47] The British political classes were already anxious about Britain's status as a fading power, with science and technology a potent symbol of this decline in the nuclear age. While the Soviet Union launched Sputnik, Britain had no space programme to speak of.[48] The pharmaceutical industry was one area where Britain might be able to compete.

Not all of the limited British supplies therefore went to the "front line", and because of the economic and political incentives to buy British, the government refused to import the American Salk vaccine at all for its programme in 1956, even when there were major shortages.[49] While the insistence on British supplies was defensible on medical grounds, the government had committed to a programme that required far more vaccine than it could realistically produce. That the government would persist with the press conference and the introduction of the programme, despite the warnings from its medical civil service and other commentators, is indicative of the perceived demand from the electorate for vaccination. Polio vaccine was emblematic of modern, technical and scientific medicine. The potential conquest of polio was heralded by commentators and the public as one of the great achievements of the modern world.[50] For any advanced nation that wanted to do so, the risk of polio could now be managed.[51] Seeing itself as an advanced nation, Britain wanted the vaccine. The Conservative government had made pledges to fund polio research in its 1955 manifesto.[52] The specific timing of the polio programme was born of pre-emptive demand on the part of the party-political side of the government. But it also reflected years of research and preparation by staff within the Ministry of Health and co-opted advisory groups such as the MRC. Private industry in the form of Glaxo and Burroughs Wellcome was also part of this process, to say nothing of the coverage afforded to the topic in the press. The issue was that in attempting to placate a potential or inferred demand for polio vaccination in the short term, the government had committed itself to a course of action that it was not yet materially prepared for.

American IPV and the Coventry polio epidemic

These difficulties were exposed further in the summer of 1957 in the wake of a polio epidemic in Coventry, Warwickshire.[53] The city's MOH, Thomas Morris Clayton, had requested extra supplies of vaccine to help deal with the epidemic and clear the backlog of registrations that had built up in the city.[54] The Ministry of Health refused. There was no stockpile of IPV (since there was still a waiting list), so IPV was distributed batch by batch as soon as it passed MRC testing. John Vaughan-Morgan, the acting Minister of Health, explained that each local authority would continue to receive a percentage of new batches of vaccine, as they became available, relative to the number of people in each district who had registered for the programme. The decision to continue vaccination over the summer months from 1957 onwards meant that this would (theoretically) allow all authorities to provide for those still waiting to be vaccinated; for the Ministry, it was more important to keep the national programme intact. The MRC was still in the process of collecting statistics to evaluate the potency of IPV, and the government was mindful of the political disaster that could follow the redirection of supplies from an area that subsequently developed an epidemic.[55] For the people of Coventry, however, vaccination appeared to be a common-sense solution to an epidemic of infectious disease. Just as towns had seen queues outside doctors' surgeries for smallpox vaccine during local outbreaks, it seemed logical that the newly discovered IPV could provide a similar public health function. The cause was taken up by the media-savvy Member of Parliament for Coventry North, Maurice Edelman. He telephoned the Ministry to ask for more supplies of the vaccine, and told the press that the government was about to send more vaccine to Coventry, constituting a policy U-turn.[56] Internal documents suggest that Edelman was, at best, mistaken, possibly as the result of a miscommunication about the timing of the next batch of vaccine. (Coventry was about to receive a new delivery of vaccine, but not over and above what it would ordinarily have received as part of its quota.)[57] When the Ministry clarified its position the following Monday morning, it appeared as if government policy was muddled and inconsistent. Over the following weeks, Vaughan-Morgan and Clayton both explained to the people of Coventry and the rest of the country that IPV was not a useful prophylactic in a mass vaccination campaign. It took six weeks to confer immunity, meaning it could provide lasting protection for individuals and communities only as part of a routine vaccination programme, established before epidemic polio reached a particular location.[58] The local press continued to ask for more help, arguing that even with a six-week delay it could help the city by the end of the summer if supplies were available immediately; however, the national press appeared to broadly accept the Ministry's arguments with regard to domestic IPV supplies.[59]

Public demand for the vaccine in Coventry may not have been entirely compatible with epidemiological knowledge or public health professionals' experience with IPV, but it was entirely consistent with the process for immunisations against other diseases. As seen in the previous two chapters, clinics were opened when there were local outbreaks of smallpox and diphtheria, as those vaccines worked relatively quickly and could act both as a long-term preventative and as a short-term prophylactic. In Coventry, the local and national media stopped demanding IPV to help end the current epidemic. Public responses through the newspapers appeared to show that the general population also bowed to medical expertise, demonstrating an understanding that IPV was a technology unlike smallpox or diphtheria immunisation.[60] What the public found less explicable or excusable was why, eighteen months after Turton's announcement, British IPV manufacturing capacity continued to lag behind demand. Coventry's registration rate was reasonably high – around 40 per cent as compared to the national average for England and Wales of 29 per cent. Scotland's registration rate was slightly higher, at 42 per cent, but even so this represented a fraction of the eligible population that were entitled to vaccination.[61] Coventronians' other major demand was therefore much more difficult to rebuff: why did the government not import extra supplies from other countries to clear its backlog and provide a more comprehensive service?[62] Two years had passed since the Cutter incident. The cause of that disaster had been found, and millions of doses of the Salk vaccine had been administered across the world without incident. When Coventry was presented with offers from Denmark, France and the United States to use foreign-made vaccine, these were rejected in no uncertain terms by the Ministry of Health.[63] Nevertheless, chronic shortages were beginning to take their toll, and the government became concerned that the entire programme was at risk of losing public confidence if it could not deal with the demands being placed upon it.

Up to this point, MRC guidance had forbidden imports of Salk-formula vaccine, protecting British IPV and the pharmaceutical companies that supplied it. The relationship between the pharmaceutical companies and the public sector had been a key part of the vaccination programme. Burroughs Wellcome had supplied many of the diphtheria and pertussis vaccines during the 1940s and 1950s, for example.[64] Stuart Blume argues that these relationships were mutually beneficial, key to ensuring innovation and supply.[65] The British government was still keen to maintain the good will and financial stability of a useful resource, but circumstances had overtaken it. Given that British capacity had not improved as quickly as had originally been hoped, the Ministry of Health went back to the JCPV and MRC to ask them to re-examine the question of importation.[66] The MRC continued to favour British IPV where at all possible, since it was still the safest and most potent version available. Yet it was unwilling to make political decisions on behalf of the government. Concerned that the Ministry was simply passing responsibility onto its shoulders, the MRC carefully worded its advice so that it would be ministers that made the final decision on how to proceed. The scientific evidence still favoured the British vaccine; but the MRC changed its guidance so that it no longer objected to American imports, provided that these were used only to augment supplies. It would be up to ministers to decide how much to buy, when, and how to use it. This protected the interests of British manufacturers, as their vaccine would form the backbone of the programme and continuing contracts from central government would be guaranteed; but it also meant that if there were problems in the supply chain the stock could be supplemented by foreign imports. As a caveat, the MRC also recommended that parents be informed if they were to be offered the Salk vaccine.[67] Although both types of vaccine were considered to be potent and safe enough for use on the British public, the MRC continued to assert that the British one was still the superior product.

Provided that parents were informed and willing to take the risk, their children could either be vaccinated immediately or remain on the waiting list until British IPV became available.

As in 1956, the government's immediate problem was that demand had outstripped supply. In that instance, overall registration rates had been higher than the amount of IPV that could be produced, leading to delays of service. The summer of 1957 presented a new challenge: how to deal with the surges in demand created by the immediate fear of polio infection. A vaccination programme based on registration and a gradual rollout was unable to coexist with a public who responded to epidemics by presenting themselves to health authorities to be immunised, following established precedent. Similarly, registration gave the government a more concrete measure of how much IPV it was likely to need. And on this basis, the demand for polio vaccine was actually too low. The *Manchester Guardian* noted that the public needed to take some responsibility for the acute shortages, given how reluctant they had been to register for the scheme during the previous year. Only with a localised epidemic and the subsequent criticism in the national press did parents appear to present their children for the procedure. The *Manchester Guardian* used the metaphor of blowing 'hot and cold' on the subject.[68] Meanwhile the *British Medical Journal* believed that the health authorities and the medical profession had not done enough to explain the benefits of vaccination to the public, resulting in extremes of reaction that had little basis in epidemiology.[69] It was thus the swings in demand that had created political embarrassment and medical anxieties during 1957. The government's attempt to equalise demand across the financial year to prevent surges, through the use of the registration system, had been upset by events out of its control.

Giving parents the choice of whether to take British IPV or the American Salk vaccine had the result of complicating demand. From an administrative point of view, the general demand could still be measured, and there is little evidence that many parents in practice opted *en masse* to boycott the Salk vaccine. The more subjective side of demand is more difficult to analyse. Clearly, the disquiet over the supply shortage showed that people were upset that they were not able to access the vaccine. But were they demanding British IPV, or simply any form of polio vaccine? Did the surges in demand perhaps suggest that the public looked to the government to protection from a threatening disease and were willing to accept anything that they believed would help? The speed at which the demand for IPV as a form of epidemic control dissipated in the wake of medical evidence supports the view that the public were broadly willing to accept expert opinion and that their demands were driven by other understandings of disease. In any case, it seems that, as with diphtheria and smallpox, the British public broadly accepted that vaccinations were a useful form of disease control. However, the government was unable to control the outside events that triggered people to apply this understanding to a concrete action of registering and presenting their children for vaccination.

Young adults and IPV: the death of Jeff Hall

The ability to import vaccine from the USA took some stress out of the system, but supply problems continued to occur. Registration rates across 1957 increased more quickly than the Ministry had anticipated. In February, the Cabinet Home Affairs Committee discussed suspending the national advertising campaign. Any more increases in registrations would be pointless, given that there would not be enough vaccine to meet the demand.[70] The Ministry, on the advice of the JCPV, had expected 50 per cent uptake, but 60 per cent had registered, leaving a shortfall of around 2.5 million doses of IPV. Further production problems with the British manufacturers meant that a new batch of Salk vaccine needed to be ordered immediately so that it could be brought into circulation before the end of the summer. The new Minister, Derek Walker-Smith, was acutely aware that 'such a situation will greatly intensify the already considerable volume of criticism about the slowness of progress in the vaccination programme', and so it proved.[71] *The Times* ran an editorial accusing the Minister of misleading the public by consistently making announcements on IPV based on best-case scenarios with regard to British manufacturing. Since this had been a recurring problem, why was the government not more honest? 'To have raised the hopes of parents … is unpardonable', *The Times* argued, 'and in view of the fiasco last year – which only a low incidence of poliomyelitis prevented from becoming a tragedy – the country is entitled to a clear statement from the Minister.'[72] At least one member of the MRC found it 'difficult to be sympathetic at this stage'.[73] The Council had advised the government consistently to ensure that there was a stockpile of

British vaccine and that there should be a proper contingency plan in place against the relatively high likelihood of lost batches.[74]

Orders of American Salk vaccine allowed the programme to muddle through, and even though there were some issues with a batch of vaccine from the US firm Parke-Davis and continued problems with the British manufacturers, the general situation improved.[75] Indeed, supplies were considered robust enough that in September 1958 the Ministry made the decision to extend the scheme to young adults under the age of 26; and offered a third dose of the vaccine to everyone else in order to secure greater immunity among the population.[76] At the same time, the government became concerned at the low overall registration rate and the variable uptake among local authorities. Only 54 per cent of Scottish under-15s had been fully vaccinated up to the end of August 1958, while rates in England and Wales varied from as high as 87 per cent to as low as 20 per cent. Plans were therefore put in place for a publicity campaign, under the belief that the most of the major supply problems were at an end.[77] Ironically, by early 1959 it seemed that there would be too much IPV in circulation. Pfizer's UK branch had begun production of British-style IPV and was planning, in the words of the Ministry of Health, to 'flood the market' in an attempt to convince the British and foreign governments to buy their stock. The Ministry was in a bind, since if it did not purchase the IPV in bulk and use it as part of the vaccination programme, Pfizer would market the drug on prescription to individuals outside the scope of the existing scheme. The NHS would cover most of the cost of the prescriptions, potentially costing the Treasury three times more than the public health scheme.[78] The Ministry therefore considered extending the scheme even further to encompass all people under the age of 40. However, events beyond the Ministry's control would cause the government to reassess this position.

Demand for vaccination among young adults spiked dramatically following the well-publicised death of England and Birmingham City footballer Jeff Hall. The 28-year-old had been taken ill after a game with Portsmouth on 21 March 1959. He died in hospital sixteen days later, on 4 April.[79] That a young, healthy man could be struck down so quickly shocked the British public. Now that adults under the age of 26 were eligible for the scheme, the case served as a 'fortuitous' advertisement to raise acceptance rates. Walker-Smith recorded messages to be played at all Football League matches to take advantage of the situation.[80] However, the sheer volume of demand overwhelmed local health authorities, and in turn put impossible demands on the Ministry to supply the vaccine.[81] It appeared that the government would be embarrassed again: having tried so hard to promote the scheme to young adults and been frustrated at low uptake, it now faced the prospect of the system again having to delay vaccinations due to a shortage of IPV. MOHs in England and Wales were reminded of the importance of registration rather than providing IPV on demand, while Scottish authorities attempted to vaccinate as many as possible before the traditional holiday month of July.[82]

Once again, the unpredictability of demand hampered the government's ability to plan its polio vaccination programme. The Ministry had felt that young adults had been too apathetic during the initial registration process, leading to under-estimation of how much IPV would be needed for the coming financial year. In the wake of a high-profile case, demand had then surged to the point that local and national authorities were unable to cope. The government's frustrations at its inability to control and spread vaccination evenly across the year were expressed by Walker-Smith following criticism in the House of Commons:

> There has been no maldistribution on the part of my Department at all. I have already pointed out that both the original requests and the supplementary requests have been met. As for any delays in delivering vaccine, these have been very slight, and those who have had to wait at all for vaccine could have been vaccinated months ago if they had registered when I asked them.[83]

The public had, as in 1957, blown hot and cold on polio vaccination. The reaction to the Jeff Hall case had again shown the reliance of the system on registration and keeping demand even. The demand following this case was slightly different, however, due to the different demographics involved. The 1957 spike in demand in Coventry had been caused by a local increase in cases that brought home to parents the threat to their children. By contrast, Jeff Hall's was an individual tragic story which resonated with young adults who were making their own decisions about the risks to their own health. To be sure, many young adults would also have been parents, and so a clear distinction between these groups cannot be drawn. This level of demand, though, was both administrative and subjective. In the short term, football clubs got their players vaccinated in front of the press and television cameras. In the slightly longer term, the Ministry tried to push forward its plans to extend the programme to everyone under the age of 40. Part of the Ministry's argument was that Hall, aged 29 at the time of his death, would not have been eligible for the existing scheme. The Treasury was unconvinced that supply problems had been adequately addressed, and initially refused to fund extension of the programme.[84] Regardless, the Conservative Party pledged to provide IPV for under 40s in its 1959 general election manifesto, and confirmed the extension in February 1960.[85]

Oral polio vaccine

The year 1960 passed without any major crises. By 30 June 1960, 77 per cent of children had been fully vaccinated with IPV, as also had been half of young adults in the 16–26 age category.[86] While the registration rate remained less than ideal among older groups, the fact that such a backlog of cases had been cleared meant that the Ministry scaled back its orders of IPV for 1960/61, causing Pfizer to gradually withdraw from the British market.[87] The long-term future of the programme appeared to rest not on securing IPV supplies, but on whether the time was now right to switch to a new technology being trialled in the Soviet Union – Albert Sabin's live vaccine (or oral poliomyelitis vaccine; OPV).

OPV used attenuated forms of the poliovirus to confer immunity through a similar transmission form as the naturally occurring virus. Taken by mouth, the vaccine entered the gut like the natural infection and could confer immunity much more quickly than IPV. Salk had managed to produce a safe version of IPV quicker than his competitors. The speed and extent to which this was adopted in the American population meant that Sabin and others were forced to test their vaccines in virgin populations abroad. Although based in the US, Sabin had been born in the Russian Empire (in latter-day Poland) and his relationships with Soviet scientists helped him convince the Soviet Union to allow trials of his OPV. These were a success and, despite initial Western scepticism, by the early 1960s the potential advantages of OPV were recognised by the United States and its allies[88] As with IPV, the British medical establishment was initially cautious.[89] Experiments with Hilary

Koprowski's OPV in Belfast in 1956 had been 'disastrous', as Lindner and Blume have described.[90] The trials, overseen by Professor George Dick, showed that the virus could revert back to an infectious form, and this dented the reputation of OPV considerably in the United Kingdom.[91] But by the early 1960s attitudes had softened significantly. Sabin's vaccine held a number of advantages for mass and routine vaccination programmes. First, it was much cheaper and easier to manufacture, promising an end to the supply issues that had plagued the British programme thus far. Second, parents found the use of an oral vaccine, requiring only a drop of vaccine on a sugar cube, more attractive, since it caused less distress for their children and eliminated the need for injections.[92] Third, it was fast acting. Because it produced immunity much more quickly than IPV, it could be used on a mass scale as a form of epidemic control. And fourth, although controversially, OPV could theoretically vaccinate other members of the community passively, since it could be spread to people in the same way as poliovirus.[93] This led to a number of ethical questions about whether this amounted to vaccination without consent, but by the early 1960s the medical community was largely agreed that OPV offered the best opportunity to truly eradicate polio.[94] IPV had worked well in many Western nations, but only up to a point. Infection rates in the United States and Canada were beginning to stagnate, after significant falls since the mid-1950s.[95] Questions about OPV's safety – since if the virus returned to virulence, it could potentially spread live polio throughout a community – were answered at a number of international conferences, most notably the Fifth International Congress on Poliomyelitis in Copenhagen in July 1960.[96] The United States Surgeon General began to recommend the use of OPV, which influenced the British authorities to purchase some vaccine, initially to control epidemics, but later as part of the routine vaccination programme.[97]

While international scientific networks may have influenced the advice given by the MRC and JCPV on the use of OPV in Britain, the Ministry was motivated to adopt it for more pragmatic reasons. It was clear that a number of pharmaceutical companies were moving towards OPV production, with Wellcome lobbying the government hard for a contract to begin trials in the United Kingdom.[98] Within the IPV programme, a relatively quiet 1960 was followed by a more difficult 1961. Demand for vaccination increased significantly after high-profile epidemics in Ipswich, West Bromwich and Liverpool.[99] Infection rates had risen after successive years of decline (see Figure 3.1), reminding the public that polio had not yet been defeated. Demand had also been boosted by a large-scale campaign from the incoming Minister for Health, Enoch Powell. While he was aware that it was impossible to say to what extent the campaign had made an impact on vaccination rates, Powell noted that it was politically difficult for the government to be in yet another supply crisis, after having spent so much effort trying to engender support among the population.[100] Even though gross demand for the vaccine was now lower, due to the clearing of the backlog of cases from the 1950s, it was still much higher than the Ministry had been expecting. A number of supply problems then hit the Ministry at once. First, a batch of Pfizer's British IPV failed; then a batch of Canadian IPV from Connaught also failed to pass MRC safety tests. This coincided with a shortage in the United States which led the US government to ban exports of Salk vaccine. The spike in demand created by the epidemics left Britain in a situation where it did not have enough stockpiles to meet demand, nor was it able to import enough in the short term to tide it over.[101]

The Ministry received a number of complaints via Members of Parliament and local councils.[102] The BMA also forwarded concerns from general practitioners who were angry that they were the ones who faced criticism from the public when there were shortages.[103] The only way to help this situation was to purchase more IPV once supplies from the USA became accessible again, but the Ministry knew that it would face pushback from the Treasury, which had become increasingly concerned at the lack of accuracy in the Ministry's predictions for vaccine demand. While it understood that demand was elastic and impossible to judge with exactitude, the consistent requests for more money were trying its patience.[104] The Ministry had already been asked to set out the scientific case for IPV, and evidence that it had actually worked in Britain, during the negotiations over extending the programme to the under-40s.[105] More importantly, the Ministry believed that any request for large amounts of cash to purchase IPV would inevitably lead to questions from both the Treasury and the press about why so much was being spent on the older technology when OPV appeared to be the way forward in terms of both the epidemiology and public acceptability.[106]

In this situation, the demand for OPV was driven by a number of administrative and subjective factors. Western opinion on OPV had shifted dramatically and quickly over the course of 1960 and 1961. This was further helped when OPV was used to help to deal with an epidemic in Kingston upon Hull, East Yorkshire, in late summer 1961. Hundreds of thousands of people were immunised during the outbreak, and the vaccine's apparent success in containing the spread cemented its reputation.[107] The subjective demand for the state to provide protection against poliomyelitis was evident. Even in the absence of an oral alternative, people were still demanding IPV during the summer epidemics. Nevertheless, administrative pressure, driven by public opinion, appeared to be pushing toward OPV in the long term. Despite variations in the exact administrative demand within the programme over time, the issue was not over whether polio immunisation should be provided but over the form that it should take.

Conclusion

In September 1961 a civil servant noted: 'obviously we have miscalculated [demand for vaccination] ... The question is whether the miscalculation is defensible.'[108] It seems to be difficult to defend the Ministry of Health's long-term policy on IPV. From the outset it promised to vaccinate many more people than were within its capacity. It began the programme before its major manufacturers were able either to build a stockpile of vaccine or to produce enough *en masse* to meet even the more limited demand of the first registration wave. It tied its own hands by simultaneously demanding the use of British IPV and either banning or severely limiting the use of American Salk vaccine. When it did allow importation, it waited until supplies were almost gone before ordering more Salk vaccine, rather than anticipating growing demand. There were some mitigating circumstances. The Ministry may have been criticised by the Treasury for under-estimating the amount of vaccine required in any given year, but the political cost of overspending during a period of financial retrenchment was considered even riskier. In late 1958, some local authorities had supplies of American IPV that was about to expire, writing off thousands of pounds' worth of stock.[109] Moreover, the field of immunisation was in a constant state of flux – planning from year to year was difficult, and if the government over-ordered one type of vaccine and suddenly found the next year that it would require a different formula, even more money could be wasted.[110] In effect, this had already happened with the last-minute switch from American to British vaccine in late 1955, and the Ministry was mindful of having to do this again.

Demand was thus a very difficult beast to tame. Its negative effects could be exacerbated by events outside the government's control. Administratively, consistent and predictable levels of registration were the easiest to provide for, but in reality they were seldom the case. Either specific scares caused spikes in registration, or a lack of immediate danger led to under-registration (and with it, under-ordering of IPV from suppliers). From a subjective point of view, it was also never entirely clear what, specifically, the public were demanding. Low levels of general registration suggested that the public were not particularly excited by polio vaccination as an abstract concept; yet the surges in demand during epidemics or high-profile cases also suggested that the public expected to have the option of polio vaccine whenever they wanted it. Media coverage of the Salk vaccine trials and the consistent criticisms of government mismanagement of the scheme pointed to a nation that expected a properly functioning service; yet general apathy meant that the public did not register when asked to do so in order to ensure that the service ran as smoothly as possible. These paradoxes may not have been unique to polio, but they became much more evident than they had been with smallpox and diphtheria, due to: the novelty of the technology; the scope of the programme in encompassing young adults as well as children; and the high-profile problems with manufacture and supply.

Regardless, OPV was introduced for those awaiting their first dose of polio vaccine. By 1962, the programme was fully operational, having vaccinated the majority of people under the age of 26 and continuing to provide for new-borns and older citizens.[111] This was emblematic of the new status quo in public health. Despite the problems outlined in Part I of this book, as of 31 December 1969, uptake among children born in 1967 was 80 per cent or more in England and Wales for vaccines against pertussis, diphtheria and poliomyelitis.[112] This continued to vary by region: several authorities reached 95 per cent for pertussis vaccine, while Halifax achieved only 52 per cent.[113] For the most part, however, the system appeared to be working. Parents presented their children for the various injections and sugar cubes that protected their children, and epidemics of these infectious diseases had become much rarer.

By the early 1970s, the childhood vaccination programme had expanded to include immunisations against diphtheria, tetanus, pertussis, poliomyelitis, measles, rubella and tuberculosis – and it had phased out smallpox vaccination. What Jacob Heller describes as the 'vaccine narrative' in the United States can be said to apply to Britain by this point. He argues that the public broadly believed that vaccinations are safe, effective and a sign of a modern functioning state. This was cemented through the poliomyelitis programme, which could work only through vaccination, rather than other curative or preventative measures.[114] In the United Kingdom, similar successes with polio had led the public, broadly, to support and avail themselves of vaccination services.

Present-day research suggests that such attitudes remain in most nations around the globe. However, confidence in individual vaccinations may be dented by local political factors, faith in medical authorities, attitudes towards specific diseases and the reputation of the vaccine.[115] Part II explores two incidents which exemplified this in the British context: the pertussis crisis and the MMR crisis. In both cases, disagreements within the medical community about vaccine safety were seized upon by the press and caused confusion for the general public and government alike. The debates that followed were embedded in the contemporary political climate, and so were manifested in different ways.

Notes

1 David M. Oshinsky, *Polio: An American Story* (Oxford: Oxford University Press, 2005); Gareth Williams and Ray Loadman, *Paralysed with Fear: The Story of Polio* (Basingstoke: Palgrave Macmillan, 2013); Paul A. Offit, *Vaccinated: One Man's Quest to Defeat the World's Deadliest Diseases* (New York: Smithsonian Books, 2007); Naomi Rogers, *Polio Wars: Sister Elizabeth Kenny and the Golden Age of American Medicine* (Oxford: Oxford University Press, 2014); Naomi Rogers, *Dirt and Disease: Polio Before FDR* (New Brunswick: Rutgers University Press, 1992).

2 On the creation of "scandals", see Mark Drakeford and Ian Butler, *Scandal, Social Policy and Social Welfare*, 2nd edn (Bristol: Policy Press, 2006).

3 Ulrike Lindner and Stuart S. Blume, 'Vaccine innovation and adoption: Polio vaccines in the UK, the Netherlands and West Germany, 1955–1965', *Medical History*, 50:4 (2006), 425–46.
4 See especially Williams and Loadman, *Paralysed with Fear*.
5 One of these, type-II has subsequently been declared eradicated by the World Health Organization. Global Polio Eradication Initiative, 'Global eradication of wild Poliovirus Type 2 declared' (20 September 2015) http://polioeradication.org/news-post/global-eradication-of-wild-poliovirus-type-2-declared/ (accessed 23 August 2017).
6 Jennifer Hamborsky, Andrew Kroger and Charles Wolfe (eds), *Epidemiology and Prevention of Vaccine-Preventable Diseases*, 13th edn (Washington, DC: Centers for Disease Control and Prevention, 2015), pp. 297–310.
7 "Poliomyelitis" comes from the Greek for "inflammation of the grey marrow", in reference to the colour that spinal tissue displays in autopsies of poliomyelitis victims. For simplicity, the disease will henceforth be called "polio" in this chapter, unless in a direct quotation from the source material. See John Rodman Paul, *A History of Poliomyelitis* (New Haven, CT: Yale University Press, 1971), p. 8; Hamborsky, Kroger and Wolfe (eds), *Epidemiology and Prevention of Vaccine-Preventable Diseases*, p. 297.
8 J. N. Hays, *Epidemics and Pandemics: Their Impact on Human History* (Santa Barbara: ABC-CLIO, 2005), p. 414.
9 Rogers, *Polio Wars*; Williams and Loadman, *Paralysed with Fear*; Offit, *Vaccinated*.
10 Matthew Smallman-Raynor and Andrew D. Cliff, 'The geographical spread of the 1947 poliomyelitis epidemic in England and Wales: spatial wave propagation of an enigmatic epidemiological event', *Journal of Historical Geography*, 40 (2013), 36–51.
11 On Guthrie, see George Dick, 'Obituary: Duncan Guthrie', *Independent* (20 October 1994) www.independent.co.uk/news/people/obituary-duncan-guthrie-1444138.html (accessed 24 August 2017). After polio became less common, the Fund was rebranded as The National Fund for Research into Crippling Diseases; it is now called Action Medical Research. Action Medical Research, 'History' (undated) www.action.org.uk/about-us/history (accessed 24 August 2017).
12 Thomas Francis, *Evaluation of the 1954 Field Trial of Poliomyelitis Vaccine. Final report* (Ann Arbor: University of Michigan, 1957); Offit, *Vaccinated*.
13 Hunter Heyck and David Kaiser, 'Introduction', *Isis*, 101:2 (2010), 362–6.
14 Marcia Meldrum, '"A calculated risk": The Salk polio vaccine field trials of 1954', *British Medical Journal*, 317:7167 (1998), 1233–6.
15 Dora Vargha, 'Between East and West: Polio vaccination across the Iron Curtain in Cold War Hungary', *Bulletin of the History of Medicine*, 88:2

(2014), 319–42. On media coverage see 'New vaccine may end polio menace', *Daily Mail* (27 January 1953), p. 1; Chapman Pincher, 'Drive for polio vaccine', *Daily Express* (26 April 1954), p. 5; 'Rome conference on poliomyelitis', *The Times* (7 September 1954), p. 6; 'Conquest of polio in sight?', *Manchester Guardian* (7 December 1954), p. 12.
16 TNA: MH 55/2458, S. A. Heald, Announcement in U.S.A. of results of Polio Vaccine Trials 12 April, 7 April; Duncan Guthrie [Director, National Fund for Poliomyelitis Research] to news editors of various publications, 6 April 1955.
17 HC Deb (25 April 1955) vol. 540, cc. 620–4.
18 Neal Nathanson and Alexander D. Langmuir, 'The Cutter Incident. Poliomyelitis following formaldehyde-inactivated poliovirus vaccination in the United States during the spring of 1955', *American Journal of Epidemiology*, 78:1 (1963), 29–60; Paul A. Offit, 'The Cutter Incident, 50 years later', *New England Journal of Medicine*, 352:14 (2005), 1411–12.
19 Per Axelsson, 'The Cutter Incident and the development of a Swedish polio vaccine, 1952–1957', *Dynamis*, 32:2 (2012), 311–28; Alison Day, '"An American tragedy". The Cutter Incident and its implications for the Salk polio vaccine in New Zealand 1955–1960', *Health & History: Journal of the Australian & New Zealand Society for the History of Medicine*, 11:2 (2009), 42–61.
20 Jane Lewis, 'The prevention of diphtheria in Canada and Britain 1914–1945', *Journal of Social History*, 20:1 (1986), 163–76; Linda Bryder, '"We shall not find salvation in inoculation": BCG vaccination in Scandinavia, Britain and the USA, 1921–1960', *Social Science & Medicine*, 49:9 (1999), 1157–67. See also Chapters 1 and 2 and discussions about the legacy of Victorian anti-vaccinationism on British policy.
21 TNA: 55/2458, Medical Research Council, Poliomyelitis Vaccine (55/336), 4 May 1955.
22 The replacement strain is referred to by many names in the literature and internal documents, including "Brunhilde", "Brunden" and "Brunender". See TNA: FD 23/1028, MRC Advisory Committee on Safety Tests for Poliomyelitis Vaccine, Minutes, 16 May 1957; Memorandum on the Importance of Gaining Answers to Two Questions Concerning the British Salk-Type Poliomyelitis Vaccine (late 1956), 1–6; Poliomyelitis Vaccines Committee (Medical Research Council), 'Assessment of the British vaccine against poliomyelitis', *British Medical Journal*, 1:5030 (1957), 1271–7; Anon, 'British poliomyelitis vaccine', *British Medical Journal*, 1:5030 (1957), 1291–2.
23 The debates over IPV would continue to make a distinction between the British formula and the American one. Henceforth, the US vaccine will be

referred to as "Salk", with IPV representing the British version. See TNA: FD 23/1028, MRC Advisory Committee on Safety Tests for Poliomyelitis Vaccine, Minutes, 16 May 1957; Memorandum on the Importance of Gaining Answers to Two Questions Concerning the British Salk-Type Poliomyelitis Vaccine (late 1956), 1–6.

24 MH 55/2458, C.H.S.C.(PV)(55)1, Central and Scottish Health Services Councils, Joint Committee on Poliomyelitis Vaccine, June 1955. The JCPV would eventually be repurposed as a general vaccination advisory body – see Chapter 2.

25 'British poliomyelitis vaccine in use this summer', *The Times* (20 January 1956), p. 8.

26 TNA: MH 55/2464, Ministry of Health, Circular 20/58, Poliomyelitis Vaccination, 2 September 1958.

27 TNA: MH 55/2461, Press Office, Ministry of Health, Polio Vaccine, January 1957.

28 'Town's boycott of vaccine scheme', *The Times* (8 March 1956), p. 10; 'Decision not to use vaccine', *The Times* (15 March 1956), p. 6; 'Parents' plea on vaccine fails', *The Times* (27 March 1956), p. 6; 'Polio drug ban angers parents', *Daily Mail* (9 March 1956), p. 7.

29 'Vaccine scheme accepted', *The Times* (12 April 1956), p. 6. See also 'Reply on vaccine to Burton parents', *The Times* (10 April 1956), p. 13; 'Town changes mind on polio', *Daily Mail* (12 April 1956), p. 7.

30 'City tilts at minister', *The Times* (8 April 1958), p. 5.

31 TNA: FD 23/1028, MRC, Advisory Committee on Safety Tests for Poliomyelitis Vaccine, Minutes, 16 May 1957.

32 TNA: FD 23/1031, Brief for meeting with Scientific Correspondents. History of Batch 10 (for conference held 27 February 1957).

33 TNA: MH 55/2461, Circular 2/56, Poliomyelitis Vaccine, 19 January 1956; TNA: FD 23/1028, The use of poliomyelitis vaccine in 1957. A memorandum by Professor A. Bradford Hill (late 1956); and *ibid.*, A. Bradford Hill to Sir John Charles, 12 October 1956.

34 See Chapter 1 and A. Bradford Hill and J. Knowelden, 'Inoculation and poliomyelitis', *British Medical Journal*, 2:4669 (1950), 1–6.

35 TNA: MH 55/2461, Circular 6/57, Poliomyelitis Vaccination, 14 May 1957; Ministry of Health, Polio vaccination to go on, 15 May 1957.

36 Ministry of Health, *Report of the Ministry of Health for the Year Ended 31st December, 1955. Part II on the State of the Public Health* (Cmnd 16) (London: HMSO, 1956), p. 79; Ministry of Health, *Report of the Ministry of Health for the Year Ended 31st December, 1956. Part II on the State of the*

Public Health being the Annual Report of the Chief Medical Officer for the Year 1956 (Cmnd 325) (London: HMSO, 1957), p. 78.
37 TNA: MH 55/2469, Announcement of developments in poliomyelitis scheme, 14 November 1960.
38 TNA: MH 55/2461, Circular 2/56, Poliomyelitis Vaccine, 19 January 1956.
39 TNA: MH 55/2458, Russell-Smith to Armer, Poliomyelitis vaccine, 7 September 1955.
40 TNA: MH 55/2458, Poliomyelitis Vaccine, Production and Supply, [undated, probably April 1955].
41 TNA: FD 23/1031, Brief for meeting with Scientific Correspondents. History of Batch 10 (for conference held 27 February 1957).
42 'Vaccine issue held up', *The Times* (28 February 1957), p. 8.
43 Anon, 'Polio fantasies', *British Medical Journal*, 1:5018 (1957), 571–2.
44 TNA: MH 55/2458, Poliomyelitis Vaccine, internal memorandum draft, December 1955.
45 TNA: MH 55/2458, H. Jephcott [Glaxo] to H. Wilkinson [Ministry of Health], 23 April 1955; TNA: FD 23/1058, Glaxo Ltd. and Polio Vaccine (1957).
46 TNA: MH 55/2458, Poliomyelitis Vaccine, Production and Supply, [undated, probably April 1955]; Sir Hilton Poynton [Colonial Office] to Sir Frederick Armer [Ministry of Health], 7 May 1955.
47 TNA: FD 23/1058, Copy of extract of Cabinet Conclusions C.C.(57)66th Conclusions of Tuesday 16th September 1957, Item No. 1; Glaxo Ltd. and Polio Vaccine (1957). On Anglo-American relations and tensions see Kevin Ruane and James Ellison, 'Managing the Americans: Anthony Eden, Harold Macmillan and the pursuit of "power-by-proxy" in the 1950s', *Contemporary British History*, 18:3 (2004), 147–67.
48 Jean-Baptiste Gouyon, 'Making science at home: Visual displays of space science and nuclear physics at the Science Museum and on television in postwar Britain', *History & Technology*, 30:1/2 (2014), 37–60; Allan Jones, 'Elite science and the BBC: A 1950s contest of ownership', *British Journal for the History of Science*, 47:4 (2014), 701–23.
49 See FD 23/1058, Note of H.A.(57)79, 3 July 1957.
50 Offit, *Vaccinated*; Williams and Loadman, *Paralysed with Fear*.
51 On risk management and obligations see Chapter 4 and Jakob Arnoldi, *Risk: An Introduction* (Cambridge: Polity, 2009).
52 Iain Dale, *Conservative Party General Election Manifestos 1900–1997* (Abingdon: Routledge, 2000), p. 121. The manifesto specifically mentions research on polio and cancer.

53 For a more in-depth appraisal of the Coventry epidemic, see Gareth Millward, '"A matter of commonsense": The Coventry poliomyelitis epidemic 1957 and the British public', *Contemporary British History*, 31:3 (2017), 384–406.
54 'Polio: Coventry vaccine plea fails', *Coventry Evening Telegraph* (3 August 1957), p. 1.
55 Anon, 'Poliomyelitis vaccine', *British Medical Journal*, 2:5041 (August 1957), 405–6. "Polio vaccine: M.P.'s protest to Ministry', *Coventry Evening Telegraph*, 5 August 1957, 1; and '"Coventry must wait," Minister tells M.P.', *Coventry Evening Telegraph* (7 August 1957), p. 3.
56 The story broke on the Saturday evening in 'Coventry to get more polio vaccine', *Coventry Evening Telegraph* (3 August 1957), p. 1. Reports also appeared in the *Daily Express*, *Daily Telegraph* and *Birmingham Evening Dispatch*. TNA: MH 55/2460, Polio Vaccine – Coventry, 6 August 1957, 4.
57 TNA: MH 55/2460, Polio Vaccine – Coventry, internal memorandum, 6 August 1957; Polio vaccine for Coventry, Press handout given over telephone by Mr. Heald this afternoon, 5 August 1957.
58 'Polio: Lord Mayor holds conference', *Coventry Evening Telegraph* (7 August 1957), pp. 1, 12; 'Why Coventry cannot have extra vaccine', *Coventry Evening Telegraph* (8 August 1957), p. 9; 'Civic talks on poliomyelitis', *The Times* (8 August 1957), p. 2; 'It's bad to inoculate for polio at present', *Coventry Standard* (9 August 1957), p. 5; Anon, 'Poliomyelitis vaccine'.
59 'Help needed now', *Coventry Evening Telegraph* (7 August 1957), p. 6; 'No extra vaccine for polio towns', *Daily Express* (8 August 1957), p. 5.
60 Millward, '"A matter of commonsense"'.
61 'Coventry not worst-affected district', *Coventry Evening Telegraph* (7 August 1957), p. 1; TNA: MH 55/2461, R. G. Forrest [Scottish Office], Poliomyelitis Vaccine, 14 May 1957.
62 Margaret Agerholm letter to *The Times* (31 August 1957), p. 11; Margaret Agerholm, 'Importation of poliomyelitis vaccine', *The Lancet*, 270:6986 (1957), 150.
63 'Danish 5000 "shots" campaign fails', *Coventry Evening Telegraph* (8 August 1957), p. 8; TNA: MH 55/2460, Edelman to Vaughan-Morgan, 28 August 1957; TNA: FD 23/1058, MRC Memorandum, 28 August 1957; 'Polio city says "no"', *Daily Mirror* (9 August 1957), p. 3; 'Health Ministry officers in city for polio talks', *Coventry Evening Telegraph* (9 August 1957), p. 1. On other nations' IPV products, see Eric A. Engels, Hormuzd A. Katki, Nete M. Nielsen, Jeanette F. Winther, Henrik

Hjalgrim, Flemming Gjerris, Philip S. Rosenberg and Morten Frisch, 'Cancer incidence in Denmark following exposure to poliovirus vaccine contaminated with simian virus 40', *Journal of the National Cancer Institute*, 95:7 (2003), 532–9; María Isabel Porras and María Victoria Cabellero, 'Vaccines and vaccination against smallpox and poliomyelitis: Economies and values', Conference paper (European Association for the History of Medicine and Health Conference, University of Cologne, September 2015); Stuart Blume, *Immunization: How Vaccines Became Controversial* (London: Reaktion, 2017), pp. 79–81.

64 See especially the discussions between the government and Burroughs Wellcome in TNA: MH 134/151.

65 Blume, *Immunization*; see also Farah Huzair and Steve Sturdy, 'Biotechnology and the transformation of vaccine innovation: The case of the hepatitis B vaccines 1968–2000', *Studies in History & Philosophy of Biological & Biomedical Sciences*, 64 (2017), 11–21.

66 TNA: FD 23/1058, See Himsworth to Home, 18 July 1957; Cabinet Home Affairs Committee H.A.(57) 17th meeting, 19 July 1957, 10am; *ibid.*, Lord Home to Vaughan-Morgan, 15 July 1957.

67 Poliomyelitis Vaccines Committee, 'Assessment of the British vaccine against poliomyelitis'; Anon, 'American polio vaccine', *British Medical Journal*, 1:5029 (1957), 1229–30; TNA: FD 23/1058, Himsworth to Wilson, 23 July 1957; Vaccination against Poliomyelitis, Considerations relating to the possible use of American Salk vaccine in this country, Himsworth to Lord Home, 25 July 1957, 5.

68 'Vaccine and epidemic', *Manchester Guardian* (12 August 1957), p. 4.

69 Anon, 'American polio vaccine'.

70 TNA: FD 23/1059, H.A.(58)2nd Meeting, Cabinet Home Affairs Committee, 7 February 1958, 11am.

71 TNA: FD 23/1059, H.A.(58)42, Cabinet Home Affairs Committee, Poliomyelitis Vaccine, Memorandum by the Minister of Health, 16 April 1958.

72 'A cautionary tale', *The Times*, 23 April 1958, p. 11.

73 TNA: FD 23/1059, W. L. M. Perry to Sir Harold Himsworth, 16 April 1958.

74 TNA: FD 23/1059, Himsworth to Lord Hailsham, 27 April 1958; Statement by the Medical Research Council on the Current Position, April 1958; Himsworth to Hailsham, 1 May 1958.

75 TNA: FD 23/1059, Polio Vaccination (Great Britain), July 1958; Himsworth to Simpson, 30 June 1958.

76 TNA: MH 55/2464, Ministry of Health, Circular 20/58, Poliomyelitis Vaccination, 2 September 1958.

77 TNA: MH 55/2464, Poliomyelitis Vaccine, Note of Meeting on 16 September 1958; Ministry of Health, *Report of the Ministry of Health for the Year 1958. Part II on the State of the Public Health being the Annual Report of the Chief Medical Officer* (Cmnd 871) (London: HMSO, 1959), pp. 80–3.
78 TNA: MH 55/2464, E. J. Prideaux to J. P. Dodds, Polio Vaccine – Messrs. Pfizers, 6 March 1959; C. W. Hales-Hunt, Poliomyelitis Vaccine, 5 March 1959; J. P. Dodds, 18 March 1959.
79 Simon Burnton, 'The forgotten story of … Jeff Hall, the footballer whose death turned the tide against polio', *Guardian* (9 December 2016) www.theguardian.com/football/blog/2016/dec/09/fogotten-story-jeff-hall-death-polio-birmingham-city (accessed 24 August 2017); Nick McCarthy, 'Polio campaigning widow of Blues legend Jeff Hall dies after cancer battle' (7 June 2016) www.birminghammail.co.uk/news/midlands-news/polio-campaigning-widow-blues-legend-11437906 (accessed 24 August 2017); AP Archive, 'Polio inoculations' (original video clip dated 13 April 1959) www.aparchive.com/metadata/youtube/4bdf81b34ff4492ea60082787a97e807 (accessed 24 August 2017).
80 TNA: MH 55/2464, Polio vaccination, 14 April 1959.
81 TNA: MH 55/2464, E. T. Prideaux to Principal Regional Officers, 14 April 1959; TNA: FD 23/1060, Derek Walker-Smith to R. A. Butler [Home Office], Lord Hailsham [Cabinet Office] and J. E. S. Simon [Treasury], 15 April 1959.
82 MH: 55/2464, Sir John Charles to MOsH (England and Wales), 16 April 1959; *ibid.*, N. W. Graham [Scottish Office] to J. P. Dodds, 25 May 1959.
83 HC Deb (27 April 1959) vol. 604, col. 880.
84 TNA: MH 55/2464, Poliomyelitis Vaccination, 9 May 1959; *ibid.*, A. S. Marre to P. M. Rossiter [Treasury], 1 July 1959 and reply, 6 July 1959.
85 Dale, *Conservative Party Manifestos*, p. 135; TNA: 55/2468, Ministry of Health Press Release, Extension of Anti-Polio Vaccination, Age limit now to be 40, 1 February 1960.
86 MH 55/2469, Ministry of Health internal memorandum, 27 July 1960.
87 MH 55/2469, John Hegarty [Health] to E. V. Hambrook [Treasury], 12 July 1960.
88 On acceptance of OPV in Western Europe, see Lindner and Blume, 'Vaccine innovation and adoption'. On the Cold War rivalry, see Vargha, 'Between East and West'.
89 MH 55/2469, Internal memo to George Godber, 30 August 1960.
90 Lindner and Blume, 'Vaccine innovation and adoption'.
91 Dick's experiences had made him cautious about the risk of vaccine damage in general, as seen in Chapter 2 in his advice on smallpox

Poliomyelitis 145

vaccination. See also G. W. A. Dick and D. S. Dane, 'Live poliomyelitis vaccine', *British Medical Journal*, 1:5125 (1959), 853–4; G. W. A. Dick and D. S. Dane, 'Vaccination against poliomyelitis with live virus vaccines', *British Medical Journal*, 2:5106 (1958), 1184–6.

92 TNA: MH 55/2472, J. M. Douglas [Treasury] to C. W. Hales-Hunt, 29 May 1961.
93 On these general benefits, as argued in Cabinet, see FD 23/1060, Cabinet Home Affairs Committee, H.A.(59)23rd Meeting, 11 December 1959.
94 Lindner and Blume, 'Vaccine innovation and adoption'. TNA: MH 55/2469, Note on live poliomyelitis vaccine, 2 September 1960; Dr Roden, Note on immunisation against poliomyelitis with particular reference to live poliomyelitis vaccine, September 1960.
95 TNA: FD 23/1060, R. H. L. Cohen to Hailsham, Poliomyelitis Vaccination, 2 December 1959.
96 There was also a major conference in Moscow in May, and a Pan American Health Organization/World Health Organization joint conference in Washington in June. See TNA: MH 55/2469, L. E. Burney [US Surgeon General] to Sir John Charles, 1 September 1960.
97 Lindner and Blume, 'Vaccine innovation and adoption'; TNA: MH 55/2469, Statement by L. E. Burney; Recommendation of the [US] Public Health Service Committee on Live Poliovirus Vaccine, 24 August 1960.
98 TNA: MH 55/2469, M. W. Perrin [Chair, Wellcome Foundation] to Enoch Powell, 12 August 1960; Enoch Powell memorandum, 29 August 1960.
99 TNA: MH 55/2472, Inactivated poliomyelitis vaccine, Meeting, 31 May 1961; George Godber to MOsH (England and Wales), 29 May 1961; '100,000 immunized in Liverpool', *The Times* (3 May 1961), p. 8.
100 TNA: MH 55/2472, New Drive Against Polio – Minister of Health appeals for 100 per cent immunisation of children and young people, 12 June 1961; Enoch Powell to Dodds, 12 September 1961.
101 TNA: MH 55/2472, Supply of polio vaccine, 17 July 1961.
102 See correspondence in TNA: MH 55/2472, including letters from Southwell, Essex, Gosport and West Hartlepool.
103 TNA: MH 55/2472, Walter Hedgecock [BMA] to Judd, 26 September 1961; 'Doctors angry over polio jabs hold-up', *Daily Mirror* (6 October 1961), p. 6.
104 TNA: MH 55/2472, Douglas to Hales-Hunt, 16 June 1961; O'Brien, Inactivated Polio Vaccine, 28 June 1961.
105 TNA: MH 55/2464, P. M. Rossiter to A. S. Marre, 15 April 1959 and replies 1 July 1959, 6 July 1959; Poliomyelitis Vaccination, 9 May 1959.

106 TNA: 55/2472, O'Brien, Inactivated Polio Vaccine, 28 June 1961; Douglas to Hales-Hunt, 29 May 1961.
107 TNA: MH 55/2473, Poliomyelitis Vaccine, Emergency Reserves of Monovalent Sabin Vaccine for Control of Outbreaks, 25 October 1961; 'Polio: city alert', *Daily Express* (13 October 1961), p. 1; '23 polio cases at Hull', *The Times* (12 October 1961); Lindner and Blume, 'Vaccine innovation and adoption'.
108 TNA: MH 55/2472, Shortage of polio vaccine, 25 September 1961.
109 TNA: MH 55/2464, Poliomyelitis Vaccine, 16 October 1958. The Ministry would have lost £4,000 in Birmingham alone, but was able to mitigate against this with some internal transfers to other local authorities and seeking permission to extend the shelf life of certain batches.
110 TNA: MH 55/2472, Dr Thomson, Oral Poliomyelitis Vaccine, 5 June 1961.
111 Lindner and Blume, 'Vaccine innovation and adoption'.
112 TNA: BN 35/57, DHSS, Local Authority Immunisation and Vaccination Statistics as at 31 December 1969.
113 *Ibid.*
114 Jacob Heller, *The Vaccine Narrative* (Nashville, TN: Vanderbilt University Press, 2008), pp. 3–8.
115 Heidi J. Larson, Caitlin Jarrett, Elisabeth Eckersberger, David M. D. Smith and Pauline Paterson, 'Understanding vaccine hesitancy around vaccines and vaccination from a global perspective: A systematic review of published literature, 2007–2012', *Vaccine*, 32:19 (2014), 2150–9; SAGE Working Group on Vaccine Hesitancy, *Report of the SAGE Working Group on Vaccine Hesitancy* (Geneva: World Health Organization, 2014).

II
Vaccination crises

4
Pertussis

Part II of this book signifies a shift in emphasis for the British vaccination programme. Some of this was due to maturity. By the 1970s, many of the fundamental questions about which vaccines to include and whether the state had a role in protecting the British public had been answered. Citizens had come to accept vaccination for themselves and demand it of others. Other changes were due to political and historical circumstances. Whereas MOHs had played a key role in the administration of immunisation from the 1940s to the 1960s, these functions were subsumed by the Department of Health and Social Security (DHSS) in the 1974 reorganisation of the NHS. The DHSS and its predecessor, the Ministry of Health, had attempted to exert more central control over and unification of the vaccination programme. This was seen in the surveillance of local authority uptake statistics; a growing role for the medical civil service through bodies such as the JCVI; and national control over the provision and funding of vaccine supplies to the regions.

These issues of localism did not disappear. General practitioners took ever greater responsibility for ensuring that their areas met centrally determined targets for vaccination rates. However, with a mature programme and a tried and tested vaccination bureaucracy, the major concerns were different. No longer were there regular surges in demand to cause supply issues. Nor was apathy so acute in a system that could better monitor and follow up with parents who did not vaccinate their children. Rather, the key crises for the national vaccination programme came when the new status quo was challenged. This was exemplified in two key incidents in which faith in specific vaccines was damaged. Chapter 5 will examine the MMR vaccine crisis and the subsequent sociological debates about vaccine confidence and health education at the turn of the millennium. This chapter deals with pertussis.

In the mid-1970s, some doctors questioned the safety of the pertussis (or whooping cough) vaccine, claiming that it could cause brain damage in young children. Despite protestations from the majority of the medical community, public confidence in the vaccine dropped significantly. Pertussis vaccination rates fell from 78.5 per cent of children born in England and Wales in 1971 to 37 per cent in 1974.[1] As a result, the whooping cough outbreak in the winter of 1978–79 was worse than any since the 1950s. It was not until the mid-1980s that vaccination rates recovered and infection rates returned to pre-crisis levels.[2] To counter negative publicity, the government commissioned a report into the science behind the vaccine and embarked on an advertising campaign to encourage parents to vaccinate their children. But science and medicine formed only part of the debate. As they had been from the first vaccination programmes, questions about the boundaries and responsibilities of the state were central. In the case of pertussis, public health policy was considered alongside social security and the wider welfare state. If the hazard of brain damage was real, regardless of how small the risk, did the government not have a duty to provide support for the families adversely affected by vaccines? Similarly, if herd immunity was a crucial part of a functioning public health programme, did the health authorities not have a duty to ensure that uptake was as high as possible? Citizens demanded that the state should provide protections, but also that citizens should be protected against state actions.

This chapter, therefore, is about risk. We have already seen how statistical computations of risk were used in the vaccination programme. The decision to ban imports of Salk vaccine from North America had been taken because it was felt that the British vaccine was less likely to cause damage. Routine infant smallpox vaccination ended when the risk of damage from the vaccine was considered higher than the risk of an unvaccinated population actually catching the disease. Diphtheria immunisation was hailed as a success because immunised children were less likely to contract the disease, and if they did they were much less likely to get a serious form of it. Such statistical calculations had become the foundation of epidemiology and chronic disease management by the 1970s, building on the research that had established the link between tobacco smoking and lung cancer.[3] Although elements of these can be seen in the chapters in Part II, this chapter focuses more on the sociological concept and how it manifested in debates around the pertussis crisis. Studies of risk usually take three forms.[4] First, they explore how societies have come to create, identify and manage new risks as they become more technologically advanced. Modern societies have created new hazards – things that can go wrong – with ever greater destructive power (e.g. the potential meltdown of a nuclear power plant). Regulatory frameworks manage the risk – the statistical likelihood that the hazard will actually occur – so that the benefits of these modern technologies outweigh the dangers.[5] Second, risk studies look at the social and cultural conditions that make certain individuals or organisations prioritise certain risks over others. These approaches tend to focus on the meaning and social construction of risk, with a focus on decision-making processes and politics.[6] Third, risk can be viewed through a Foucauldian lens. We can analyse how power identifies and manages risks through governance. Risks are managed by the state as well as being internalised by citizens.[7] Together, these analyses stress the centrality of risk to modern states, especially since the early twentieth century. Thus, we can analyse not just what risks were identified but also how different societies focused on specific risks and how those were integrated into systems of governance.

This chapter does not seek to explain why parents chose to eschew whooping cough vaccination during the crisis. Instead, it puts the pertussis debate in context by showing how it was inherently tied up in wider public concerns over risk. These risks were partly to do with the vaccine. The medical deliberations over the relative risks of vaccine damage and infectious disease were clearly the catalyst for the crisis. More importantly, however, these debates were rooted in anxieties about the role of the welfare state. The most prominent discussions were over the provision of financial compensation to the victims of vaccine damage. This was a product of renewed political interest in groups whose risks of poverty had not been successfully managed by the 1948 welfare state.[8] The public demanded protection from the risks of vaccine damage – that is to say, they wanted to prevent damage from happening and to have an adequate safety net for those who became disabled. But they also demanded protection from infectious disease, as evidenced by the queues outside clinics for vaccination when the epidemic broke out. Moreover, the levels of risk and the importance attached to them varied by constituency. This was a policy debate in which there were multiple actors, including parliamentarians, voluntary organisations, the medical profession, the DHSS, the Treasury and the press.

These concerns were an extension of a classic problem in decision making around vaccination: omission versus commission.[9] A child who catches a disease when they have not been vaccinated can be said to be a victim of an 'error of omission'. An act was not taken (whether deliberately or not), leading to an unwanted event. A child who suffers an allergic reaction to a vaccine may be a victim of an 'error of commission'. This is the opposite of 'omission', since an action was deliberately taken.[10] Parents and individuals tend to be better at rationalising acts of omission, where a negative event can be attributed more to chance than to an active, harmful decision on the part of the individual. As this chapter will show, this dilemma was present throughout the pertussis crisis. The potential negative outcomes (or hazards) to individual families of either brain damage or whooping cough were catastrophic. While medical experts debated the acceptable odds of these events happening (risk), the lay public found it difficult to find a clear answer.[11] This debate was fuelled and reflected by the ample press coverage which the crisis received.[12] But it was not just parents caught in this bind. As risks became both visible and manageable through technological change, certain obligations were placed upon individuals and organisations to manage them.[13] For supporters of vaccination, parents were expected to vaccinate their children as part of their duty towards themselves and their fellow citizens (as seen in Chapter 1).[14] For critics, the government's slow response meant that it had failed to manage the risks of either vaccine damage or infectious disease adequately. Neither omission nor commission alone would give the DHSS an easy policy option. The risks of continuing to use a vaccine that might prove to be dangerous were obvious. At the same time, doing nothing about the impending epidemic was also unacceptable.

This chapter explores these themes by outlining the key events of the pertussis crisis. It then focuses on the two main areas of debate. First, the passage of the Vaccine Damage Payments Act 1979 was predicated on the idea that individuals who were vaccinated for the good of society should be compensated for taking that risk if things went wrong. This argument was generally accepted by the major policy actors from an early stage. The second debate came over how likely vaccine damage was, especially in relation to the benefits of the pertussis vaccine. As doubts about the safety of the vaccine declined, new concerns arose over the likelihood of widespread whooping cough in a now under-vaccinated population. In both cases, the government came under sustained criticism for not taking decisive action to reduce doubt over the vaccine, thus increasing uncertainty and making it more difficult for parents to make the – by public health standards – correct decision. To conclude, the chapter explores another vaccination debate rooted in both the omission/commission dilemma and contemporary concerns over disability. Voluntary organisations had become concerned that the DHSS had not done enough to vaccinate against rubella, and thus prevent Congenital Rubella Syndrome. Although this was not as high profile as the pertussis crisis, it shows that the debates over risk were widespread in 1970s public health policy.

The pertussis crisis

Pertussis is an infectious disease that can lead to violent coughing, especially in children. Complications can include pneumonia and encephalitis. While only around 1 per cent of cases in the 1940s were fatal in Britain, the unpleasantness of the disease and its disproportionately damaging effect on children under the age of 2 years meant that parents had long feared it.[15] It affected communities in epidemic cycles, meaning that national notifications tended to spike every two to three years.[16] A vaccine against pertussis had been developed before the Second World War, but it was not until the 1950s that it became part of the routine childhood vaccination schedule in Britain. Despite this, many local authorities chose to administer it alongside diphtheria immunisation to take advantage of parents' concerns about the disease before its national introduction in 1957.[17] A large-scale MRC trial had confirmed both the effectiveness and the safety of the vaccine in 36,000 children.[18] By the 1970s, the trivalent diphtheria-tetanus-whole-cell-pertussis vaccine (DTwP) was used routinely throughout the country, although separate diphtheria-tetanus (DT) and whole-cell pertussis vaccines were available.[19] The whooping cough vaccine was successful. Pertussis morbidity dropped significantly over the 1960s, from an average of 122,000 cases (and 374 deaths) per year in the ten years

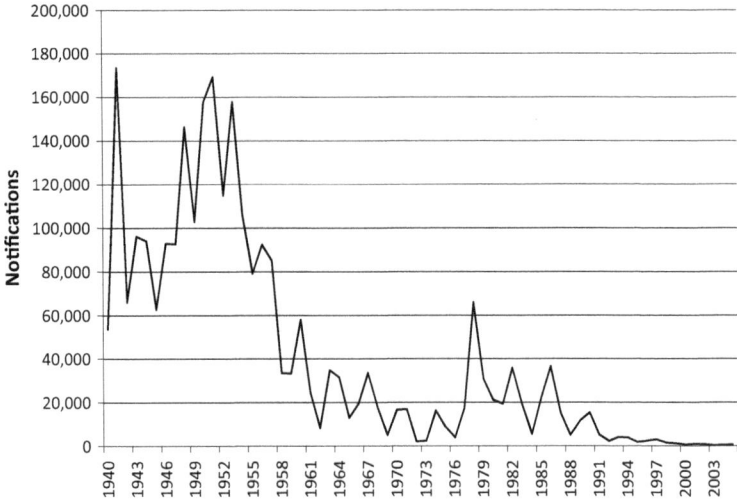

Figure 4.1 Pertussis notifications, England and Wales, 1940–2005. After 2005, improvements in laboratory testing and notifications mean that data are not comparable.
Source: Public Health England, 'Table 6: Pertussis notifications and deaths, England and Wales: 1940–2014' (5 May 2016). www.gov.uk/government/uploads/system/uploads/attachment_data/file/521438/Table_6_Pertussis_notifications_and_deaths__E_W__1940_-_2015.pdf (accessed 5 August 2017).

ending 1956, to just 20,400 cases (and 24 deaths) per year for the ten years ending 1970 (Figure 4.1).[20]

In 1974, doctors from Great Ormond Street Hospital published a paper claiming that there might be a link between the pertussis vaccine and brain damage.[21] The resultant media attention and public debate saw a rapid reduction in the number of parents presenting their children for DTwP vaccination. Jeffrey Baker has described this crisis and its significance for public health as beginning around 1974 and ending in the mid-1980s, after the final court cases against the government brought by parents of children with brain injuries collapsed.[22] He rightly argues that the crisis needs to be put into historical rather than simply epidemiological context. For public health professionals, the crisis – or the event which must be remembered and studied – is the drop in vaccination rates and subsequent rise in infections. It has become a lesson from history, and was referenced regularly during the later MMR crisis.[23] Studies have therefore tended to focus on public attitudes towards the pertussis vaccine. While these were clearly important, we can learn more from extending our view of the crisis and putting it into the wider context of debates around the welfare state and the role of the government.

The risks of this brewing crisis can be separated into three broad issues. The first was the government's duty to protect the public from pertussis. Since it was now possible to manage the risk of infectious diseases through vaccination, public health authorities were obliged to do so.[24] The second issue was protection from damage. If, as the Great Ormond Street doctors implied, there was a risk of damage from vaccines, then the government was failing in its obligation to provide a *safe* vaccine against pertussis. But it was a third issue that drove the majority of press coverage and public debate around pertussis vaccine: the government's responsibility to provide welfare support for those affected by failures in the first two policy areas. The 1960s and 1970s had seen extensive debate about and attention drawn to the increased risk of poverty associated with impairment and disability.[25] The thalidomide scandal (in which a number of children were born with significant injuries due to the ingestion of the thalidomide drug by their mothers while they were pregnant) had recently resurfaced when it was shown that the British distributors had not paid adequate compensation to the victims.[26] In the wake of this, the Conservative government of Edward Heath established the Family Fund to provide social security payments to families with 'congenitally disabled children', and the subject of medical negligence had been added to the remit of the Royal Commission on Civil Liability and Compensation for Personal Injury.[27] In this environment, vaccine damage became a potential special case for additional compensation, especially if the health authorities could be shown to be at fault.[28]

For the government, then, these three issues required three different approaches. Its goal was to restore confidence in the pertussis vaccine and in the vaccination programme. First, it needed to establish that the vaccine was effective. Second, it needed to show that the vaccine was safe. And third, it needed to provide assurances that if any children were adversely affected they would receive adequate support. Each of these approaches became relatively more important than the others at different points of the crisis. At first, arguments about compensation dominated the popular press coverage and were the subject of much discussion in the medical press, Parliament and government departments. Once this principle had been accepted, the debate moved into a second phase, driven by fears that the anticipated 1978/79 epidemic would lead to unnecessary deaths because the government had allowed the vaccination rate to drop too far.

Compensation

The basic principle of vaccine damage payments was accepted, with little opposition from a number of constituencies.[29] The debates began to gain political traction in 1973. Two mothers, Rosemary Fox and Rene Lennon, were featured in the *Birmingham Post*. Their children, Helen and Joanne, had become disabled after vaccinations, and they called for parents with similar experiences to join a campaign for compensation for vaccine damage. The organisation that grew from this was the Association of Parents of Vaccine Damaged Children (APVDC).[30] Fox and Lennon received letters from hundreds of parents, around two-thirds of whom blamed their children's impairment on pertussis vaccine. Despite their own children becoming disabled after the poliomyelitis vaccine, Fox chose to focus attention on this emerging potential scandal, amplifying it through interviews and media appearances.[31] The APVDC drew on the sort of campaigning that had characterised the small but respected groups of the "poverty lobby" that had successfully convinced the Heath government to institute the first disability benefits.[32] These organisations articulated the lived experience of their members through the growing mass media, allying it with sociological research and professional organisational structures to influence government policy. During the 1970s, at least, governments of both parties were receptive to such overtures, given that they both spoke the language of policy makers and exerted enough pressure on public opinion to make elected representatives take notice.[33] APVDC in particular made allies with key parliamentary advocates such as the disability campaigner Jack Ashley, and quickly asserted its position. The two core aims were to 'establish the reality of vaccine damage' and to demand compensation for those affected.[34] It argued that since the government recommended vaccination for the public good, the state should also provide for the individuals whose health was damaged in the pursuit of personal and herd immunity to infectious disease. Because the government's position was so dominant and even doctors (let alone parents) were often not fully informed of the potential risks of vaccination, there was a moral imperative for a compensation scheme within the public health or social security system.[35] By basing these arguments on the existence rather than the extent of vaccine damage, the APVDC was in an advantageous position. It did not have to necessarily prove that vaccine damage was widespread, nor to concern itself with relative weightings of the risks of vaccination versus the disease itself. All that was required was proof that the hazard of vaccine damage was real, and that the number of cases in the country was above zero. The Royal Commission, Family Fund and general attitude towards the welfare state meant that the case for compensation was readily accepted. As the *British Medical Journal* argued soon after the APVDC was established:

> The moral justification for compensation ... is based on the social contract. National immunization programmes not only aim to protect the individual but also to protect society. ... If individuals are asked to accept a risk (even a very small one) partly for the benefit of society then it seems equitable that society should compensate the victims of occasional unlucky mishaps.[36]

Enough stories had emerged in the media and medical press at this time to guide the APVDC's campaign and highlight both the risk and existence of vaccine injury. Although the mere existence of vaccine injury was enough for the moral argument, showing that there were a number of cases helped to turn this into a scandal which the press could parse as a news story.[37] Drs J. V. T. Gosling and J. H. Moseley wrote to the *Guardian* weeks after the APVDC had been created, claiming that DTwP was not effective enough to be worth continuing and could cause brain damage.[38] George Dick, the member of the JCVI who had been cautious over oral polio and smallpox vaccines, also alleged that up to eighty cases of brain damage could be caused by pertussis vaccine each year.[39] Then, more forcefully, the Great Ormond Street doctors M. Kulenkampff, J. S. Schwartzman and J. Wilson published their case studies in *Archives of Disease in Childhood*.[40] After this point, concerns with DTwP appeared credible, even if they were not completely provable or supported by medical consensus. Parliament became interested in the story, and backbenchers from both major parties tabled a number of questions and Early Day Motions calling for inquiries into the vaccine and support for the potential victims.[41] Doctors were, according to Fox, worried that they might have another 'thalidomide episode' on their hands.[42]

The APVDC may have borrowed from the disability poverty lobby in its demands for compensation, but its arguments also resonated with the growing consumer rights movement around health in the 1970s.[43] It was telling that the Consumers' Association lent its support to compensation while still recommending that vaccines were a safe and effective choice for parents wishing to protect their children. The issue surrounded informed consent, with the implication both from supporters and critics of the vaccination programme that parents were capable of making the right choices.[44] When select cases were presented to the Parliamentary Commissioner Sir Idwal Pugh, the final report did not make judgements on the statistical risk or causation of vaccine damage. Instead, it found that the British health departments had 'failed to make available to parents all the information that they should have taken into account' and that doctors appeared to have been poorly advised about the contra-indications that meant children should not be immunised against pertussis.[45] Advice was sent out to doctors to re-emphasise the need to check for contra-indications – a direct way of managing the risk of vaccine damage by further decreasing the likelihood that a susceptible person would be vaccinated.[46]

The DHSS accepted the argument that financial payments to vaccine-damaged children should happen, and began to make preparations. The only questions were about how to make the scheme affordable, how to make it acceptable to the Treasury and how to try to head off potential claims from other special-case groups that could potentially unbalance the social security system.[47] The government slowed down the process by referring the issue to the Royal Commission on Civil Liability and Compensation for Personal Injury. Yet the DHSS also knew that it had to be seen to be doing something, and repeatedly promised that vaccine-damage payments would be enacted as soon as practically possible. 'Political considerations favour an early announcement', Labour Secretary of State for Social Services David Ennals told the Cabinet, lest the administration undermine its reputation 'as a caring government'.[48]

It was not just a moral exercise, however. Restoring confidence in the vaccination programme by providing a safety net for the few affected by vaccine damage was 'vital ... especially because of an outbreak of poliomyelitis this summer – an event for which many people would lay responsibility at the Government's door'.[49] To show that they accepted the principle of compensation, an exchange of correspondence was engineered between Prime Minister James Callaghan and the chair of the Commission, Lord (Colin) Pearson, confirming that it would consider vaccine injury and was very likely to recommend a payment scheme.[50] When the report was published in March 1978 it concluded that 'there is a special case for paying compensation for vaccine damage where vaccination is ... undertaken to protect the community'.[51] Legislation to enact Vaccine Damage Payments went through Parliament quickly, with no opposition, weeks before the vote of no confidence in Prime Minister Callaghan and the subsequent 1979 General Election.[52]

Despite expansions of pension and disability provision under the previous Prime Minister, Harold Wilson, and Secretary of State for Social Services Barbara Castle (both in office 1974–76), Callaghan's premiership was marked by restrictions in spending following the 1973 oil crisis and subsequent loan from the International Monetary Fund in 1976.[53] That the Vaccine Damage Payments Bill 1979 could be passed so quickly said much both about attitudes towards compensation for supposed victims and about the low number of potential claimants. It also demonstrated how seriously the government considered the consequences of a critical lack of confidence in the vaccination programme. The legislation was passed not because vaccine damage was a common occurrence but because the hazard of vaccine damage had become politically unacceptable to multiple constituencies. On the population level, the financial and political benefits of protecting the population from pertussis vastly outweighed the risk of damage in a limited number of children.[54] From a clinical and administrative point of view, then, the advantages and moral imperative to provide support could be justified on the relatively low financial cost of such a scheme – one that was additionally kept low by strict qualification criteria and payment levels that were generally considered to be somewhat parsimonious.[55] For the public, considerations about the real or statistical risk were not so important. The question was a moral one, based on the way that debates about the role of the welfare state had emphasised and prioritised certain risks over others.

Safety

In 1977, the general principle of and preparations for a damage payment scheme had been established. This was aided by the general acceptance of the argument that vaccination worked – that is to say, that it was safe for the vast majority of people and was clearly a technology that protected children and the wider public from deadly diseases. This vaccination narrative had never truly been broken, and while the negative publicity around pertussis vaccination had seen a dramatic fall in the uptake of DTwP vaccination, the uptake of immunisation against diphtheria and tetanus remained relatively robust. This suggested that many parents and doctors had decided to make alternative arrangements to ensure that children were otherwise fully immunised.[56] Once the principle of vaccine payments had been accepted, attention turned towards the danger posed by pertussis itself.

The publicity surrounding the compensation debate had clearly affected parents' confidence in the vaccine (as would also be seen with MMR – Chapter 5). This was reflected most notably in the decline in the pertussis vaccination rate. Criticism of the government's slow progress on compensation payments was largely replaced by concerns that the DHSS was working too slowly to re-establish the vaccination programme.[57] It had commissioned the JCVI and Committee on the Safety of Medicines (CSM) to investigate the science surrounding DTwP, but scheduled arrival of the final results was too late to stop a potential epidemic in the winter of 1978/79.[58] Fox and Ashley regularly had to defend their campaign against accusations of scaremongering and "anti-vaccine" sentiment. While they protested this point, they became useful targets in a new narrative that was being built around the pertussis story.[59] Too much anxiety had been caused by talk of damage, and now there would be a new group of victims – those who would otherwise have been immunised.

Majority medical opinion had consistently extolled the virtues of DTwP and the safety of the pertussis component.[60] However, while publicity about the possibility of brain damage remained, the government felt that it had to be cautious. Thalidomide and other medical tragedies had shown that medical opinion could be wrong. Despite the much more robust and long-term testing on pertussis vaccine than on thalidomide before its widespread use, the potential political fall-out could be catastrophic if the government was mistaken. Thus, much as the hazard of vaccine damage was central to the APVDC's argument, the risk that safety-testing procedures might have failed loomed over the DTwP programme. This reflected the traditional caution showed by the British government and medical establishment with regard to immunisation technology. Like BCG, the whole-cell pertussis vaccine had been developed in the 1920s, but it was not used on a national scale in Britain until the 1950s.[61] In the 1970s, the concern was that if pertussis vaccine was shown to be unsafe, the lack of faith shown in it would spread to other parts of what, up to that point, had been a successful vaccination programme.[62] Gordon Stewart, Professor of Public Health at Glasgow University, made these points repeatedly during the 1970s and 1980s and was a key ally in the case being made by the APVDC against the government in Parliament, in the European Court of Human Rights and in subsequent lawsuits during the 1980s.[63] As a professor with an air of authority and an ability to give the press a good quotation, he maintained an air of doubt in the public mind throughout the 1970s.[64] Over-publicising pertussis vaccination during a time of crisis was therefore thought to be unwise, as it might draw attention to the debate; but without a publicity programme, reinforcing messages about the need for and safety of the vaccine would leave many children unprotected. The Secretary of State, David Ennals, eventually chose to run a national campaign, but ran into problems in doing so.

The DHSS asked medical advisers from the JCVI and the CSM to produce a report on the safety and efficacy of pertussis vaccine. This, it was hoped, would re-establish the vaccine's legitimacy by means of concrete medical statistics and expertise; it also allowed the DHSS to delay making a firm decision on DTwP, as it could argue that it was awaiting scientific confirmation. An interim report came from the JCVI in 1977, while the full details of the investigation were released in 1981.[65] However, the advice to the Secretary of State was not unanimous, and made it difficult to begin a campaign in 1977. The JCVI, whose responsibility was to advise on vaccination policy, firmly believed that the evidence of harm was slight and the evidence in favour of the efficacy of the vaccine was indisputable. The JCVI's data also suggested that an epidemic would occur in 1978/79, and that many more children would be infected due to years of under-immunisation.[66] The CSM, whose responsibility was to ensure that drugs were safe and used in an appropriate manner, wanted to wait until the full results of safety testing were available. While the causation relationship between pertussis vaccine and brain damage was very difficult to prove, it was also impossible to disprove (or at least show that there was no evidence for it) until a full investigation had been completed.[67] Once the Vaccine Damage Payments Bill had been used to 'mollify' the APVDC's campaign, however, the government as a whole became more willing to promote DTwP in the light of growing evidence that the vaccine was indeed safe and effective.[68] The risk of the anticipated epidemic and possible damage to other areas of the vaccination programme far outweighed the likelihood that the campaign would face a negative reaction from anxious parents. Adverts were placed in major daily newspapers outlining the risks and benefits of vaccination. The emphasis was on choice, but with a clear message that the most logical choice was to have one's child vaccinated. 'Vaccination protects', explained the headline. 'These facts will help you make your decision – but your doctor is there to advise you.' While no exact figure was given for vaccination injuries (either as a percentage of all vaccines or as an absolute), the full-page advertisement quoted the decrease in morbidity of pertussis and diphtheria since the vaccination programmes against the diseases began.[69] It marked a distinct change in tone from the diphtheria and smallpox campaigns described in Chapters 1 and 2. Rather than focusing on the potential catastrophic consequences of failing to follow government advice, the adverts were presented as more sober reflections on the benefits of vaccination over the risk of catching the diseases against which they protected.

With the campaign running and the Vaccine Damage Payments Bill going through Parliament, the bulk of negative media coverage was now over. Some areas saw a large increase in demand, causing supply shortages of the pertussis vaccine reminiscent of the strains put on poliomyelitis vaccine supplies during the Jeff Hall incident and the outbreak in Liverpool.[70] Doubts about whole-cell pertussis vaccine did not disappear entirely. Court cases against the DHSS with regard to pertussis vaccine damage occasionally surfaced in the 1980s, although negligence was never proved and vaccination rates recovered.[71] Outbreaks in 1982 and 1986 showed that pertussis was still a threat, but 1990 was the last year in which there were over 10,000 cases.[72] What this entire episode had exposed was that the government's protection role was complex, and public attitudes towards vaccination were not straightforward. Both the government and parents juggled multiple risks, weighing up their relative importance based on a range of factors. Parents appeared to avoid DTwP, but were able and willing to have their children immunised with DT. The press shifted its focus from the risks of damage without compensation to the risks to a population without adequate immunisation coverage. Medical advisers produced conflicting advice depending on their remit and specialisation – from the JCVI, which became most concerned with the risk of an infectious disease outbreak to the CSM, which was preoccupied with the risk of vaccine damage. The medical profession focused on statistics regarding safety and efficacy, advocating widespread use of DTwP to stave off pertussis outbreaks, yet paying close attention to contra-indications so as to manage the risk of vaccine damage. Voluntary organisations concerned themselves with the financial and social risks to all vaccine-damaged children, regardless of how many or few there were.

Rubella "crisis"

At the same time as this public debate surrounding vaccine damage, a lower-profile argument was brewing between the DHSS and voluntary organisations. The APVDC's compensation campaign had gained political traction by emphasising the problems associated with uncompensated disability and the government's inability to recognise the specific needs of children damaged as a direct result of government policy. Another disease also carried with it the potential for disability. In this case the issue was not that the government could cause disability by commission; rather, while a vaccine existed but was not widely administered to at-risk groups, the government could allow disability to occur through omission.

In 1978 there was a rubella epidemic across Britain. In itself, this was not considered to be a great problem. Rubella (or German measles) is a mostly harmless childhood disease. It causes a rash, mild fever and swollen glands. Although in rare cases it can cause complications, symptoms can be so mild that many people catch it and do not realise that they have been infected. However, rubella can be dangerous in pregnant women. It can lead to Congenital Rubella Syndrome (CRS), which can cause blindness, deafness and problems in the functioning of key organs such as the brain and the heart in new-borns.[73] Such were the risks that it was standard practice to recommend termination to women who contracted rubella in early pregnancy. To combat CRS, the government began the routine vaccination of teenage girls in schools in 1970, so that gradually the cohort of child-bearing women would be fully protected from rubella.[74] Women were also offered the vaccine, but they had to undergo blood tests to determine whether or not they were immune to the disease beforehand. Since there was a risk of damage to the foetus if a woman became pregnant within three months of being vaccinated, authorities did not want to risk vaccinating women who would not directly benefit. Because of the inconvenience of this testing system, it was less common for non-school-age girls to be vaccinated.[75] The 1978 epidemic therefore came too soon for the programme to achieve a high degree of coverage. The first group of girls to be vaccinated would have been around 21 years old in 1978, leaving the majority of fertile women unprotected and therefore potentially at risk of their babies developing CRS. It would be an exaggeration to call this debate a crisis, since it gained nowhere near the public attention of damage payments and pertussis. Yet it was significant, and worrying enough to force the DHSS into action.

The Spastics Society and the National Association for Deaf/Blind and Rubella Children (NADBRC) both had an interest in preventing CRS. Both were charities established in the 1950s to provide services for disabled people. The latter submitted evidence to the Royal Commission's chapter on ante-natal injury in 1975, arguing for a compensation scheme similar to that for the thalidomide children and (later) vaccine-damaged children.[76] Along with the children's committee of the Central Health Services Council, they urged the government to embark on a campaign of mass immunisation of young women to improve protection against the disease. On the current policy of focusing on vaccinating only in schools, it would take until the end of the century to fully immunise all females who might go on to bear children.[77] The DHSS also wanted to increase the population of immune women, but there were barriers to mass immunisation. First, the goal of the programme was not to eliminate rubella, as was the case with other diseases; it was to prevent pregnant women from becoming infected. Thus, the target population was only teenage girls and women of child-bearing age rather than the entire public. Second, the mass vaccination of all females in the target population could exacerbate the problem. Women were advised not to get pregnant within three months of receiving the vaccine. A mass programme would, of course, vaccinate more women – meaning that there was an increased chance of vaccinating pregnant or soon-to-be-pregnant women. This would lead to an increase in abortions and/or children born with CRS. Such a risk would have been politically damaging both to the reputation of vaccination programmes in general and to the government's electoral chances, given the sensitivity around the subject of abortion. This was closely related to a third problem, the pertussis vaccine crisis. Any attempts to run a mass advertising campaign while doubts had been expressed about other parts of the programme and while the DHSS was still uncertain about its publicity efforts was politically challenging.[78]

As with pertussis, the DHSS took the JCVI's advice that it should intensify the anti-CRS campaign, but that it should do so by getting local Area Health Authorities to work with women, rather than through a 'crash' national campaign.[79] Implementation was delayed by the general election, but the plans were carried through by the new Thatcher administration in June 1979.[80] As an interim measure, the government tried to ensure that immunisation rates remained as high as possible among school girls by distributing information leaflets through the Health Education Council in November 1978.[81] The DHSS also made a concerted effort to target immigrant communities where the rates of rubella were known to be higher and potential mothers were much less likely to have come through the school system or to have been in contact with health services before and during the early stages of pregnancy. Advertisements were placed in Urdu, Hindi and Punjabi newspapers read by the South Asian diaspora in Britain, urging women to visit their local health centre and ask about rubella vaccination.[82]

These developments came too late for the Spastics Society led by General Secretary James Loring. Frustrated at the slow progress made by the JCVI and the DHSS, in November 1978 the Society ran its own campaign to increase the number of women presenting for vaccination. It had been approached by parents worried by recent media coverage about the rubella epidemic and increased risk of CRS, and wrote to the Minister of State (Health) Roland Moyle to tell him that it would launch a campaign if the DHSS did not already have one planned to start soon. It accused the government of 'gross neglect'.[83] Its newspaper advert led with the headline 'Urgent Warning – German Measles can damage your unborn baby', before encouraging women to present for testing and possible vaccination.[84] Backed by prominent London Labour politician Peggy Jay, this form of activism caused frustration for the Chief Medical Officer, Sir Henry Yellowlees.

> Any campaign by the Spastics Society would be premature and embarrassing. ... Overworked staff in the Department are trying their best to prepare for the extension [to rubella vaccination] ... At present, this work is being held up while the staff deal with approaches from Mrs Peggy Jay and from the Spastics Society to several different parts of the Department and now to Ministers.[85]

Neither the DHSS nor the BMA was concerned about a lack of vaccine supply (unless there was an unprecedented surge in demand). They were worried about the blood testing service's ability to cope with the screening required before giving women the vaccine.[86] Since the government planned to begin its own publicity programme over the coming months, the Spastics Society's approach could create a large-scale advertising campaign that the JCVI had been keen to avoid.[87] There was also a high risk of misinformation. The Society reported a positive response to its campaign from family planning centres, with requests for reprints of its press advertisements and other material. Yet it also received complaints from women who were told by their general practitioners that the vaccine was not necessary or were given conflicting advice about how long after vaccination they should avoid pregnancy. As with pertussis, the argument was that a lack of education on the part of doctors, rather than the public, was an impediment to good protection. Loring wrote to the Secretary of State:

> It appears that the public when given the facts is willing to act responsibly to protect their health, but this action cannot be successful if doctors are not fully aware of the correct procedures and the advice that they should be giving.[88]

The annotations made by a DHSS civil servant on a copy of Loring's letter suggest that some of these criticisms appeared to be out of context. Nonetheless, the lack of a harmonised government campaign, including education for the public and for medical professionals, appeared to bear out the BMA's and Yellowlees' concerns. The risks of CRS needed to be managed through central coordination, as the vaccination programme included more than simply the availability of vaccine. Organised public activism of the type being pushed by the Spastics Society could, as far as the DHSS was concerned, cause a different set of issues around public confidence in the system. It may well have been that the only material difference between the Society and the Department was over timing;[89] but, as the Minister was advised to answer on the radio in the event of being asked why the campaign was not launched sooner:

> You know, I am beginning to think we are wrong whatever we do. It is, for example, the case that, towards the end of last year, the Faculty of Community Medicine warned the Department against having a rubella vaccination campaign because of the attitude of the public which, at the time, was against vaccination generally.[90]

The epidemic appeared to have brought attention to CRS and increased demand for rubella vaccination – but from and for whom? The campaign being led by the Spastics Society touched on an area that the DHSS was acting upon following advice from the Central Health Services Council and the JCVI. For the most part, debate in the medical community appears to have focused on how best to improve uptake and efficiency of vaccination in women, although some argued that universal routine childhood vaccination would help to eliminate the disease entirely, rather than simply immunising individuals to prevent CRS.[91] NADBRC and the Spastics Society were both what the disability rights movement would call traditional charities, often staffed and run by middle-class people concerned with the medical aspects of impairment rather than with tackling structural inequalities that made discrimination against disabled people worse.[92] Class had shown itself to be a factor in rubella immunisation before. Girls in private schools, for instance, had been shown to be far less likely to get the vaccine than those from state schools.[93] Now, one DHSS civil servant wondered, were the women writing to the Spastics Society becoming concerned because of reports in the *Sunday Times*? If so, 'it will be interesting to see the response of the "Mail" and "Express" readership'.[94]

As with vaccine damage, it is striking how relatively few people were potentially at risk of disability. In 1975, NADBRC claimed a membership of 424, representing some 196 deaf/blind people.[95] Similarly, the

APVDC told Lord Pearson that it had amassed 356 cases of serious vaccine damage.[96] This was not a problem on the scale of poliomyelitis in the 1950s or diphtheria in the 1940s. It was about a smaller number of people in serious need, made visible by campaigning for expanded welfare state provision, and the relative importance of these cases now that other serious infectious diseases had been reduced to negligible levels. As the state's duty to protect and care for serious disability increased, the need to reduce the risk of the onset of serious impairment also rose. Long-term health problems were becoming the main focus of health systems during this period of the twentieth century, and the Labour government had given much thought to how preventative medicine could reduce the burden on welfare services.[97] Vaccination had a role to play in this epidemiological transition. Even though the DHSS could not provide the Treasury with an exact cost-to-benefit figure, from 1971 to 1974 there were, on average, forty-two cases of CRS per year and 801 terminations.[98] The expanded anti-rubella programme was therefore 'highly desirable … both in terms of the avoidance of human suffering and of savings to the health and social services.'[99]

The rubella vaccination debate might not have become a public crisis on the level of pertussis, but it did reflect certain sections of the public demanding protection from the government in the form of increased vaccination coverage. For financial and moral reasons, the government broadly accepted its obligation to manage this risk, although there were disagreements about how quickly and to what extent such protection should be offered. We must be cautious about arguing that the Spastics Society and NADBRC were representative of the general public. They did, however, show wider concerns about the role of the government and the welfare state in protecting people against the risks of disability that were seen in other areas of policy. When we look at the drop in the number of CRS cases and terminations, attempts to improve coverage did broadly work. In the four years up to the introduction MMR in 1988, there were an average of twenty-two cases a year and seventy-three terminations.[100]

Conclusions

In 1978, Michael Church of the Health Education Council wrote to the *British Medical Journal* calling for 'an index of health risks, meaningfully related and straightforwardly stated'. Quoting the recent lecture by Lord Rothschild on broadcast on BBC1, he proclaimed that 'there is no such thing as a risk-free society'. 'What we need' is 'some guidance as to when to flap and when not'.[101] Both pertussis and rubella vaccination policy, however, showed that "flapping" depended on the constituency and the information available. The risk of vaccine damage to any one person in the population may have been slight, but the consequences for the family that became affected were total.[102] CRS and vaccine damage were small-scale problems in terms of the gross numbers affected, but the difficulties faced by those affected compelled the government to demonstrate that it was able to offer protection for these groups.

To say that the pertussis vaccine crisis constituted a crisis of faith in vaccination is too simplistic. The contemporary campaigns for rubella immunisation, as well as the shift in tone of the press towards providing adequate levels of whooping cough vaccination demonstrate that the vaccination narrative was alive and well. Rather, for a brief period, segments of the public lost faith in the government's ability to manage risk. Once the safety of the vaccine had been re-asserted and a damage payments scheme had been promised, immunisation rates began to recover and the overall programme was kept intact. The crisis must therefore be understood within the wider context of anxieties over the role of the welfare state in the late 1970s. The financial crisis had led to political debates about what financial protections the state could offer through social security, a fully funded health service and so on. Public health was not isolated from such matters. Both pertussis and rubella vaccination were part of the state's role as protector of the nation's health both from infectious disease and from medical neglect. The DHSS had to address the concerns of parents over vaccine damage while providing a comprehensive vaccination programme backed by high immunisation rates. Collective risks of infectious disease were weighed against the individual risks of disability. Throughout, it received conflicting messages from parliamentarians, different expert groups, medical advisers and the public (whose voice was refracted through the press and voluntary organisations).

The pertussis crisis is now used as a "lesson from history" by public health professionals. It is seen as a good example of how a mature vaccination programme in a high-income setting can undergo a loss in public confidence. Similar incidents in Japan, the United States and elsewhere have shown how individual vaccines can be doubted at times, while national vaccination systems remain largely robust.[103] Global public health research now monitors and theorises vaccine confidence and vaccine hesitancy to try to anticipate and avoid such problems.[104] In the United Kingdom context, the pertussis vaccine crisis became a guiding example in the management of a crisis which was not adequately anticipated – MMR.

Notes

1 Swansea Research Unit of the Royal College of General Practitioners, 'Effect of a low pertussis vaccination take-up on a large community', *British Medical Journal (Clinical Research Edition)*, 282:6257 (1981), 23–6.
2 Jeffrey P. Baker, 'The pertussis vaccine controversy in Great Britain, 1974–1986', *Vaccine*, 21:25–26 (2003), 4003–10.
3 Virginia Berridge, *Marketing Health* (Oxford: Oxford University Press, 2007).
4 For a summary of these approaches, see Jakob Arnoldi, *Risk: An Introduction* (Cambridge: Polity, 2009), esp. pp. 38–66; Baruch Fischoff and John Kadvany, *Risk: A Very Short Introduction* (Oxford: Oxford University Press, 2011).
5 See Ulrich Beck, *Risk Society: Towards a New Modernity* (London: Sage, 1992).
6 Mary Douglas and Aaron Wildavsky, *Risk and Culture* (Berkeley: University of California Press, 1983).
7 Michel Foucault, *The Birth of the Clinic: An Archaeology of Medical Perception* (London: Tavistock, 1973); Michel Foucault, *Discipline and Punish: The Birth of the Prison* (New York: Pantheon Books, 1977).
8 Brian Abel-Smith and Peter Townsend, *The Poor and the Poorest: A New Analysis of the Ministry of Labour's Family Expenditure Surveys of 1953–54 and 1960* (London: Bell, 1965); Paul Whiteley and Steve Winyard, *Pressure for the Poor: The Poverty Lobby and Policy Making* (London: Methuen, 1987).
9 Katrina F. Brown, J. Simon Kroll, Michael J. Hudson, Mary Ramsay, John Green, Charles A. Vincent, Graham Fraser and Nick Sevdalis, 'Omission bias and vaccine rejection by parents of healthy children: implications for the influenza A/H1N1 vaccination programme', *Vaccine*, 28:25 (2010), 4181–5; Jacqueline R. Meszaros, David A. Asch, Jonathan Baron, John

C. Hershey, Howard Kunreuther and Joanne Schwartz-Buzaglo, 'Cognitive processes and the decisions of some parents to forego pertussis vaccination for their children', *Journal of Clinical Epidemiology*, 49:6 (1996), 697–703; Abigail L. Wroe, Angela Bhan, Paul Salkovskis and Helen Bedford, 'Feeling bad about immunising our children', *Vaccine*, 23:12 (2005), 1428–33.

10 Katrina F. Brown, J. Simon Kroll, Michael J. Hudson, Mary Ramsay, John Green, Susannah J. Long, Charles A. Vincent, Graham Fraser and Nick Sevdalis, 'Factors underlying parental decisions about combination childhood vaccinations including MMR: A systematic review', *Vaccine*, 28:26 (2010), 4235–48; Andrea Kitta, *Vaccinations and Public Concern in History: Legend, Rumor, and Risk Perception* (New York: Routledge, 2012); Julie S. Downs, Wändi Bruine de Bruin and Baruch Fischhoff, 'Parents' vaccination comprehension and decisions', *Vaccine*, 26:12 (2008), 1595–607.

11 On the historical narratives surrounding vaccination decision making, see Kitta, *Vaccinations and Public Concern in History*.

12 Baker, 'The pertussis vaccine controversy'.

13 Arnoldi, *Risk*.

14 On this, see the introduction to this book and: Dorothy Porter, *Health Citizenship: Essays in Social Medicine and Biomedical Politics* (Berkeley: University of California Press, 2011); Frank Huisman and Harry Oosterhuis, 'The politics of health and citizenship: Historical and contemporary perspectives', in Frank Huisman and Harry Oosterhuis (eds), *Heath and Citizenship: Political Cultures of Health in Modern Europe* (London: Pickering and Chatto, 2014), pp. 1–40.

15 See Centers for Disease Control and Prevention, 'Pertussis (whooping cough)' (27 June 2016) www.cdc.gov/pertussis/about/index.html (accessed 6 June 2017); Anne Hardy, *The Epidemic Streets: Infectious Disease and the Rise of Preventive Medicine, 1856–1900* (Oxford: Oxford University Press, 1993), pp. 9–27.

16 Public Health England, 'Table 6: Pertussis notifications and deaths, England and Wales: 1940–2014' (5 May 2016) www.gov.uk/government/uploads/system/uploads/attachment_data/file/521438/Table_6_Pertussis_notifications_and_deaths__E_W__1940_-_2015.pdf (accessed 6 June 2017).

17 See Chapter 1 and TNA: INF 12/238, Specification Sheet – Campaigns – 14 February 1953; Ministry of Health, *Report of the Ministry of Health for the Year 1957. Part II on the State of the Public Health being the Annual Report of the Chief Medical Officer* (Cmnd 559) (London, 1958).

18 Medical Research Council, 'Vaccination against whooping-cough; relation between protection in children and results of laboratory tests; a report to the Whooping-cough Immunization Committee of the Medical Research Council and to the medical officers of health for Cardiff, Leeds, Leyton, Manchester, Middlesex, Oxford, Poole, Tottenham, Walthamstow, and Wembley', *British Medical Journal*, 2:4990 (1956), 454–62.
19 Baker, 'The pertussis vaccine controversy'.
20 Public Health England, 'Pertussis notifications and deaths'.
21 M. Kulenkampff, J. S. Schwartzman and J. Wilson, 'Neurological complications of pertussis inoculation', *Archives of Disease in Childhood*, 49:1 (1974), 46–9.
22 Baker, 'The pertussis vaccine controversy'.
23 See Chapter 5 and: E. J. Gangarosa, A. M. Galazka, C. R. Wolfe, L. M. Phillips, E. Miller, R. T. Chen and R. E. Gangarosa, 'Impact of anti-vaccine movements on pertussis control: the untold story', *The Lancet*, 351:9099 (1998), 356–61; Rachel Casiday, 'Risk communication in the British pertussis and MMR vaccine controversies', in Peter Bennett, Kenneth Calman, Sarah Curtis and Denis Fischbacher-Smith (eds), *Risk Communication and Public Health*, 2nd edn (Oxford: Oxford University Press, 2010), pp. 129–46; Maria A. Riolo, Aaron A. King and Pejman Rohani, 'Can vaccine legacy explain the British pertussis resurgence?', *Vaccine*, 31 (2013), 5903–8. On the capacity of history to teach lessons to policy makers, see Virginia Berridge, Martin Gorsky and Alex Mold, *Public Health in History* (Maidenhead: Open University Press, October 2011).
24 Arnoldi, *Risk*, pp. 9–10.
25 Jameel Hampton, *Disability and the Welfare State in Britain: Changes in Perception and Policy 1948–1979* (Bristol: Policy Press, 2016); Gareth Millward, 'Social security policy and the early disability movement – expertise, disability and the government, 1965–1977', *Twentieth Century British History*, 26:2 (2015), 274–97.
26 Sunday Times, *Suffer the Children: The Story of Thalidomide* (New York: Viking Press, 1979); Jack Ashley, *Acts of Defiance* (London: Reinhardt, 1992); Derek Kinrade, *Alf Morris: People's Parliamentarian: Scenes from the Life of Lord Morris of Manchester* (London: National Information Forum, 2007).
27 HC Deb (29 November 1972) vol. 847, col. 446. Colin Pearson, *Royal Commission on Civil Liability and Compensation for Personal Injury Vol.1* (Cmnd 7054-I) (London: HMSO, 1978).
28 On the role of disability politics in the crisis, see Gareth Millward, 'A disability act? The Vaccine Damage Payments Act 1979 and the British

government's response to the pertussis vaccine scare', *Social History of Medicine*, 30:2 (2016), 429–47. On thalidomide and general disability policy, see Claire Sewell, '"If one member of the family is disabled the family as a whole is disabled": Thalidomide children and the emergence of the family carer in Britain, c. 1957–1978', *Family & Community History*, 18:1 (2015), 37–52.
29 See in particular Pearson, *Royal Commission on Civil Liability* (Cmnd 7054-I), p. 296.
30 TNA: MH 154/1053, '"Society should compensate for brain damage"', *Birmingham Post* (26 June 1973) [page numbers omitted]; Mary McCormack, 'The hazards of health', *Guardian* (3 August 1973), p. 11; Rosemary Fox, *Helen's Story* (London: John Blake, 2006).
31 Fox effectively took the lead in the campaign, acting as the organisation's spokesperson and general secretary. On her tactics see Fox, *Helen's Story*.
32 Whiteley and Winyard, *Pressure for the Poor*; Matthew Hilton, Nick Crowson, Jean-François Mouhot and James McKay, *The Politics of Expertise: How NGOs Shaped Modern Britain* (Oxford: Oxford University Press, 2013); Hampton, *Disability and the Welfare State in Britain*; Millward, 'Social security policy and the early disability movement'.
33 Hilton et al, *The Politics of Expertise*.
34 Fox, *Helen's Story*, p. 28.
35 These arguments were brought before the Parliamentary Commissioner for Administration, see Parliamentary Commissioner for Administration, *Sixth Report for Session 1976–77: Whooping Cough Vaccination* (HC 571) (London: HMSO, 1977).
36 Anon, 'Help for victims of immunizations', *British Medical Journal*, 1:5856 (1973), 758–9.
37 On how advocates and publicity turn political issues and events into "scandals", see Mark Drakeford and Ian Butler, *Scandal, Social Policy and Social Welfare*, 2nd edn, (Bristol: Policy Press 2006).
38 J. V. T. Gosling and J. H. Moseley, 'To jab or not to jab?', *Guardian* (20 August 1973), p. 9.
39 William Breckon, 'A vaccinating question', *Guardian* (29 August 1973), p. 9. See also G. W. A. Dick, 'Letter: whooping-cough vaccine', *British Medical Journal*, 4:5989 (1975), 161. On Dick's concerns with OPV and smallpox, see Chapters 2 and 3.
40 Kulenkampff, Schwartzman and Wilson, 'Neurological complications of pertussis inoculation'.
41 TNA: MH 154/1053; PIN 35/549. For questions from MPs, especially Jack Ashley and Robert Adley (Conservative, Bristol North East), see HC Deb (17 January 1974) vol. 867, cc. 172–5W; HC Deb (1 July 1976)

vol. 914, cc. 277–8W; HC Deb (2 November 1976) vol. 918, cc. 547–8W; HC Deb (20 December 1976) vol. 923, cc. 240–59; HC Deb (17 January 1977) vol. 924, cc. 73–4W; HC Deb (7 February 1977) vol. 925, cc. 575–7W; and passim. Early Day Motion 70 (1974–75) had been signed by 'more than 50' MPs by 3 December 1974. It read, 'That this House is concerned at the lack of statistics concerning vaccine-damaged children: believes that their case for compensation is at least as just as those children suffering as a result of the thalidomide tragedy; and demands an immediate investigation into the problem.' HC Deb (3 December 1974) vol. 882, cc. 1514–26.
42 Mary McCormack, 'The hazards of health', *Guardian* (3 August 1973), p. 11.
43 Alex Mold, *Making the Patient-consumer: Patient Organisations and Health Consumerism in Britain* (Manchester: Manchester University Press, 2015).
44 Violet Johnstone, 'Common sense about whooping cough vaccine', *Daily Telegraph* (6 October 1974), p. 10; Suzanne Lowry, 'Needle points', *Guardian* (20 October 1975), p. 9; Hugh Herbert, 'Which? backs vaccine injury compensation', *Guardian* (13 January 1977), p. 7; John Stevenson, 'Who is to blame for the great vaccination fiasco?', *Daily Mail* (13 January 1977), p. 12.
45 Parliamentary Commissioner for Administration, *Whooping Cough Vaccination* (HC571), pp. 3, 17–22.
46 'Doctors get stronger code on vaccine', *Daily Telegraph* (15 April 1977), p. 8.
47 See debates over implementation in TNA: BN 13/360.
48 TNA: CAB 129/195/16, David Ennals, Payment for Vaccine Damaged Children, 2 May 1977.
49 *Ibid.*
50 TNA: BN 120/10, James Callaghan to Lord Pearson, 6 June 977 and reply 9 June 1977. See also HC Deb (14 June 1977) vol. 933, cc. 240–1.
51 Pearson, *Royal Commission on Civil Liability* (Cmnd 7054-I), p. 296.
52 Millward, 'A disability act?'
53 Chris Rogers, 'The politics of economic policy making in Britain: A reassessment of the 1976 IMF crisis', *Politics & Policy*, 37:5 (2009), 971–94; Colin Hay, 'Chronicles of a death foretold: The Winter of Discontent and construction of crisis of British Keynesianism', *Parliamentary Affairs*, 63 (2010), 446–70; Barbara Castle, *Fighting All the Way* (London: Pan Books, 1994); Bernard Donoughue, *Prime Minister: The Conduct of Policy under Harold Wilson and James Callaghan* (London: Cape, 1987).
54 This point was made in the Cabinet papers surrounding the decision to bring forward the Bill. TNA: CAB 128/61/18, CM(77) 18th Conclusions,

Cabinet minutes, 5 May 1977 10.30am, 10; CAB 129/195/14, Vaccine Damage; CAB 129/195/16, Payment for Vaccine Damaged Children; HC Deb (8 February 1977) vol. 925, cc. 1227–39.

55 The Act provided £10,000 lump sums rather than the regular payments that the APVDC had hoped for. See TNA: BN 13/360; Fox, *Helen's Story*; Millward, 'A disability act?' This continues to be contentious. See Wendy E. Stephen, 'Re: UK doctors re-examine case for mandatory vaccination', *British Medical Journal*, 358 (2017), j3414.

56 The Royal Commission's statistics showed that in 1972 81 per cent of children born in 1970 had been vaccinated against diphtheria and tetanus, 79 per cent against pertussis and 80 per cent against polio. In 1976, the equivalent figures were 75, 38 and 74 per cent. Pearson, *Royal Commission on Civil Liability* (Cmnd 7054-I), p. 293.

57 John Stevenson, 'Who is to blame for the great vaccination fiasco?', *Daily Mail* (13 January 1977), p. 12.

58 Joint Committee on Vaccination and Immunisation, *Whooping Cough Vaccination: Review of the Evidence on Whooping Cough Vaccination* (London: HMSO, 1977); Department of Health and Social Security, Committee on Safety of Medicines and Joint Committee on Vaccination and Immunisation, *Whooping Cough: Reports from the Committee on Safety of Medicines and the Joint Committee on Vaccination and Immunisation* (London: HMSO, 1981).

59 For Ashley, see especially Ashley, *Acts of Defiance*. HC Deb (5 February 1979) vol. 962, col. 33; HL Deb (12 January 1994) vol. 551, col. 124. Fox and the APVDC repeated the line that they were not anti-vaccine and framed their campaign around choice and informed consent. See Mary McCormack, 'The hazards of health', *Guardian* (3 August 1973), p. 11; 'Bringing the law up to scratch', *Guardian* (7 August 1974); Fox, *Helen's Story*, p. 248.

60 Baker, 'The pertussis vaccine controversy'; Anon, 'Whooping-cough immunisation.', *British Medical Journal*, 2:6078 (July 1977), 5–6.

61 Linda Bryder, '"We shall not find salvation in inoculation": BCG vaccination in Scandinavia, Britain and the USA, 1921–1960', *Social Science & Medicine*, 49:9 (1999), 1157–67. See also the debates on diphtheria immunisation in the 1930s and 1940s in Chapter 1.

62 Immunisation rates had fallen for other diseases, but not as dramatically as for pertussis. Pearson, *Royal Commission on Civil Liability* (Cmnd 7054-I), p. 293.

63 Baker, 'The pertussis vaccine controversy'; G. T. Stewart, 'Vaccination against whooping-cough', *Lancet*, 1:8005 (1977), 234–7; G. T. Stewart, 'The law tries to decide whether whooping cough vaccine causes brain

damage: Professor Gordon Stewart gives evidence', *British Medical Journal (Clinical Research Edition)*, 293:6540 (1986), 203–4; Fox, *Helen's Story*. For the European case, see MH 154/1057.

64 On Stewart's role in the press, see Baker, 'The pertussis vaccine controversy'. See also Alison Shaw, 'Gordon Stewart, expert in public health and colleague of Fleming who helped pioneer the use of penicillin', *Herald* (15 November 2016) www.heraldscotland.com/opinion/obituaries/14904952.Obituary___Gordon_Stewart__expert_in_public_health_and_colleague_of_Fleming_who_helped_pioneer_the_use_of_penicillin/ (accessed 19 June 2017).

65 Joint Committee on Vaccination and Immunisation, *Whooping Cough Vaccination*; Department of Health and Social Security, Committee on Safety of Medicines and Joint Committee on Vaccination and Immunisation, *Whooping Cough*.

66 Joint Committee on Vaccination and Immunisation, *Whooping Cough Vaccination*.

67 Pearson, *Royal Commission on Civil Liability* (Cmnd 7054-I), p. 298; Anon, 'Whooping-cough immunisation'.

68 TNA: CAB 128/61/18, CM(77) 18th Conclusions, Cabinet minutes, 5 May 1977 10.30am, 10; 'Vaccination campaign shelved', *Guardian* (22 November 1977), p. 4; 'Minister defers campaign to encourage vaccination', *The Times* (22 November 1977), p. 2; 'Vaccine campaign launched soon', *Guardian* (8 February 1978), p. 5.

69 See Department of Health and Social Security, 'Vaccination protects', *Daily Mail* (15 March 1978), p. 5.

70 'Cough alert over vaccine', *Daily Mail* (16 December 1977), p. 17; 'Rush for cough vaccine "could do harm"', *Guardian* (19 December 1977), p. 2.

71 Baker, 'The pertussis vaccine controversy'.

72 See Figure 4.1 and Public Health England, 'Pertussis notifications and deaths'. Due to improvements in detection and diagnosis, data after 2005 are not comparable; even so, after 1991 there was only one year in which there were more than 5,000 cases.

73 Public Health England and Department of Health, *Immunisation against Infectious Disease*, 2nd edn (London: Public Health England, 2013), pp. 343–6.

74 TNA: BS 14/28, Children's Committee CC78(2)(5), Prevention of Rubella Deformities in the Newborn.

75 A. J. Vyse, N. J. Gay, J. M. White, M. E. Ramsay, D. W. G. Brown, B. J. Cohen, L. M. Hesketh, P. Morgan-Capner and E. Miller, 'Evolution of surveillance of measles, mumps, and rubella in England and Wales:

providing the platform for evidence-based vaccination policy', *Epidemiological Reviews*, 24:2 (2002), 125–36.
76 TNA: LCO 20/1293, Summary Ev523, The National Association for Deaf/Blind and Rubella Children, July 1975.
77 TNA: BS 14/28, Brimblecombe statement on rubella, 2 November 1978; Raymond Clarke [Secretary, Children's Committee] to P. J. Fletcher [Central Health Services Council], 20 December 1978.
78 TNA: BS 14/28, Central Health Services Council, Rubella Vaccination, Paper by the Department, CHSC(79)10, December 1978; HC Deb (7 November 1978) vol. 957, cc. 110–2W.
79 TNA: BS 14/28, Rubella Vaccination Campaign Appendix, Recommendations by the Joint Committee on Vaccination and Immunisation and the Rubella Vaccination Sub-Committee of the JCVI.
80 TNA: BS 14/28, Health Circular HC(79)15/Local Authority Letter LAC(79)8, Rubella Vaccination, June 1979.
81 'Leaflet is first step in rubella campaign', *The Times* (9 November 1978), p. 4.
82 TNA: BS 14/28, Health Circular HC(79)15/Local Authority Letter LAC(79)8, Rubella Vaccination, June 1979; TNA: MH 154/1471, Advertisements for Amar Deep Weekly (18 July 1979), Navin Weekly (29 July 1979), Punjab Times (17 July 1979) and Mashriq Weekly (26 July 1979 to 1 August 1979).
83 TNA: MH 154/1466, A. W. Jones, Rubella – Radio 4 interview 8 November 1978.
84 See for example, Spastics Society, 'Urgent warning', *Guardian* (2 November 1978), p. 11.
85 TNA: MH 154/1465, Yellowlees to Moyle, Immunisation against rubella, 23 October 1978.
86 TNA: MH 154/1466, Yellowlees to R. A. Keable-Elliot [BMA], 13 November 1978.
87 TNA: MH 154/1464, M. J. Lowe [BMA assistant Secretary] to Yellowlees, 2 November 1978.
88 TNA: MH 154/1466, Loring to Ennals, 18 December 1978.
89 TNA: MH 154/1466, Ennals to Loring, 1 November 1978.
90 TNA: MH 154/1466, A. W. Jones, Rubella – Radio 4 interview 8 November 1978.
91 L. A. Crawford, 'Rubella vaccination', *British Medical Journal*, 1:6125 (1978), 1485; W. M. Styles, 'Rubella immunisation', *British Medical Journal*, 2:6140 (1978), 834.
92 Michael Oliver, *The Politics of Disablement* (London: Macmillan Education, 1990); Hilton et al, *The Politics of Expertise*.

93 'Vaccination less likely for girls at private schools', *The Times* (18 October 1977), p. 6.
94 TNA: MH 154/1465, J. B. Benwell, Rubella Immunisation, 20 October 1978.
95 TNA: LCO 20/1293, Summary Ev523, The National Association for Deaf/Blind and Rubella Children, July 1975.
96 Pearson, *Royal Commission on Civil Liability* (Cmnd 7054-I), p. 294.
97 Department of Health and Social Security, Department of Education and Science, Scottish Office and Welsh Office, *Prevention and Health* (Cmnd 7047) (London: HMSO, 1977). See also George Weisz, *Chronic Disease in the Twentieth Century* (Baltimore: Johns Hopkins University Press, 2014); Berridge, *Marketing Health*. See also the work of Peder Clark on public health responses to heart disease, '"Problems of today and tomorrow": prevention and the National Health Service in the 1970s', *Social History of Medicine* (forthcoming).
98 Vyse et al, 'Evolution of surveillance of measles, mumps, and rubella in England and Wales'.
99 TNA: BS 14/28, Central Health Services Council, Rubella Vaccination, Paper by the Department, CHSC(79)10, December 1978.
100 Reductions from 42 and 801, respectively, in the period 1971–74. Vyse et al, 'Evolution of surveillance of measles, mumps, and rubella in England and Wales'.
101 M. Church, 'Return of whooping cough', *British Medical Journal*, 1:6157 (1979), 195. Lord Rothschild's lecture was part of the *Richard Dimbleby Lecture* series. See BBC, 'The Richard Dimbleby Lecture (original broadcast 23 November 1978) www.bbc.co.uk/programmes/p00fr9fs (accessed 19 June 2017).
102 See David Ennals at the Vaccine Damage Payments Bill second reading: 'The Bill seeks to alleviate the cruel paradox that, because the great majority benefit, a minority, albeit a very small minority, has suffered.' HC Deb (5 February 1979) vol. 962, col. 38.
103 Mikio Kimura and Harumi Kuno-Sakai, 'Pertussis vaccines in Japan – a clue toward understanding of Japanese attitude to vaccines', *Journal of Tropical Pediatrics*, 37:1 (1991), 45–7; James Colgrove, *State of Immunity: The Politics of Vaccination in Twentieth-century America* (Berkeley: University of California Press, 2006); Baker, 'The pertussis vaccine controversy'; Gangarosa et al, 'Impact of anti-vaccine movements on pertussis control'; Casiday, 'Risk communication in the British pertussis and MMR vaccine controversies'; Riolo, King and Rohani, 'Can vaccine legacy explain the British pertussis resurgence?'

104 Larson et al, 'Understanding vaccine hesitancy around vaccines and vaccination from a global perspective'; Heidi J. Larson, Alexandre de Figueiredo, Zhao Xiahong, William S. Schulz, Pierre Verger, Iain G. Johnston, Alex R. Cook and Nick S. Jones, 'The state of vaccine confidence 2016: Global insights through a 67-country survey', *EBioMedicine*, 12 (2016), 295–301.

5

MMR

As the pertussis crisis faded into memory, it appeared that Britain had once again bought into the vaccine narrative. Immunisation rates increased over the 1980s, and new vaccines offered the British public even greater protection from infectious disease. Parents were well aware of the vaccines on offer, and broadly considered these to be safe and effective.[1] The iconic new public health threat, HIV, did not yet have a vaccine; but there was great optimism that one would eventually be found.[2] Then, in the late 1990s, another crisis threatened to dent confidence yet again. This time, the culprit was another trivalent vaccine – MMR. In 1998, Andrew Wakefield and colleagues published a paper in the medical journal *The Lancet* which alleged a possible link between MMR and a rare form of autism. While the journal itself took the unusual step of printing a repudiation alongside the paper, Wakefield used the press conference to launch the edition to claim that MMR was dangerous and parents should immediately seek separate measles, mumps and rubella vaccines until further safety testing had been completed. Medical consensus was always against Wakefield and his small group of allies – but the controversy made for a great media story. Over the following years, uptake of MMR dropped. Multiple studies showed that there was no evidence for a link between MMR and autism, and in 2004 ethical violations and poor research practices were exposed in Wakefield's work. After that point, vaccination rates recovered once more. But the crisis has become infamous as an example of how public health authorities can struggle in the modern, digital world to overcome misinformation.

MMR led to a reappraisal of public health researchers' and practitioners' approaches to parents who refused vaccination for their children. It had been traditional to reassert the facts, relying on scientific authority and health statistics to prove the worth of vaccination and the errors of its opponents. This approach did not die in the early years of the twenty-first century, but there was a more concerted effort to borrow from the research of those engaging with sociological conceptions of risk and health. Just as new technologies, such as the internet and twenty-four-hour news networks, changed the way that members of the public received, consumed and interpreted information about health risks, the authorities began to make use of those same media to communicate with the public in different ways. By the 2010s, the memory of the MMR crisis and similar concerns about the progress of vaccination schemes in other countries led researchers not just to focus on parents who refused vaccines, but to begin to investigate the various trends in society that affected decision making, either pro- or anti-vaccine.

This chapter is about the concept of hesitancy within the MMR crisis. The concept of hesitancy used by the WHO in the 2010s argues that parents' choices are affected by confidence, convenience and complacency.[3] As the British experience shows, confidence was rocked by reports that MMR might have caused autism in some children. Yet major reforms in public health over the 1980s and early 1990s meant that vaccination was more convenient than ever for both parents and administrators. Similarly, while there had been some complacency about whether measles, mumps or rubella were serious diseases, the immunisation rates against all three dropped nowhere near as significantly as pertussis had done in the 1970s.[4] Instead, British parents appeared to be unsure about what to do for their children at the turn of the millennium. Despite the popular conception of British parents during the MMR crisis, they were not, for the most part, anti-vaccine.[5] Average uptake of MMR in England fell from 91.8 per cent in 1996 to 79.9 per cent in 2004; but it dropped below 80 per cent in only three English regions, and rates remained robust elsewhere in the United Kingdom (Figure 5.1).[6] There was instead a public debate about whether MMR was specifically the right vaccine to be giving to children. Potential alternatives such as separate measles, mumps and rubella vaccines offered compromise solutions that were shut down by the government, leading to disquiet. To follow the WHO model, parents were hesitant primarily because confidence in MMR had been substantially

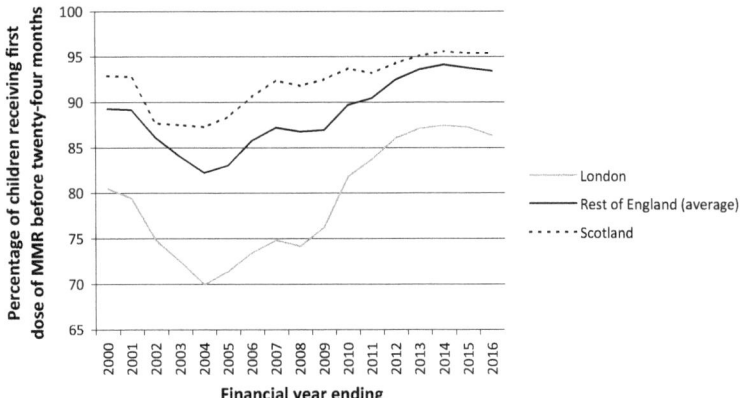

Figure 5.1 Percentage of children receiving first dose of MMR before 24 months in London, rest of England and Scotland, 1999–2000, 2015–16.
Source: England 1999–2000 to 2004–5: Health and Social Care Information Centre, 'NHS Immunisation Statistics: England, 2004–05' http://content.digital.nhs.uk/catalogue/PUB00176 (accessed 23 August 2017); England 2006–16: NHS Digital, 'NHS Immunisation Statistics: England, 2015–16' (London, September 2016). Scotland: Information Services Division Scotland, 'Trends in immunisation uptake by quarter, calendar and financial year – Scotland' (Edinburgh, June 2016).

weakened. This chapter examines why that was the case by looking at the crisis in the wider historical context of the events discussed elsewhere in this book. British public health authorities had engendered broad support for vaccination, overcoming apathy, protecting the nation from outside threats, sating demand for protection from infectious disease and managing the risks to individuals and the nation as a whole. The MMR crisis was significant not because of how widely confidence was dented, but in the depth of the damage done to those who were unsure of the best way to protect their children.

First, this chapter explains how MMR came to be used in Britain. The trivalent vaccine was part of a number of reforms to health care in Britain in the late 1980s. The DHSS was split into two separate departments, and greater emphasis was placed on preventative health. Better monitoring systems, WHO targets and remuneration for general practitioners meant that vaccination rates improved significantly over this period, giving a greater degree of protection than hitherto enjoyed by the British population. Parents were placed under more extensive surveillance by local health authorities, allowing better follow-up, more convenient appointments and more successful vaccinations. Yet the nature of those reforms stored up potential political dilemmas that came to the fore during the MMR crisis. The chapter then goes on to describe the chronology of the crisis and explain the role of the major players. Focusing primarily on the years 1998 to 2004, it shows how and why the case against MMR was made by its opponents. This leads to a discussion of the main issues of the crisis and just how the MMR–autism link took hold. In short, it was believable. Faith in medical and political authorities in Britain had been rocked by a succession of crises, most notable the bovine spongiform encephalopathy (BSE) and variant Creutzfeldt-Jackob (vCJD) scare and subsequent investigation into what the government knew before the people. There was little concrete research into autism's causes and aetiology, and doubts about vaccine safety had been raised in other parts of the world. The government responded through traditional educational campaigns, but these did little to persuade parents. The chapter details how the government launched new websites to speak to the public through "risk communication". By outlining various choices and the potential impacts of those decisions, the government hoped that it could restore confidence. Finally, the chapter shows how public health researchers have used the memory of MMR as part of their analyses of how members of the public make decisions about vaccination. Rather than focusing solely on events where parents show hesitancy, there has been more focus on both a lack of and an adequate supply of confidence. It is just as instructive to ask why, as a nation, we usually *do* vaccinate our children as why we might not.

Vaccination policy in the 1980s

The late 1980s saw a shift in emphasis in vaccination policy, reflecting other trends in health care and public health.[7] The problems of low pertussis vaccine uptake faded over the course of the Thatcher administration.[8] As the decade wore on, the Conservative government looked to preventative health care as a way of managing the demands on the health services, the financial costs of health care and lost productivity and to emphasise moral values surrounding personal and parental responsibility. For public health, the 1987 White Paper *Promoting Better Health* included government plans for how this might be achieved UK-wide, bolstered by the publication of the Acheson Report on the state of English public health a year later.[9] Personal responsibility and vaccination featured prominently in the White Paper. Among a list of key statistics to show the extent to which public health interventions might reduce the burden on other health services, it noted that there were 90,000 measles cases in 1986 and over 1,000 hospital admissions. Parents who did not present their children for measles vaccination were placed implicitly in the same category as people making poor dietary choices ('obesity: a quarter of young people are overweight'), smokers ('100,000 deaths a year ... 50 million working days lost ... £400 million in [NHS] treatment costs') and drug users ('the number of addicts newly notified in 1986 exceeded 5,000').[10] But while this responsibility rhetoric was a key part of managing the risk of measles and its attendant economic impacts, the report also recognised the government's obligation to make services available for individuals and to promote them properly so that people were able to make the "right choices". Vaccination was therefore also in the same category as cancer screening – citizens were expected to present themselves for medical surveillance so that symptoms could be caught early and treatment outcomes would be both more successful and cheaper in the long run.[11] These problems could be overcome by reforming primary care:

> The Government intends positively to encourage family doctors and primary health care teams to increase their contribution to the promotion of good health. These professional workers as well as dentists and pharmacists are in daily contact with large numbers of the public and represent the front line of health care; they are therefore very well placed to persuade individuals of the importance of protecting their health; of the simple steps needed to do so; and of accepting that prevention is indeed better than cure.[12]

In promoting health, the UK was not acting alone. Increased monitoring of health statistics from the 1970s, including the rise of health economics and related disciplines, had led to a greater understanding of Britain's place relative to other nations. Global public health was firmly on the political agenda, as reflected in the Alma Ata conference and subsequent regional and worldwide programmes run by the WHO to achieve 'Health For All' by the year 2000.[13] International comparisons were nothing new. The British government had gathered information on the use of smallpox vaccine in other countries when deliberating over whether to cease routine vaccination. Similarly, the entry into the European Economic Community in the 1970s had led to the use of regular comparisons with other member states when considering policy on vaccination, vaccine compensation and other areas of DHSS activity. WHO goals and targets did, however, place a new political imperative to improve certain metrics and increased the overlaps between public health and foreign policy.[14]

The WHO's goal of 90 per cent immunisation in Europe against common childhood diseases was considered to be a challenge, but not an impossible one for the British programme.[15] Many Area Health Authorities had already achieved this by the late 1980s. Yet the national average still lagged some way behind, and rates varied between vaccine types.[16] To incentivise higher uptake, the Department of Health announced that it would begin to pay general practitioners a bonus if they achieved high vaccination rates in their area. This performance-related pay was part of a number of changes designed to shift the focus of general practice towards preventative medicine and to make primary health care run more efficiently, while also reflecting the increased marketisation within the NHS.[17] The new general practitioner contract faced significant opposition from the BMA, but Health Secretary Kenneth Clarke forced it through in 1990.[18] This was linked to the economic and social imperatives of what might broadly be called the New Right or Thatcherism during the 1980s and early 1990s.[19] Managerialism and the internal market in the NHS were designed to deliver efficiency savings and improve quality and choice.[20] Similarly, individuals partaking in healthy and responsible behaviours would decrease the demand on the system, aided by properly incentivised primary health care professionals to make those "correct" decisions. Vaccination was an ideal public health measure in this context. As Jennifer Stanton has argued, vaccines themselves are 'high-demand, low-cost' technologies, especially for common childhood diseases such as poliomyelitis or whooping cough.[21] During the late twentieth century they were also technologies that could be developed by private pharmaceutical companies with public sector support, creating both supply from profit-making bodies and demand from public health programmes looking to reduce the financial burden of infectious disease.[22] But there were limits to what health departments would fund, based on the perceived gains relative to cost. Stanton shows that in the case of hepatitis B – a relatively rare disease associated with stigmatised groups and behaviours such as homosexual men and intravenous drug-taking communities – the government was not willing to fund and implement a routine childhood vaccination programme in the 1980s.[23]

Structural reforms to the general practitioner contract could go only so far. The other major innovation of the 1980s was the introduction of MMR. Measles vaccination had remained low in comparison to other countries, including some in the developing world. WHO targets, combined with a sense of embarrassment, led to a change of approach.[24] As with multivalent vaccines in previous decades – like DTwP – the hope was that the vaccine would be easier to administer for health authorities and more acceptable to parents because it reduced the number of injections their children had to endure and the number of trips needed to be made to the clinic.[25] Experiences in other countries appeared to bear this out. Indeed, in the trials in the United Kingdom, uptake had been much better than for the single measles vaccine even though participants had been inconvenienced by asking them to fill out a diary of any possible side-effects for three weeks afterwards.[26] The vaccine was given in two doses, one before the second birthday and the second before the child started school. Since around 90 per cent of MMR vaccinations confer immunity, two doses gave a 99 per cent chance of success.[27]

Authorities had reasons to be concerned by all three diseases. Measles was explicitly cited in *Promoting Better Health* because of its high morbidity and the number of hospital visits it necessitated. A vaccine had been recommended in Britain since 1968.[28] However, uptake had remained stubbornly low; and while the number of cases had dropped from 236,000 in 1968 to 86,000 in 1988, the Department of Health wished to go further. This was problematic, as measles is an unusually infectious disease. Herd immunity requires a vaccination rate upwards of 95 per cent. The disease itself can be relatively mild, resulting in a rash and a fever. In some cases symptoms can be much more severe, leading to swelling of the inner ear (1 in 11–14 cases) convulsions (1 in 200) and even death (1 in 5,000).[29] Because there were so many cases of measles per year, even this small percentage led to a high number of complications. As discussed in the previous chapter, rubella vaccine was used to prevent CRS. Although CRS rates had declined, it remained a concern for the Department of Health, which hoped that MMR would increase the vaccination rate in females as well as interrupting disease transmission by creating a cohort of immune males.[30] Like measles, CRS was part of the WHO's immunisation targets.[31]

The final component, mumps, was not a specific WHO target but was still thought to be serious enough to be included in the overall programme.[32] Mumps could also be a mild disease – many who contract it do not realise they have done so – but when it presents it commonly results in hospitalisation, accompanied by painful swelling of the glands and, in boys, the potential for infertility. Deafness is another possible side-effect.[33] Uptake of mumps vaccine before MMR was poor, compounded by the perception that mumps was a boys' disease.[34] The trivalent vaccine was therefore not simply about reducing the number of visits and injections needed to make vaccination more convenient for parents. It was designed to increase the immunisation rates against the three diseases by protecting boys against rubella, girls against mumps and everyone against measles, despite the fact that parents might have previously expressed less enthusiasm for one vaccine over another.[35]

One final element of the changes during the Thatcher and Major governments concerns the measurement of vaccination levels. In order to remunerate general practitioners properly, authorities needed reliable and comparable measures of uptake. Moreover, the Department of Health had tried to learn lessons from the pertussis crisis. In 1987, Public Health Laboratory Services established Cover of Vaccination Evaluated Rapidly (COVER) to produce nation-wide statistics on a quarterly basis.[36] This replaced other forms of local reporting of vaccination numbers which had evolved since before the 1940s (see Part I). COVER was supplemented in 1991 by the creation of six-monthly surveys of parental knowledge and attitudes towards vaccination.[37] These tools were designed to be able to monitor if vaccination rates were dropping and/or if parents were expressing doubts about a particular vaccine at any given time. With the pertussis crisis, one of the major issues that the vaccine's opponents had been able to draw upon was the relative scarcity of hard evidence that there was no link between brain damage and the vaccine at the population level.[38] Therefore, research had also begun on new, active monitoring systems for adverse events. The existing passive reporting system required general practitioners to submit information on possible reactions to vaccines on "yellow cards" to the health authorities. These could be unreliable, and tended towards under-reporting of incidents and damage to the credibility of drug safety administration.[39] Increasing computerisation during the 1980s and 1990s offered the possibility of monitoring indicators such as hospital admissions for certain conditions in children of specific ages and mapping these onto vaccination coverage in a particular area.[40]

Despite these top-down reforms in the late 1980s and early 1990s, the government did not simply impose vaccination on the population from above. As in the 1970s, it was clear that the vaccine narrative was broadly accepted and uptake was relatively high as compared to previous decades, albeit with the same problems of local variation as before. Vaccination had proved its worth. It had eradicated smallpox worldwide, and once-common childhood diseases had been virtually eliminated in high-income countries. All of these issues reflected the topics covered in previous chapters of this book. If apathy was a product of low engagement, the inconvenience for parents and lack of access to vaccines, then incentive payments and combination vaccines were designed to prompt local doctors to solve these issues.[41] The protection of the nation was to come not simply through vaccinating the population, but from regional cooperation with other European countries through the WHO.[42] The popularity of the MMR vaccine in the trial areas appeared to show demand for this new technology from some constituencies – in any event, increased surveillance and monitoring of parents would ensure compliance. All of this, however, was refracted through the lens of risk: the risk to the state of the costs and burdens of infectious disease, and the outlining of personal responsibility for ensuring that risky behaviours did not put the nation's health or finances at risk. Official and public confidence in the vaccine rested on whether it would be convenient for parents, protect children from disease and be more cost-effective than the public health measures that had preceded it.

The MMR crisis

These developments improved vaccination rates. It was now easier for local authorities to monitor and follow up on parents of unvaccinated children, and doctors had a direct financial incentive to do so. The single vaccine, given in two doses, was also much more convenient. However, this system still required parents to choose to vaccinate. This caused problems during the MMR crisis itself. For while there was little counter information or other options available to parents, there was only one obvious choice. When the MMR–autism link became more widely talked about and an alternative action was considered possible – separate vaccinations – choice became a major issue. The rise of the rhetoric around choice and growing health consumerism meant that citizens were more likely to seek out and demand alternative forms of care.[43] This was compounded by the fact that the political context of the late 1990s and early 2000s made the claims of anti-government voices sound credible. It was because of this that confidence could be damaged and parents could become more hesitant.

For public health professionals and researchers, the MMR crisis refers to the period in which significant doubt was expressed over MMR's safety, leading to a drop in immunisation rates. While this decline was not as striking as it had been over the pertussis scandal in the 1970s, the level of coverage devoted to MMR in popular media, coupled with the circulation of vaccine-sceptic information through growing internet usage meant that convincing the public of the vaccine's safety was a much more difficult task. Most accounts of the crisis place its beginnings in the *Lancet* paper published by Wakefield and colleagues in 1998. This acts as a useful starting point for tracing the public debate about MMR, particularly in the popular and medical press. The most intense period of press activity began around 2001 (Figure 5.2).[44] By late 2004, the main crisis was over. Brian Deer's exposés were published in this year, and ten of the twelve co-authors of the Wakefield *Lancet* paper retracted their conclusions.[45] However, as with all historical periodisations, we should be aware that concerns with MMR permeate these clean boundaries. Immunisation rates had been falling for a couple of years before 1998, and Wakefield's research (as detailed below) exposed a number of concerns in a minority of parents, rather than simply appearing *ex nihilo*. Similarly, quoting an end date for the crisis is complicated by the fact that many of the debates of that time continued to be felt among some communities in the United Kingdom and elsewhere in the world.[46]

It is therefore worth briefly exploring this timeline. Wakefield was the key figure for MMR sceptics. A clinical researcher working at the

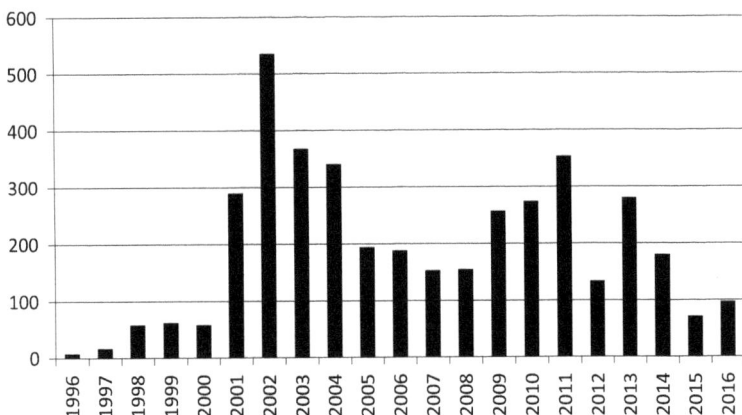

Figure 5.2 Mentions of MMR in major daily newspapers, 1996–2016.
Source: Search for string 'MMR' in ProQuest European Newsstream on selected newspapers. Newspapers chosen were major dailies in the database with full text searchable from 1 January 1996 onwards: *The Times, Daily Mirror, Independent, Guardian* and *Sun* (accessed via Senate House Library, University of London, 28 June 2017).

Royal Free Hospital, University College London, he and his team had studied a particular form of autism which was associated with problems in the gut. The 1998 paper described this syndrome in twelve children, but also claimed a temporal link with the onset of their symptoms and MMR. While the article itself made it clear that the authors 'did not prove an association between measles, mumps, and rubella vaccine and the syndrome described', Wakefield himself was far less reserved.[47] At a press conference organised by *The Lancet* at the Royal Free Hospital to explain the paper and its wider context, Wakefield declared MMR to be dangerous and asserted that it would be safer to give separate vaccines until more was known about its effects. The media covered this as a potential medical scandal, but there were clear reservations.[48] The authors had failed to prove an association, as the critical commentary printed alongside the paper in *The Lancet* had argued.[49] And while the volume of newspaper stories on MMR for 1998 compared to subsequent years would suggest that the *Lancet* article was not hugely significant in itself (Figure 5.2), it provided the basis for debate in the medical and popular press. The tabloid press was more sensationalist than the broadsheets, as might be expected. In particular, the *Sun*, *Daily Mail* and *Daily Express* gave the matter significant coverage – in the case of the latter two even after most had accepted that the MMR–autism link was unfounded.[50]

While co-authors John Walker-Smith and Simon Murch both continued to claim that MMR was still safe and recommended parents to vaccinate their children, Wakefield was more strident in his opposition.[51] In December 2000 he and Scott Montgomery published a critique of the testing procedures for the vaccine during its initial licensing stage.[52] The national media gave this new paper a new round of attention. To assuage doubts and combat declining vaccination rates, the Department of Health began a publicity campaign for MMR in January 2001.[53] In the meantime, epidemiological and public health studies continued to find no evidence of a link between MMR and autism.[54] It was in early 2002 that the crisis reached its peak, however. Over Christmas 2001 and the New Year, Prime Minister Tony Blair refused to answer questions from Members of Parliament or journalists about whether his young son Leo had received the vaccine.[55] The BBC's *Panorama* documentary series publicised the work of MMR-sceptic John O'Leary on 3 February 2002.[56] While it too did not prove an autism link, the media seized upon the story. Vaccination rates continued to drop, and measles cases were on the rise, including an outbreak in London.[57] The drip of newspaper articles questioning MMR became a flood, with the bulk of the torrent coming in February 2002. The government was again forced into a defensive campaign to restore faith in MMR.[58]

While the crisis rumbled on over 2003, newspaper mentions of MMR declined. Parents of autistic children had begun legal proceedings against the Department of Health, claiming that MMR had caused their children's conditions. Initially it had secured legal aid, but in September 2003 the Legal Services Commission withdrew its support. The weight of evidence suggested very little chance of success.[59] For the most part, the mainstream debate ended in 2004 following the work of investigative reporter Brian Deer. He had returned to the original 1998 *Lancet* paper to reassess Wakefield and colleagues' claims about the twelve children. He uncovered a number of issues which called into question the integrity of the researchers and the scientific validity of their findings. The claims included: that ethics approval had not been given for some procedures (such as lumbar punctures and colonoscopies); that ethics approval had been sought for a different project to the one eventually carried out; that there was bias in the selection of cases for the study (including accusation that Wakefield had paid children for blood samples at a birthday party); that legal aid funding had been used for supposedly independent research; and that findings were used for legal cases prior to peer review and publication.[60] When these claims were aired in a Channel 4 *Dispatches* documentary and printed as a series of exposés in the *Sunday Times*, Wakefield's credibility was destroyed. Ten of the paper's twelve co-authors retracted their conclusions, stating:

> We wish to make it clear that in this paper no causal link was established between MMR vaccine and autism as the data were insufficient. However, the possibility of such a link was raised and consequent events have had major implications for public health. In view of this, we consider now is the appropriate time that we should together formally retract the interpretation placed upon these findings in the paper, according to precedent.[61]

Declining confidence

It is overly simplistic to attribute the MMR crisis solely to the *Lancet* paper. However, the debate it sparked raised a number of issues about the vaccine and vaccination that were difficult for the government to counter effectively. It was the interplay between these that chipped away at the public's confidence. It is worth highlighting five of these issues. First, autism rates had been increasing for some years with no definitive explanation. Second, Japan had banned MMR on safety grounds, leading to questions about the reliability of the UK's safety testing procedures. Third, the quality of the government's medical advice and the role of the medical profession were complicated further by other scandals reported at the same time as MMR, such as "mad cow disease" (BSE). Fourth, the changes to the general practitioner contract led to a debate over whether doctors were recommending MMR for the money or because they genuinely believed that it was in their patients' best interests. Fifth, and finally, the apparent compromise position of administering separate measles, mumps and rubella vaccinations was attractive to parents but was denied out of hand by the government. These interrelated debates meant that the British public had every reason to be sceptical about MMR.

The first major issue, and the one with the longest life beyond the crisis, was the alleged link between MMR and autism. Autism, like brain damage in the pertussis crisis, was seen as the main potential hazard of MMR. Wakefield's work centred on establishing a connection between the two, while the majority of scientific evidence presented in favour of MMR mobilised to show that there was no provable statistical correlation.[62] One of the reasons why this debate was so potent was because so little was known about autism around the turn of the millennium. Even if there was no evidence of a link between MMR and the syndrome, there were also no clear answers about what did cause it. It was common knowledge that autism diagnoses had increased significantly over the previous twenty years. For concerned members of the public, any explanation was worth exploring. The *Daily Mail* was particularly interested in these questions.[63] 'It would be a gross insult to the intelligence of … parents', wrote David Goldberg, a doctor and the father of an autistic son, 'if their collective view was explained as an emotional response to media hyperbole.'[64] Parents of autistic children were a key part of Wakefield's campaign against the vaccine, just as parents of children damaged by the pertussis vaccine had been key to the 1970s campaign. The mother of an autistic child, Jackie Fletcher, had founded the group Justice Awareness and Basic Support (JABS) in the mid-1990s.[65] Fletcher eventually won vaccine damage payments for her son, albeit for severe epilepsy rather than autism.[66] The group was much more overtly anti-vaccine than the APVDC, and made use of the visibility afforded by the internet to spread their message directly (through their website) and indirectly (through responses in the press).[67] It and the Society for the Autistically Handicapped were involved in litigation against the Department of Health, and successfully secured legal aid to help them with the case.[68] For parents weighing up the risks of vaccination, the publicity given to the possibility of autism had an impact on their decision.

Although the weight of scientific evidence of MMR's safety eventually resulted in the withdrawal of legal aid funding in 2003, the existence of the case contributed to the debate's credibility.[69] Other evidence further complicated this picture. Concerns had been raised about MMR's safety before. In Japan, MMR was withdrawn completely because the mumps component produced a higher-than-acceptable risk of meningitis. Britain responded to concerns about the Urabe strain of mumps vaccine by replacing it entirely with the more expensive but safer Jeryll-Lynn strain. Most other nations did likewise. In Japan, however, legislation meant that its public health system could use only Japanese-made vaccine. The vaccine had been withdrawn not because it was dangerous per se, but because no Japanese manufacturer was yet able to produce it.[70] To supporters of vaccination, this proved how robust testing systems were. It had caught a potential problem early, and the increased rate of measles in Japan following the withdrawal showed that the vaccine was effective.[71] To critics, it showed that even in a modern advanced nation potentially dangerous medications could slip through the cracks. Wakefield was keen to emphasise this point.[72] Again, however, medical consensus supported the testing procedure. *Adverse Drug Reactions and Toxicological Reviews* took the unusual step of publishing Wakefield and Montgomery's article alongside the peer review reports, emphasising the journal's support for freedom of scientific expression, but also its reservations about the legitimacy of Wakefield and Montgomery's conclusions.[73] Still, given the lack of information on autism and the Japanese withdrawal of the vaccine, the possibility of MMR being dangerous remained plausible. The British government said that it wanted to protect the nation from infectious disease – but was it capable of doing so?

For the public this was not the first time in recent memory that medical professionals had been wrong, had withheld information or had actively attempted to deceive. Just as the pertussis crisis occurred in the shadow of thalidomide, the BSE and vCJD scandal loomed heavily over discussions of MMR. As Tammy Speers and Justin Lewis have argued, it also served as a narrative framing for press coverage and public understanding of the crisis.[74] Even in the medical press, it was acknowledged that the fall-out of the BSE crisis meant that medical experts could not be seen to dismiss criticism of MMR out of hand.[75] Nevertheless, this was not the only example of government and medical establishment incompetence. In a 2003 study of the role of the media in attitudes towards science, 24 per cent said that their 'trust in science' had decreased as a result of BSE, the most-quoted single reason.[76] As the autism lawsuit was building up, the victims of contaminated blood transfusions won their case against the Department of Health, using legal aid.[77] The reports of the inquiries into the Bristol heart scandal (in which a number of children had died unnecessarily due to a poorly staffed hospital department) and the Alder Hey scandal (where dead children's organs had been retained without parental consent) were also published at this time.[78] Trust was dented both in whether doctors could be believed in and whether, even if they were not trying to deceive, they were capable of finding the truth. In an article in the *British Medical Journal* radio journalist Sharon Alcock described a programme she had made with the Warburton family in 2002. The Warburtons were chosen as a "typical" family who were unsure about whether or not to vaccinate their children. The parents debated the issues surrounding MMR throughout the week with selected "experts", before declaring their decision on the Friday. The BSE issue had left the family feeling especially sceptical.[79]

While there were clearly reasons to distrust the official government line, confidence in general practitioners had also been shaken. It was well established that patients and parents were more predisposed to trust medical advice from general practitioners than from government advertising or other sources of information.[80] As we saw with the campaigns of the 1940s and 1950s, the government had long emphasised the role of face-to-face contact with medical professionals in convincing parents to have their children vaccinated. Changes to the NHS contract, however, meant that GPs now had a direct financial incentive to convince parents to accept MMR. The Warburtons found the relationship between GPs, money and the government problematic. 'They couldn't really decide where to draw the lines between government and medical professionals' advice,' wrote Alcock. 'They wanted to trust their doctor and health visitor, but felt they were being spun a political line.' The government had made vaccination policy decisions based on cost-benefit analyses before, notably over hepatitis B.[81] One correspondent to the *British Medical Journal* argued that there was an inherent conflict between offering the patient choice and following government evidence and guidelines.[82] Doctors insisted that they supported MMR regardless, and that the financial payments were simply to formalise actions that ought to be taken anyway.[83] Such was the strength of feeling on this point that the BMA recommended that performance-related pay on vaccination should be abandoned.[84] By the time the new general practitioner contract was rolled out in 2004, other priorities had arisen and worries over MMR had faded.[85] The concern was not that doctors would favour cash over patient safety; indeed, since vaccination was an epidemiologically proven preventative health measure, it was clearly in both the doctor's and child's best interests. Rather, it was that physicians *could be perceived to be* compromised in their decision making. Certain sections of the public health profession, therefore, understood that building trust was also an exercise in presentation as well as hard numbers.

When taken together, there were clear reasons for parents to be cautious about MMR. For those worried both about the vaccine and about infectious disease, however, Wakefield had offered a solution. At the press conference to announce the 1998 *Lancet* paper, he had urged parents to seek out separate measles, mumps and rubella vaccines so as to reduce the risks to the child. As with the pertussis crisis and compensation, this appeared to be a compromise position between two entrenched viewpoints. It was known from a study in the United States that parents were more willing to take risks with errors of omission (i.e. the risks associated with not vaccinating) than with errors of commission (i.e. the risk that something could go wrong with their active decision to vaccinate).[86] Helen Bedford, a researcher into child health, lamented that 'natural infection is somehow thought of as being out of our control, but immunisation is something that parents have to decide to take up, so they feel more responsible'. One of the more-strident critics of Wakefield, a London GP and the father of an autistic son, Michael Fitzpatrick, also placed this debate in political context. The New Labour government had championed choice in public services, including health care.[87] While this was designed to begin to equalise the doctor–patient relationship, improve satisfaction and improve outcomes, vaccination was, paradoxically, an area in which the government offered very little choice.[88] It could not countenance separate vaccines. No individual immunisations were licensed for use in the United Kingdom – and, as the government repeatedly stated, no country which used MMR offered separate vaccines.[89] There was no evidence that the individual immunisations were safer. Indeed, pre-MMR experience in Britain suggested the opposite. Since child vaccination rates against the three diseases were lower before the trivalent vaccine became available, separate vaccines (on the population level at least) placed the public at greater risk of infection.[90]

Again, while this was epidemiologically justifiable, it appeared to some to be too draconian. Private clinics began to offer separate vaccinations to concerned parents, drawing the ire of the Department of Health.[91] Separate vaccines were strictly forbidden on the NHS, and individual doses were technically not licensed for use in the United Kingdom. General practitioner Peter Mansfield offered this service to his patients through his private practice, leading the Director of Public Health in Worcestershire to refer him to the General Medical Council.[92] The case was eventually dropped, but the apparent lack of flexibility on the part of the government made some parents suspicious. The *Daily Mail*, a notable critic of the government throughout the crisis, published a series of letters about the decision. One nurse 'fully support[ed]' the 'right to choose' of the parents of her grandchildren. Another questioned whether this was a matter for the General Medical Council, which was surely 'supposed to be saving us from the Dr Shipmans[93] of this world not stopping us having the treatment that's right for us'. Many emphasised the choice element, concluding that it was better for children to get some protection through unconventional practice than receive no vaccination at all.[94] Back at Alcock's radio programme, the Warburtons were especially puzzled on this point. Having spoken to the "experts" in the BBC programme – including Wakefield and Mansfield – they opted for the separate vaccines. The head of the Public Health Laboratory Service, Elizabeth Miller, and Scope (previously called the Spastics Society) had convinced them that measles, mumps and rubella were dangerous and that vaccination would protect their child. But they still questioned whether MMR was the right solution. They told the BBC that their decision to vaccinate would have been much easier if separate injections were available on the NHS.[95]

Risk communication

As vaccination rates continued to decline and press interest remained, the government made attempts to re-establish confidence in MMR. The scientific position was much clearer than it had been with the pertussis crisis, and so the Department was quicker to begin a new publicity campaign. While some funds were directed into increased research in autism to build a body of evidence for other causes for the syndrome, £3 million was set aside in 2001 to educate parents.[96] At the launch, Chief Medical Officer Liam Donaldson declared that 'on each occasion that these scares have been raised they have been thoroughly examined and on each occasion MMR has been given a clean bill of health.'[97] Yet it appeared to have little impact. The government was forced to re-launch the campaign in 2002 in the wake of yet more negative publicity, mostly stemming from the BBC *Panorama* documentary and Tony Blair's refusal to confirm his son Leo's vaccination status.[98] This was mainly an attempt to draw media attention to the campaign rather than a major change in tack, although it is clear that risk communication took a more central role from this point forward. Authorities had been accused of taking a 'patronising, high-handed and arrogant' approach to parents.[99] The medical press also criticised public health authorities' responses.[100] While organisations from the BMA to the Scottish Government produced guidance and reports on MMR and its safety, nothing appeared to be working.[101] The approach of giving information and answering questions was not enough on its own, as Richard Horton, editor of *The Lancet* later noted:

> Wider public trust is best fostered neither by referring to abstract evidence alone nor by official pronouncements of reassurance, but by explaining face-to-face in transparent, human, even anecdotal terms with personal stories, why a particular course of action is being advocated.
>
> Persuading the public to support vaccination is not only a matter of winning an argument. It is also about understanding the reasons why parents are and are not inclined to take their children for immunisation. The complexity of this decision demands a more nuanced response from the public-health community than it has so far received.[102]

In searching for alternative approaches, social science work on decision making and risk began to gain traction with public health professionals. This built on the growing professionalisation of health education, beginning in the 1980s.[103] The Medical Research and Economic and Social Research Councils funded a study into how the recent body of scholarly work on risk could help in public health. As the lead researchers noted, the education and persuasion approach:

> assumes that the target audience is made up of individuals who rationally review evidence to identify and choose the best course of action – that

is, the one that will maximise health benefit. There is little evidence that these approaches have made a major impact, despite the investment in health promotion and public health targeted in particular 'at risk' groups.[104]

The authors identified five aspects that affected how publics receive public health messages. First, the extent to which the source of the information is trusted; second, 'the relevance of the information to everyday life'; third, 'the relation to other perceived risks'; fourth, 'the fit with previous knowledge and experience'; and fifth 'the difficulty and importance of the choices and decisions'. The authors were critical of medical authorities that had appeared slow to incorporate this approach into their attempts to change population behaviours.[105] In some ways this was justified. The government publicity campaign had been a traditional advertising affair, with regular pronouncements about the safety of the vaccine, backed by epidemiological studies. As the Alcock documentary demonstrated, however, there was a perception that "the Lady doth protest too much":

> Halfway through their journey, Darren and Carol [Warburton] said that the more insistent the government became, the more they distrusted its advice. So when Professor Liam Donaldson called a press conference to endorse MMR, flanked by the great and the good of the medical world, it was the last straw. If more measles outbreaks are to be avoided, parents have to feel as though the medical profession isn't pulling rank and dismissing their concerns.[106]

The Department of Health was acutely aware of criticisms. At the time of the 2002 relaunch, a spokesman explained that research had shown how anxious parents were, and so the government had continued to focus on facts and 'the message' of 'individual choice'.[107] But it could do more to communicate risk in the way advocated by contemporary researchers.

One way of doing this in a less 'highhanded' way was to make use of growing access to the internet. According to World Bank statistics, web usage among Britons increased dramatically in the early years of the twenty-first century. The United Kingdom had a number of internet users broadly comparable to the Organisation for Economic Cooperation and Development average, but significantly behind the United States, in the late 1990s. In 2001, 33.4 per cent of the UK population was online, compared to 49.1 for the United States. By 2003, Britain had overtaken the United States.[108] Public health professionals noted how the internet had changed their interactions with certain sections of the public. Patients appeared to be armed with more knowledge – albeit the quality and relevance of this knowledge was contested – and the volume of vaccine-sceptic data available to parents raised questions that professionals found it difficult to answer without preparation.[109] Parents have always sought and received information from sources other than the government and medical professionals. Folk knowledge, self-care guides and informal networks had existed for centuries, and continued to do so even as the power of biomedicine increased.[110] What was different was the amount of information and the speed at which it could be delivered through this new communication network. Anti-MMR campaigners had used the internet to deliver previously obscure academic journal papers to journalists to help fuel the evidence for their cause and keep the debate in the popular press.[111] While we must be careful not to overstate the reach of the web – only 5 per cent of respondents in a 2003 study said that they got their science news mainly from the internet – this was undoubtedly a new issue for public health professionals to deal with.[112] It also offered a platform for solutions.

The government therefore sought to inform the public and communicate the risks and benefits of MMR through a new website called 'MMR The Facts'.[113] Hosted on the nhs.uk domain, it used an interactive map feature to show how MMR was used safely across the world. Britain's place as a modern nation in a global public health network was an important selling point. According to NHS information, only less-developed and obscure nations did not trust MMR. The map also provided ample statistics on MMR usage in different countries, and how many cases statistical modelling estimated could be prevented if non-adopting nations were to use the vaccine.[114] This type of risk communication extended to the 'myths and truths' section of the site, which used WHO data and published papers to dispel the 'Top 10 Myths about MMR'.[115] The main content of these static pages did not change over the course of the crisis. However, there was an element of interactivity in the 'Your questions answered' section. Site users could fill in a form, and a team of experts at the NHS would reply. The top questions were kept on the main 'questions' page. The Internet Archive has captured around forty of these questions, covering a wide range of topics from specific enquiries about personal circumstances to broader requests for more data on vaccination and autism.[116] Although it was clearly curated and mediated through the form of the website, this did at least represent an attempt by central government to speak directly to parents on issues about vaccination in the same medium through which they consumed other information about health decisions.

However, it was not just parents who needed access to reliable information. Researchers had found that many health workers' knowledge about MMR was poor. For example, many did not understand the reasons for the second dose, believing it to be a booster to the first dose rather than an important element in ensuring herd immunity.[117] NHS staff themselves acknowledged that it was difficult when presented with vaccine-sceptic material for the first time to respond to parents in a meaningful and reassuring way.[118] And, as members of the public, medical professionals were affected by the scares too. Very few were experts in immunology, and clear information was difficult to obtain.[119] The government's main advice to practitioners, the 'Green Book' on immunisation, was a rather weighty document and could not be readily updated to reflect the ever-changing field of vaccination science and public debate. In Scotland, specific information was sent to general practitioners in 'discussion packs' so that they could speak to parents and 'explore related concerns together'.[120] In England, the Department of Health set up a sister site to 'MMR The Facts' to include up-to-date information on MMR and all the other childhood immunisations. The MMR section included a succinct explanation of why the government refuted the paper by Wakefield and colleagues, what extant literature there was on the link with autism and the statistical details on why the risks of not vaccinating far outweighed the risks of MMR. It then made the political case, refuting suggestions that it was simply looking to cut costs, "bully" parents or deny people choice. It concluded by setting out the moral case for the vaccine:

> There is no doubt that parents always face real dilemmas when it comes to protecting their children's health. All want to do what is right by their children. ... However, it is the Government's responsibility to ensure that the care and treatment it makes available is the best possible. ... All the experts advise that MMR is the safest and best option and that single vaccines are definitely second best. For this fundamental reason, the Government does not support the use of separate vaccines.[121]

Talking about risks was by no means new. In the 1940s the government's main defence of diphtheria immunisation was that children were twenty times more likely to die of diphtheria if they were not immunised.[122] But the focus on risk communication in this way was a product of its time. The growing popularity of risk as a category of sociological analysis was born out of and in turn influenced the rhetoric around health and society at the turn of the millennium.[123] The venue for the communication outlined here, the World Wide Web, was certainly new, reflecting the growing access to the technology and its increasing influence on parents' decision making. The major turning point in the MMR narrative, however, was the detective work and subsequent publications of Brian Deer, the freelance investigative journalist. He published damning reports on Wakefield and his work in the *Sunday Times*, *British Medical Journal* and Channel 4's *Dispatches* documentary series. After this point, the public debate on the MMR–autism link appeared to be relatively settled. While some publications, including the *Daily Mail* and the satirical/investigative magazine *Private Eye*, ran pieces questioning this new consensus, the number of references to the subject dropped significantly in both the medical and popular press (see Figure 5.2).[124] It was also after this point that MMR vaccination began to recover to pre-crisis levels.

Conclusion

While the MMR vaccination rate dropped across Britain until 2004, the Department of Health saw nothing like the extremes experienced with pertussis. There, rates fell from 79 per cent to 37 per cent in three years.[125] With MMR, uptake in England fell from 92 per cent in 1996 to 80 per cent in 2004. Based on the aetiology of measles and the expectations and successes of the WHO and Department of Health over the early 1990s, this was a public health problem; but in historical context, it was relatively mild. Figure 5.3 shows that measles notifications did indeed increase, but the aggregate number of cases remained moderate by 1980s standards. In Scotland, MMR uptake remained above 87 per cent throughout the crisis. Indeed, when London is factored out of the national figures for England, it is clear that regional variation remained part of the story of vaccination rates in British public

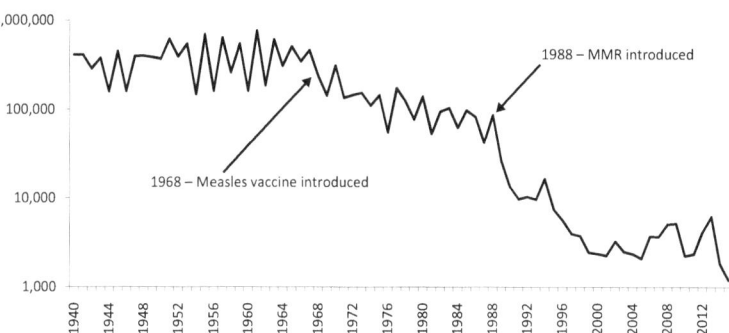

Figure 5.3 Notifications of measles in England and Wales, 1940–2015. Logarithmic scale.
Source: Public Health England, 'Measles notifications and deaths in England and Wales: 1940 to 2016', www.gov.uk/government/publications/measles-deaths-by-age-group-from-1980-to-2013-ons-data/measles-notifications-and-deaths-in-england-and-wales-1940-to-2013 (accessed 2 August 2017).

health (see Figure 5.1). It was also evident that the public had not lost its faith in vaccination. The clamour for the separate vaccines, even in MMR-sceptic newspapers such as the *Daily Mail*, indicated that even parents who wanted to avoid the trivalent vaccine were willing to go to great lengths to ensure that their children remained protected against infectious disease. However, outbreaks of measles in London at the time of the crisis, and in Swansea in 2012, showed that even these relatively small changes could have disastrous consequences.[126] In the latter case, the fear of MMR had largely dissipated, but many parents had not taken steps in the years following the crisis to ensure that their children were protected. Much like with the smallpox outbreaks seen in Chapter 2, there was a lingering problem for public health authorities in convincing parents to use vaccination as a preventative rather than epidemic control tool. As a result, when measles broke out in the Swansea area during the winter of 2012/13 there were large queues outside doctors' offices as parents sought to have their children vaccinated.[127]

MMR, then, lives on. It is a cautionary tale for public health workers, just as the generation fighting the crisis at the time looked back on pertussis.[128] As the rise in online anti-vaccination activity and growing mistrust of political authorities threaten once again to reduce uptake of vaccination among certain groups, the MMR crisis is held up as an example of how people can be misled by misinformation and how public health professionals must remain ever vigilant.[129] It even formed part of the 2011–12 Leveson Inquiry into the conduct of the press.[130]

Public health researchers' concerns have changed since the beginning of the century. MMR is not simply being used here, therefore, as a lesson from history from which direct predictions of future action can be gleaned.[131] Vaccine crises in other countries led the WHO and the Global Alliance for Vaccines and Immunization to create a Strategic Advisory Group of Experts (SAGE) to investigate how such drops in confidence could be avoided in the future. In some countries, progress towards world vaccination goals had stalled. In high-income countries, pockets of non-vaccinators caused health authorities to worry about high-risk, geographically concentrated areas with poor herd immunity.[132] SAGE identified that the main reason for these problems was vaccine hesitancy. The MMR crisis in the United Kingdom and subsequent debates in other high-income countries formed part of this analysis – especially the difficulties around convincing populations to take the vaccine against the swine flu H1N1 virus.[133]

Yet hesitancy as a concept grew out of changing ways of seeing non-vaccinators in the wake of MMR and emphases on risk communication in the previous decade. As Heidi Larson's work showed, few parents are completely pro- or anti-vaccine; rather, their attitudes towards specific vaccines at specific times can be changed. By focusing solely on individuals when they become a problem for public health authorities, this fluid state can be obscured.[134] This is a story borne out by the history of vaccination in Britain since the Second World War. Parents did not abandon or adopt vaccination as a technology wholesale. Enthusiasm for diphtheria immunisations waxed and waned over the 1940s. Smallpox vaccination was embraced as a form of epidemic control, but treated with indifference by the majority of the population in the 1950s and 1960s. Polio vaccine was hailed a modern marvel; and yet both the government and the public had an awkward relationship with it until the oral vaccine became widely available. And even at the height of the pertussis vaccine crisis, immunisation rates for other diseases remained relatively robust.

While this chapter has used the language and framework of hesitancy, this concept has been developed by researchers for investigating present-day public health problems. It must be historicised. It is itself born out of the historical period covering MMR. Convenience did not appear to be a great issue. The reforms to the general practitioner contract and the introduction of MMR meant that access to the vaccine was straightforward, and there were incentives throughout the system for following up on defaulters. While there were still issues of monitoring and access in some inner-city areas and amongst some populations,[135] public health officials did not face the same hurdles as those explored in the first section of this book. Confidence was a different matter. Declining trust in state authorities meant that anti-government voices carried an air of legitimacy. With a hostile press, the growth of twenty-four-hour news channels and increasing access to the internet, some parents' confidence shifted towards other sources of expertise.[136] Contemporaries also pointed to increased complacency and the idea that vaccination had, ironically, become a victim of its own success. As the threat of measles and other infectious diseases receded (Figure 5.3), some parents became less motivated to seek out vaccination, or felt that they could afford to wait and try out alternative vaccines and vaccination schedules.[137] This was, in some ways, the language of apathy reconstituted in a different era – albeit one that was more grounded in the sociology of risk and wider qualitative studies of parental attitudes through surveys and systematic literature reviews.

This is not to say that qualitative investigations into the issues surrounding hesitancy had not been conducted before the crisis and its aftermath. Questions about parental attitudes were being asked of pertussis vaccine and MMR going back to at least the 1980s.[138] The ways in which they are now being used to explain and measure vaccine confidence as an indicator is, however, historically intriguing.[139] SAGE has done so through breaking hesitancy into three constituent parts: confidence in a vaccine and vaccination authorities; convenience of access to vaccination; and complacency about the risks of inaction.[140] What history shows is that confidence, convenience and complacency have manifested in different ways at different times. They have not been universal, either within populations or across all types of vaccine. Moreover, the fact that imperfect levels of these three qualities have still resulted in the general public following government guidelines says much about how well established and accepted vaccination was in the post-war period.

Notes

1 Joanne Yarwood, Karen Noakes, Dorian Kennedy, Helen Campbell and David Salisbury, 'Tracking mothers' attitudes to childhood immunisation 1991–2001', *Vaccine*, 23:48–49 (2005), S670–87.
2 Patricia Thomas, *Big Shot: Passion, Politics, and the Struggle for an AIDS Vaccine* (New York: Public Affairs, 2001); Jon Cohen, *Shots in the Dark: The Wayward Search for an AIDS Vaccine* (London: Norton, 2001).
3 SAGE Working Group on Vaccine Hesitancy, *Report of the SAGE Working Group on Vaccine Hesitancy* (Geneva: World Health Organization, October 2014); Caitlin Jarrett, Rose Wilson, Maureen O'Leary, Elisabeth Eckersberger, Heidi J. Larson and SAGE Working Group on Vaccine Hesitancy, 'Strategies for addressing vaccine hesitancy – a systematic review', *Vaccine*, 33:34 (2015), 4180–90.
4 See Chapter 4.
5 It is common to see in present-day discourse, especially from lay vaccination advocates, that parents who refused MMR during the crisis were acting irrationally and were opposed to vaccination. On this debate, see Alice Dredger, 'What if not all parents who question vaccines are foolish and anti-science?', *New Statesman* (4 June 2015) https://www.newstatesman.com/2015/05/heretic-academy (accessed 29 March 2018).
6 Health and Social Care Information Centre, 'NHS immunisation statistics: England, 2014–15' (23 September 2015) http://digital.nhs.uk/catalogue/PUB18472/nhs-immu-stat-eng-2014–15-rep.pdf (accessed 23 August 2017); National Health Services Scotland, 'Childhood immunisation statistics Scotland: quarter and year ending 31 December 2015' (22 March 2016) www.isdscotland.org/Health-Topics/Child-Health/Publications/2016-03-22/2016-03-22-Immunisation-Report.pdf (accessed 23 August 2017); Public Health Agency [Northern Ireland], 'Vaccination coverage: COVER' (March 2017) www.publichealthagency.org/sites/default/files/directorates/files/24%20months%20of%20age_20.pdf (accessed 23 August 2017).

7 Alan R. Petersen and Deborah Lupton, *The New Public Health: Health and Self in the Age of Risk* (London: Sage, 2000); Rudolf Klein, *The New Politics of the NHS: From Creation to Reinvention*, 7th edn (Oxford: Radcliffe, 2013).
8 Jeffrey P. Baker, 'The pertussis vaccine controversy in Great Britain, 1974–1986', *Vaccine*, 21:25–26 (2003), 4003–10.
9 Department of Health and Social Security, *Promoting Better Health: The Government's Programme for Improving Primary Health Care* (Cm 249) (London: HMSO, 1987); Department of Health and Social Security, *Public Health in England: The report of the Committee of Inquiry into the future development of the Public Health Function* (Cm 289) (London: HMSO, 1988).
10 All statistics and quotations from paragraph 1.10: Department of Health and Social Security, *Promoting Better Health* (Cm 249), pp. 2–3.
11 *Ibid.*
12 *Ibid.*, p. 3. See also Theodore M. Brown, Elizabeth Fee and Victoria Stepanova, 'Halfdan Mahler: Architect and defender of the World Health Organization "Health for All by 2000" declaration of 1978', *American Journal of Public Health*, 106:1 (2016), 38–9.
13 On immunisation specifically, see K. Keja, C. Chan, G. Hayden and R. H. Henderson, 'Expanded programme on immunization', *World Health Statistics Quarterly*, 41:2 (1988), 59–63. See also International Conference on Primary Health Care, *Declaration of Alma-Ata* (Alma-Ata: World Health Organization, 1978); *Cm 289*, p. 65. On the role of British economist Brian Abel-Smith in the negotiations over European health targets, see Sally Sheard, *The Passionate Economist: How Brian-Abel Smith Shaped Global Health and Social Welfare* (Bristol: Policy Press, 2013).
14 N. T. Begg and N. D. Noah, 'Immunisation targets in Europe and Britain', *British Medical Journal (Clinical Research Edition)*, 291:6506 (1985), 1370–1; HC Deb (26 October 1982) vol. 29, col. 377W; I. Kickbusch, 'The development of international health policies – accountability intact?', *Social Science and Medicine*, 51:6 (2000), 979–89.
15 HC Deb (2 May 1989) vol. 152 cc. 25–80. The target diseases were measles, polio, neonatal tetanus, diphtheria and congenital rubella. Begg and Noah, 'Immunisation targets in Europe and Britain'.
16 N. Klein, K. Morgan and M. H. Wansbrough-Jones, 'Parents' beliefs about vaccination: the continuing propagation of false contraindications', *British Medical Journal*, 298:6689 (1989), 1687.
17 Klein, *The New Politics of the NHS*.
18 Jane Lewis, 'The medical profession and the state: GPs and the GP contract in the 1960s and the 1990s', *Social Policy & Administration*, 32:2

(1998), 132–50; Bonnie Sibbald, Ian Enzer, Cary Cooper, Usha Rout and Valerie Sutherland, 'GP job satisfaction in 1987, 1990 and 1998: Lessons for the future?', *Family Practice*, 17:5 (2000), 364–71.

19 Norman Johnson, *The Welfare State in Transition: The Theory and Practice of Welfare Pluralism* (Amherst: University of Massachusetts Press, 1987); Norman Barry, 'Neoclassicism, the New Right and British social welfare', in Robert M. Page and Richard Silburn (eds), *British Social Welfare in the Twentieth Century* (London: Macmillan, 1999), pp. 55–79; Stuart Hall, 'The great moving right show', in Stuart Hall and Martin Jacques (eds), *The Politics of Thatcherism* (London: Lawrence & Wishart, 1983), pp. 19–39.

20 Klein, *The New Politics of the NHS*; Department of Health, *The Health of the Nation: A Strategy for Health in England* (Cm 1986) (London: HMSO, 1992).

21 Jennifer Stanton, 'What shapes vaccine policy? The case of hepatitis B in the UK', *Social History of Medicine*, 7:3 (1994), 427–46.

22 Farah Huzair and Steve Sturdy, 'Biotechnology and the transformation of vaccine innovation: The case of the hepatitis B vaccines 1968–2000', *Studies in History & Philosophy of Biological & Biomedical Sciences*, 64 (2017), 11–21. Although this relationship has become more strained in recent years as private companies pull out of the vaccine market. For a longer history of this process, see Stuart Blume, *Immunization: How Vaccines Became Controversial* (London: Reaktion, 2017).

23 Jennifer Stanton, 'What shapes vaccine policy?'.

24 T. Smith, 'Measles and the government', *British Medical Journal (Clinical Research Edition)*, 294:6578 (1987), 989–90; A. Nicoll and D. Jenkinson, 'Decision making for routine measles/MMR and whooping cough immunisation', *British Medical Journal*, 297:6645 (1988), 405–7; J. Badenoch, 'Big bang for vaccination', *British Medical Journal*, 297:6651 (1988), 750–1.

25 See Chapter 1 and Nicoll and Jenkinson, 'Decision making for routine measles/MMR and whooping cough immunisation'; David Elliman and Helen Bedford, 'Safety and efficacy of combination vaccines', *British Medical Journal*, 326:7397 (2003), 995–6.

26 Badenoch, 'Big bang for vaccination'.

27 Marko Petrovic, Richard Roberts and Mary Ramsay, 'Second dose of measles, mumps, and rubella vaccine: Questionnaire survey of health professionals', *British Medical Journal*, 322:7278 (2001), 82–5.

28 Ministry of Health, *Annual Report of the Ministry of Health for the year 1967* (Cmnd 3702) (London: HMSO, 1968), p. 20.

29 Public Health England and Department of Health, *Immunisation against Infectious Disease* (London: Public Health England, 2nd edn, 2013), p. 209.
30 Badenoch, 'Big bang for vaccination'.
31 Begg and Noah, 'Immunisation targets in Europe and Britain'.
32 Public Health England and Department of Health, *Immunisation against Infectious Disease*, p. 343.
33 Estimates of the risk of deafness range from 1 in 3,400 to 1 in 20,000 cases. See Public Health England and Department of Health, *Immunisation against Infectious Disease*, p. 255.
34 M. Evans, H. Stoddart, L. Condon, E. Freeman, M. Grizzell and R. Mullen, 'Parents' perspectives on the MMR immunisation: a focus group study', *British Journal of General Practice*, 51:472 (2001), 904–10.
35 *Ibid.*; Klein, Morgan and Wansbrough-Jones, 'Parents' beliefs about vaccination'; Badenoch, 'Big bang for vaccination'.
36 Norman T. Begg, O. N. Gill and Joanne M. White, 'COVER (cover of vaccination evaluated rapidly): Description of the England and Wales scheme', *Public Health*, 103:2 (1989), 81–9.
37 Mary E. Ramsay, J. Yarwood, D. Lewis, H. Campbell and J. M. White, 'Parental confidence in measles, mumps and rubella vaccine: evidence from vaccine coverage and attitudinal surveys', *British Journal of General Practice*, 52:484 (2002), 912–16.
38 Baker, 'The pertussis vaccine controversy'.
39 Stephen A. Goldman, 'Limitations and strengths of spontaneous reports data', *Clinical Therapeutics*, 20 (1998), C40–C44.
40 P. Farrington, M. Rush, E. Miller, S. Pugh, A. Colville, A. Flower, J. Nash and P. Morgan-Capner, 'A new method for active surveillance of adverse events from diphtheria/tetanus/pertussis and measles/mumps/rubella vaccines', *The Lancet*, 345:8949 (1995), 567–9.
41 See Chapter 1. On the role of doctors as levers for change in 1980s and 1990s health reforms, see Martin D. Moore, *Managing Diabetes, Managing Medicine: Chronic Disease and Clinical Bureaucracy in Post-War Britain* (Manchester: Manchester University Press, 2019).
42 See Chapter 2.
43 Alex Mold, *Making the Patient-consumer: Patient Organisations and Health Consumerism in Britain* (Manchester: Manchester University Press, 2015); Mike Fitzpatrick, 'Choice', *The Lancet*, 363:9409 (2004), 668; Department of Health, *Building on the Best: Choice, Responsiveness and Equity in the NHS* (Cm 6079) (London: TSO, 2003); Kenneth C. Calman, 'Communication of risk: Choice, consent, and trust', *The Lancet*, 360:9327 (2002), 166–8.

44 See Tammy Speers and Justin Lewis, 'Journalists and jabs: Media coverage of the MMR vaccine', *Communication & Medicine*, 1:2 (2004), 171–81; Ian Hargreaves, Justin Lewis and Tammy Speers, *Towards a Better Map: Science, the Public and the Media* (London: Economic and Social Research Council, 2003).

45 Simon H. Murch, Andrew Anthony, David H. Casson, Mohsin Malik, Mark Berelowitz, Amar P. Dhillon, Michael A. Thomson, Alan Valentine, Susan E. Davies and John A. Walker-Smith, 'Retraction of an interpretation', *The Lancet*, 363:9411 (2004), 750; Brian Deer, 'Reflections on investigating Wakefield', *British Medical Journal*, 340 (2010), c672.

46 Heidi J. Larson, Alexandre de Figueiredo, Zhao Xiahong, William S. Schulz, Pierre Verger, Iain G. Johnston, Alex R. Cook and Nick S. Jones, 'The state of vaccine confidence 2016: Global insights through a 67-country survey', *EBioMedicine*, 12 (2016), 295–301.

47 A. J. Wakefield, S. H. Murch, A. Anthony, J. Linnell, D. M. Casson, M. Malik, M. Berelowitz, A. P. Dhillon, M. A. Thomson, P. Harvey, A. Valentine, S. E. Davies and J. A. Walker-Smith, 'RETRACTED: Ileal-lymphoid-nodular hyperplasia, non-specific colitis, and pervasive developmental disorder in children', *The Lancet*, 351:9103 (1998), 637–41.

48 Sarah Boseley, 'Doctors' dilemma', *Guardian* (27 February 1998), p. 5; Celia Hall, 'Vaccination may trigger disease linked to autism', *Daily Telegraph* (27 February 1998), p. 2; Ian Murray, 'Measles vaccine's link with autism studied', *The Times* (27 February 1998), p. 6.

49 Robert T. Chen and Frank DeStefano, 'Vaccine adverse events: Causal or coincidental?', *The Lancet*, 351:9103 (1998), 611–12.

50 Richard Horton, *MMR: Science and Fiction – Exploring a Vaccine Crisis* (London: Granta, 2004), pp. 139–72; Speers and Lewis, 'Journalists and jabs'; Lord Leveson, *An Inquiry into the Culture, Practices and Ethics of the Press. Report, Volume II* (HC 780-II, 2012–13) (London: TSO, 2012).

51 John Walker-Smith, 'Autism, bowel inflammation, and measles', *The Lancet*, 359:9307 (2002), 705–6; Simon Murch, Mike Thomson and John Walker-Smith, 'Autism, inflammatory bowel disease, and MMR vaccine', *The Lancet*, 351:9106 (1998), 908; Susan Mayor, 'Researcher from study alleging link between MMR and autism warns of measles epidemic', *British Medical Journal*, 327:7423 (2003), 1069.

52 A. J. Wakefield and S. M. Montgomery, 'Measles, mumps, rubella vaccine: through a glass, darkly', *Adverse Drug Reactions and Toxicological Reviews*, 19:4 (2000), 265–83; discussion 284–92.

53 Sarah Ramsay, 'UK starts campaign to reassure parents about MMR-vaccine safety', *The Lancet*, 357:9252 (2001), 290.

54 Jacqui Wise, 'Finnish study confirms safety of MMR vaccine', *British Medical Journal*, 322:7279 (2001), 130; Haroon Ashraf, 'US expert group rejects link between MMR and autism', *The Lancet*, 357:9265 (2001), 1341; Claudia E. Kuehni, Adrian M. Brooke, Anthony Davis and Michael Silverman, 'Vaccinations as risk factors for wheezing disorders', *The Lancet*, 358:9288 (2001), 1186.
55 Speers and Lewis, 'Journalists and jabs'.
56 V. Uhlmann, C. M. Martin, O. Sheils, L. Pilkington, I. Silva, A. Killalea, S. B. Murch, J. Walker-Smith, M. Thomson, A. J. Wakefield and J. J. O'Leary, 'Potential viral pathogenic mechanism for new variant inflammatory bowel disease', *Molecular Pathology*, 55:2 (2002), 84–90; A. Morris and D. Aldulaimi, 'New evidence for a viral pathogenic mechanism for new variant inflammatory bowel disease and development disorder?', *Molecular Pathology*, 55:2 (2002), 83. The journal *Molecular Pathology* released the paper early after it appeared on BBC1's *Panorama*. See the press release: Journal of Molecular Pathology, 'Pre-published Molecular Pathology paper', *Journal of Molecular Pathology* (3 February 2002) http://jcp.bmj.com/content/55/1/suppl/DC1 (accessed 5 January 2017).
57 Roger Dobson, 'Parents' champion or loose cannon?', *British Medical Journal*, 324:7334 (2002), 386.
58 Zosia Kmietowicz, 'Government launches intensive media campaign on MMR', *British Medical Journal*, 324:7334 (2002), 383.
59 Legal Services Commission, 'Decision to remove funding for MMR litigation upheld on appeal' (captured 10 October 2003, 11:25:31) https://web.archive.org/web/20031010112531/ http://www.legalservices.gov.uk/misl/news/press/press-13-03.htm (accessed 5 January 2017).
60 Richard Horton, 'A statement by the editors of The Lancet', *The Lancet*, 363:9411 (2004), 820–21. Wakefield would be investigated and eventually struck off the medical register in 2010 for his involvement. Murch and Walker-Smith were investigated but eventually exonerated. General Medical Council, *Dr Andrew Jeremy Wakefield: Determination on Serious Professional Misconduct (SPM) and Sanction* (London: General Medical Council, 2010); Iain Chalmers and Andy Haines, 'Commentary: Skilled forensic capacity needed to investigate allegations of research misconduct', *British Medical Journal*, 342 (2011), d3977; Clare Dyer, 'Co-author of Wakefield paper on MMR vaccine wins his appeal against decision by GMC to strike him off', *British Medical Journal*, 344 (2012), e1745.
61 Murch et al, 'Retraction of an interpretation'.
62 David C. Burgess, Margaret A. Burgess and Julie Leask, 'The MMR vaccination and autism controversy in United Kingdom 1998–2005: Inevitable

community outrage or a failure of risk communication?', *Vaccine*, 24:18 (2006), 3921–8.
63 Speers and Lewis, 'Journalists and jabs'. See especially the series of articles in the paper on MMR and autism by Melanie Phillips, beginning: Melanie Phillips, 'MMR the truth', *Daily Mail* (11 March 2003), p. 42.
64 David Goldberg, 'MMR, autism, and Adam', *British Medical Journal*, 320:7231 (2000), 389.
65 An interview with the Scottish newspaper the *Herald* suggests JABS was formed around 1994 or 1995. Marian Pallister, 'Now break down those walls', *Herald* (25 January 2000), p. 12. The group was definitely active in 1995. JABS, 'Fair warning' (captured 25 October 2001, 14:41:25) http://web.archive.org/web/20011025144125/ http://www.jabs.org.uk:80/jabsinformation.htm (accessed 1 July 2017).
66 Sarah-Kate Templeton, 'Mother wins MMR payout after 18 years', *Sunday Times* (29 August 2010), p. 12.
67 The website focused heavily on MMR and autism. The first capture in the Internet Archive is in April 2001. See JABS, 'Welcome to JABS on the internet' (captured 5 April 2001, 03:52:43) http://web.archive.org/web/20010405035243/ http://www.jabs.org.uk (accessed 1 July 2017). For the group's press activities, see Melanie Phillips, 'Are we facing an autism epidemic?', *Daily Mail* (13 March 2003), p. 68; Marian Pallister, 'Now break down those walls', *Herald* (25 January 2000), p. 12; Kate Foster, 'Injection fears that linger on', *Scotsman* (3 November 2001), p. 6.
68 JABS, 'Welcome to JABS on the internet'; Society for the Autistically Handicapped, 'Vaccines fact sheet' (captured 2 September 2000, 06:08:43) http://web.archive.org/web/20000902060843/ http://www.autismuk.com:80/index1sub4.htm (accessed 28 July 2017); Michael Fitzpatrick, 'Parents: Jabs and junk science', *Guardian* (8 September 2004), G2 supplement, p. 9; Brian Deer, 'How the case against the MMR vaccine was fixed', *British Medical Journal*, 342 (2011), c5347.
69 Legal Services Commission, 'Decision to remove funding for MMR litigation upheld on appeal'; Clare Dyer, 'Commission withdraws legal aid for parents suing over MMR vaccine', *British Medical Journal*, 327:7416 (2003), 640.
70 Farrington et al, 'A new method for active surveillance'; Kohji Ueda, Chiaki Miyazaki, Yasufumi Hidaka, Kenji Okada, Koichi Kusuhara and Ryo Kadoya, 'Aseptic meningitis caused by measles-mumps-rubella vaccine in Japan', *The Lancet*, 346:8976 (1995), 701–2.
71 Harumi Gomi and Hiroshi Takahashi, 'Why is measles still endemic in Japan?', *The Lancet*, 364:9431 (2004), 328–9.
72 Wakefield and Montgomery, 'Measles, mumps, rubella vaccine'.

73 David Elliman and Helen Bedford, 'MMR vaccine: the continuing saga', *British Medical Journal*, 322:7280 (2001), 183–4; Wakefield and Montgomery, 'Measles, mumps, rubella vaccine'.
74 Speers and Lewis, 'Journalists and jabs'.
75 Kamran Abbasi, 'Man, mission, rumpus', *British Medical Journal*, 322:7281 (2001), 306. See also Richard Horton, 'The lessons of MMR', *The Lancet*, 363:9411 (2004), 747–9; R. L. Salmon, 'Science in the face of disaster', *The Lancet*, 363:9414 (2004), 1084–5.
76 Forty-five per cent said nothing had decreased their trust. The next most popular reason was 'Foot & Mouth' (17 per cent) followed by 'GM Food' (15 per cent). MMR was fifth (12 per cent). Hargreaves, Lewis and Speers, *Towards a Better Map*, p. 30.
77 Clare Dyer, 'NHS told to pay £10m to patients infected with hepatitis C', *British Medical Journal*, 322:7289 (2001), 751.
78 Ian Kennedy, *The Report of the Public Inquiry into Children's Heart Surgery at the Bristol Royal Infirmary 1984–1995: Learning from Bristol* (Cm 5207) (London: TSO, 2001); Michael Redfern, *The Royal Liverpool Children's Inquiry Report* (HC 12-II, 2000–01) (London: TSO, 2001).
79 Sharon Alcock, 'How parents decide on MMR', *British Medical Journal*, 324:7335 (2002), 492.
80 M. Pareek and H. M. Pattison, 'The two-dose measles, mumps, and rubella (MMR) immunisation schedule: factors affecting maternal intention to vaccinate', *British Journal of General Practice*, 50:461 (2000), 969–71; Various letters to the editor under the title, 'Health professionals' attitudes to MMR vaccine', *British Medical Journal*, 322:7294 (May 2001), 1120–1.
81 Stanton, 'What shapes vaccine policy?'
82 Richard Fry, 'Debate crystallises dilemma facing many medical disciplines', in Various, 'MMR vaccine debate', *British Medical Journal*, 324:7339 (2002), 733. See also Tom Heller, Dick Heller, Stephen Pattison and Tom Heller, 'Vaccination against mumps, measles, and rubella: is there a case for deepening the debate?', *British Medical Journal*, 323:7317 (October 2001), 838–40.
83 Peter M. B. English, 'General practitioners' two roles are not in conflict with MMR immunisation', in Various, 'MMR vaccine debate'.
84 Nigel Hawkes, 'GPs want to end pay incentives for MMR targets', *The Times* (3 July 2002), p. 11; Annabel Ferriman, 'London mayor attacked for doing "irreparable damage" on MMR', *British Medical Journal*, 325:7355 (2002), 66.
85 Kate Hilpern, 'Ripping up the Red Book: A long-negotiated contract is intended to give GPs' practices greater flexibility and control', *Independent* (24 June 2004), p. 5.

86 See this discussion in Chapter 4 and: Jacqueline R. Meszaros, David A. Asch, Jonathan Baron, John C. Hershey, Howard Kunreuther and Joanne Schwartz-Buzaglo, 'Cognitive processes and the decisions of some parents to forego pertussis vaccination for their children', *Journal of Clinical Epidemiology*, 49:6 (1996), 697–703. See also Katrina F. Brown, J. Simon Kroll, Michael J. Hudson, Mary Ramsay, John Green, Charles A. Vincent, Graham Fraser and Nick Sevdalis, 'Omission bias and vaccine rejection by parents of healthy children: Implications for the influenza A/H1N1 vaccination programme', *Vaccine*, 28:25 (2010), 4181–5; Heidi J. Larson, Louis Z. Cooper, Juhani Eskola, Samuel L. Katz and Scott Ratzan, 'Addressing the vaccine confidence gap', *The Lancet*, 378:9790 (2011), 526–35.
87 Department of Health, *Building on the Best* (Cm 6079).
88 Fitzpatrick, 'Choice'.
89 Hilary Bower, 'MMR vaccine policy is backed', *British Medical Journal*, 316:7136 (1998), 955; Zosia Kmietowicz, 'Separate vaccines could endanger children', *British Medical Journal*, 323:7315 (2001), 711; British Medical Association Board of Science and Education, *Childhood Immunisation: A Guide for Healthcare Professionals* (London: British Medical Association, 2003), esp. pp. 10–11.
90 Elliman and Bedford, 'Safety and efficacy of combination vaccines'.
91 Chris Brown, 'MMR parents besiege clinic – families pay £60 for single jab', *Daily Post* [Liverpool] (2 February 2001), p. 1; 'The great MMR dilemma', *Daily Mail* (6 February 2002), p. 18; Sue Leonard, 'Edinburgh doctor is highest earner in MMR jabs bonanza', *Sunday Times* (17 February 2002), p. 4; Sue Leonard and Rosie Waterhouse, 'Doctors cash in on MMR fear with £280 charge for single jabs', *Sunday Times* (17 February 2002), p. 9.
92 Helen Barratt, 'MMR vaccine row raises questions of clinical freedom', *British Medical Journal*, 323:7308 (2001), 300; Azeem Majeed, 'Referral of Dr Peter Mansfield to the GMC', *British Medical Journal*, 323:7309 (2001), 356; Alcock, 'How parents decide on MMR'; Felicity Lawrence, 'Portrait: This might hurt', *Guardian* (7 August 2001), p. 6.
93 Harold Shipman was a GP who had killed a number of his patients, possibly as many as 250. He was convicted following a high-profile trial in 2000.
94 Various letters to the editor, 'We should praise jab GP, not hound him', *Daily Mail* (13 August 2001), p. 70.
95 Alcock, 'How parents decide on MMR'.
96 Ramsay, 'UK starts campaign to reassure parents'; Susan Mayor, 'Medical Research Council review sets research agenda for autism', *British Medical*

Journal, 324:7328 (2002), 10; Medical Research Council, *Review of Autism Research: Epidemiology and Causes* (London: Medical Research Council, 2001).
97 Ramsay, 'UK starts campaign to reassure parents'.
98 Kmietowicz, 'Government launches intensive media campaign on MMR'; Speers and Lewis, 'Journalists and jabs'.
99 Eddie Barnes, 'MMR policy relaunch backfires on Minister', *Daily Mail* (14 February 2001), p. 19.
100 Andy Alaszewski and Tom Horlick-Jones, 'How can doctors communicate information about risk more effectively?', *British Medical Journal*, 327:7417 (2003), 728–31.
101 British Medical Association Board of Science and Education, *Childhood Immunisation*; MMR Expert Group, 'Report of the MMR Expert Group', *Scottish Government* (April 2002) www.gov.scot/Publications/2002/04/14619/3779 (accessed 24 August 2017). See also Medical Research Council, *Review of Autism Research*.
102 Horton, 'The lessons of MMR'.
103 Peter Duncan, 'Failing to professionalise, struggling to specialise: The rise and fall of health promotion as a putative specialism in England, 1980–2000', *Medical History*, 57:3 (2013), 377–96.
104 Alaszewski and Horlick-Jones, 'How can doctors communicate?'
105 *Ibid.*
106 Alcock, 'How parents decide on MMR'.
107 Sarah Ramsay, 'UK government tries to control MMR panic', *The Lancet*, 359:9306 (2002), 590.
108 UNdata, 'Internet users (per 100 people)' (undated) http://data.un.org/Data.aspx?d=WDI&f=Indicator_Code%3AIT.NET.USER.P2 (accessed 22 June 2017).
109 J. Selway, 'Medical practitioners need to give more than reassurance', in Various, 'MMR vaccination and autism 1998', *British Medical Journal*, 316:7147 (1998), 1824; Richard Smith, 'Do patients need to read research?', *British Medical Journal*, 326:7402 (2003), 1307; A. Rouse, 'Autism, inflammatory bowel disease, and MMR vaccine', *The Lancet*, 351:9112 (1998), 1356.
110 Diane E Goldstein, *Once Upon a Virus: AIDS Legends and Vernacular Risk Perception* (Logan: Utah State University Press, 2004); Andrea Kitta, *Vaccinations and Public Concern in History: Legend, Rumor, and Risk Perception* (New York: Routledge, 2012); Roberta Bivins, *Alternative Medicine? A History* (Oxford: Oxford University Press, 2007).
111 Speers and Lewis, 'Journalists and jabs'.
112 Hargreaves, Lewis and Speers, *Towards a better map*, p. 23.

113 The website was taken down in the late 2000s, but is still archived. Department of Health, 'MMR the facts' (captured 8 September 2002, 12:06:49) https://web.archive.org/web/20020908120649/ http://www.mmrthefacts.nhs.uk:80/ (accessed 11 July 2017). See also: Joanne Yarwood, 'Communicating vaccine benefit and risk – lessons from the medical field', *Veterinary Microbiology*, 117:1 (2006), 71–4.
114 Sadly, the map itself has not been archived. The text is still available. Department of Health, 'MMR world map' (captured 14 December 2002, 01:46:04) https://web.archive.org/web/20021214014604/ http://www.mmrthefacts.nhs.uk:80/worldmap/ (accessed 11 July 2017).
115 Department of Health, 'MMR: myths and truths' (captured 19 October 2002, 07:32:21) https://web.archive.org/web/20021019073221/ http://www.mmrthefacts.nhs.uk:80/basics/truths.php (accessed 11 July 2017).
116 Department of Health, 'Your questions answered' (captured 3 December 2002, 00:10:27) https://web.archive.org/web/20021203001027/ http://www.mmrthefacts.nhs.uk:80/questions/ (accessed 11 July 2017).
117 Only around 80 per cent of children get immunity from one dose. A second dose ensures that the statistical likelihood of getting immunity is increased without the need for unreliable and painful blood tests. Petrovic, Roberts and Ramsay, 'Second dose of measles, mumps, and rubella vaccine'; Elliman and Bedford, 'MMR vaccine'.
118 Samuel Ghebrehewet and Catherine Quigley, 'Format of "green book" should be changed', in Various, 'Health professionals' attitudes to MMR vaccine'.
119 Yarwood, 'Communicating vaccine benefit and risk'.
120 Helen Barratt, 'Scottish GPs to be sent discussion packs on MMR vaccine', *British Medical Journal*, 323:7312 (2001), 532.
121 Department of Health, 'Measles, mumps and rubella vaccine (MMR)' (captured 13 December 2002) http://web.archive.org/web/20021213092753/ http://www.doh.gov.uk/mmr/ (accessed 11 July 2017).
122 See Chapter 1. Ministry of Health, *Summary report of the Ministry of Health for the year ended 31st March, 1943* (Cmd 6468) (London: HMSO, 1943).
123 Ulrich Beck, *Risk Society: Towards a New Modernity* (London: Sage, 1992); Petersen and Lupton, *The New Public Health*; Calman, 'Communication of risk'; Paul Bellaby, 'Communication and miscommunication of risk: understanding UK parents' attitudes to combined MMR vaccination', *British Medical Journal*, 327:7417 (2003), 725–8.

124 As examples of coverage in the *Daily Mail* and *Private Eye*, see Phillips, 'MMR the truth'; Heather Mills, *Private Eye Special Report: MMR: The Story So Far* (London: Pressdam, 2002); Phil Hammond, 'The editor asks M.D. to peer review Private Eye's MMR coverage', originally published in *Private Eye* 1256 (17 February 2010). www.drphilhammond.com/blog/2010/02/18/private-eye/dr-phil%E2%80%99s-private-eye-column-issue-1256-february-17-2010/ (accessed 11 July 2017).
125 See Chapter 4 and report from the Swansea Research Unity of the Royal College of General Practitioners, 'Effect of a low pertussis vaccination uptake on a large community', *British Medical Journal (Clinical Research Edition)*, 282:6257 (1981), 23–6.
126 David Elliman and Helen Bedford, 'Should the UK introduce compulsory vaccination?', *The Lancet*, 381:9876 (2013), 1434–6.
127 Kenneth Clarke, 'Rush for vaccine in epidemic of whooping cough', *Daily Telegraph* (16 December 1977), p. 6; Paul Cahalan, 'Hundreds queue for MMR jab as Welsh measles outbreak slows', *Independent on Sunday* (7 April 2013), p. 10.
128 Chen and DeStefano, 'Vaccine adverse events'; Sarah J. O'Brien, Ian G. Jones and Peter Christie, 'Autism, inflammatory bowel disease, and MMR vaccine', *The Lancet*, 351:9106 (1998), 906–7; Norman Begg, Mary Ramsay, Joanne White and Zoltan Bozoky, 'Media dents confidence in MMR vaccine', *British Medical Journal*, 316:7130 (1998), 561; Angus Nicoll, David Elliman and Euan Ross, 'MMR vaccination and autism 1998', *British Medical Journal*, 316:7133 (1998), 715–16; The Lancet, 'Time to look beyond MMR in autism research', *The Lancet*, 359:9307 (2002), 637.
129 Leszek K. Borysiewicz, 'Prevention is better than cure', *The Lancet*, 375:9713 (2010), 513–23; E. Richard Moxon and Claire-Anne Siegrist, 'The next decade of vaccines: societal and scientific challenges', *The Lancet*, 378:9788 (2011), 348–59. Roy Greenslade, 'Measles: Analysis: The story behind the MMR scare', *Guardian* (25 April 2013), p. 13; Chris Smyth, 'Babies at risk from MMR jab timebomb', *The Times* (30 May 2013), p. 1.
130 Helen Mooney, 'More "responsible" science reporting is needed, Leveson inquiry hears', *British Medical Journal*, 343 (2011), d8051; Leveson, *Inquiry into the Culture, Practices and Ethics of the Press* (HC 780-II, 2012–13).
131 Virginia Berridge categorically cautions against this in Virginia Berridge, 'Thinking in time: Does health policy need history as evidence?', *The Lancet*, 375:9717 (2010), 798–9.

132 World Health Organization, 'Weekly epidemiological record' (7 January 2011) http://www.who.int/wer/2011/wer8601_02.pdf (accessed 24 August 2017); Doug Campos-Outcalt, 'Measles: Why it's still a threat', *The Journal of Family Practice*, 66:7 (2017), 446–9.

133 SAGE Working Group on Vaccine Hesitancy, *Report*; Pawel Stefanoff, Svenn-Erik Mamelund, Mary Robinson, Eva Netterlid, Jose Tuells, Marianne A. Riise Bergsaker, Harald Heijbel and Joanne Yarwood, 'Tracking parental attitudes on vaccination across European countries: The Vaccine Safety, Attitudes, Training and Communication Project (VACSATC)', *Vaccine*, 28:35 (2010), 5731–7.

134 Heidi J. Larson, Caitlin Jarrett, Elisabeth Eckersberger, David M. D. Smith and Pauline Paterson, 'Understanding vaccine hesitancy around vaccines and vaccination from a global perspective: A systematic review of published literature, 2007–2012', *Vaccine*, 32:19 (2014), 2150–9; Jarrett et al, 'Strategies for addressing vaccine hesitancy'.

135 Sally Jefferies, Sylvia McShane, Juliet Oerton, Christina R. Victor and Rosemary Beardow, 'Low immunization uptake rates in an inner-city health district: fact or fiction?', *Journal of Public Health*, 13:4 (1991), 312–17; Jeremy I. Hawker, Babatunde Olowokure, Annette L. Wood, Richard C. Wilson and Richard Johnson, 'Widening inequalities in MMR vaccine uptake rates among ethnic groups in an urban area of the UK during a period of vaccine controversy (1994–2000)', *Vaccine*, 25:43 (2007), 7516–19.

136 Horton, 'The lessons of MMR'.

137 On the idea of vaccination becoming a "victim of its own success", see Begg et al, 'Media dents confidence in MMR vaccine'; Robert T. Chen and Beth Hibbs, 'Vaccine safety: Current and future challenges', *Pediatric Annals*, 27:7 (1998), 445–5.

138 Karen A. Roberts, Mary Dixon-Woods, Ray Fitzpatrick, Keith R. Abrams and David R. Jones, 'Factors affecting uptake of childhood immunisation: a Bayesian synthesis of qualitative and quantitative evidence', *The Lancet*, 360:9345 (2002), 1596–9; C. A. Peckham, Action Research for the Crippled Child, British Postgraduate Medical Federation, Institute of Child Health and Department of Paediatric Epidemiology, *The Peckham Report: National Immunisation Study: Factors Influencing Immunisation Uptake in Childhood* (London: Department of Paediatric Epidemiology, Institute of Child Health ; Horsham, West Sussex : Action Research for the Crippled Child, 1989); Richard J. Roberts, Quentin D. Sandifer, Merion R. Evans, Maria Z. Nolan-Farrell and Paul M. Davis, 'Reasons for non-uptake of measles, mumps, and rubella catch up immunisation in a measles epidemic and side effects of the vaccine', *British Medical Journal*, 310:6995

(1995), 1629–39; Rachel Casiday, 'Risk communication in the British pertussis and MMR vaccine controversies', in Peter Bennett, Kenneth Calman, Sarah Curtis and Denis Fischbacher-Smith (eds), *Risk Communication and Public Health* (Oxford: Oxford University Press, 2010), 129–46; Calman, 'Communication of risk'.
139 Larson et al, 'The state of vaccine confidence 2016'; Larson et al, 'Addressing the vaccine confidence gap'.
140 SAGE Working Group on Vaccine Hesitancy, *Report*.

Conclusion

When the National Health Service Acts were passed in 1946 and 1947, two vaccines were part of the routine infant vaccination schedule. By 2018 these had increased to seventeen.[1] Ninety-four per cent of children received the pentavalent diphtheria-tetanus-acellular-pertussis, polio-myelitis and haemophilus influenza type b vaccine before their first birthdays in England and Wales in 2014–15.[2] Polio is no longer endemic in Britain and has nearly been eradicated worldwide. There were 18,596 notifications of diphtheria in England and Wales in 1945. In 2016 there were nine.[3] For the public health profession, this has been a major achievement over a period of some seventy years. As we have seen, this progress has not been linear, nor consistent. Nevertheless, the mature vaccination system in Britain has created and reflects Jacob Heller's vaccine narrative – people believe that vaccines work, that they are safe and that they are an integral part of the modern, functioning British state.[4] Anxieties over outbreaks such as the 2012 measles outbreak in Swansea also seem to suggest that vaccination is part of being a good British citizen.[5] Vaccination is not simply imposed upon the British public. It is something which the public demands of its government and its fellow citizens.[6]

The preceding chapters have shown how the routine immunisation of children became the status quo in Britain after the Second World War. Modern vaccination programmes based on laboratory science and state-guided public health administration arrived on a national scale in the 1940s. The success of the anti-diphtheria campaign during the war showed both to the Ministry of Health and to the general public that vaccination could be an effective public health tool. Building on advertising and education techniques employed in other jurisdictions in the inter-war period, the lack of compulsion in the diphtheria immunisation campaign gave it credibility. These new health tools – born from modern vaccinology and without the baggage of the imposition and unpleasant nature of smallpox vaccination – could now be exploited. During the 1950s and 1960s, improvements in research and manufacturing techniques led to new vaccines which could be introduced to a receptive public. Indeed, for the high-profile ones (such as Salk's poliomyelitis vaccine) there was active demand from citizens. But such demand was also tempered by concerns about other risks, such as vaccine damage, convenience and financial sustainability.

Thus, the public played a key role in shaping public health authorities' priorities. The general trend was toward the increased use of vaccination, in terms both of the number of vaccines available and of percentage uptake among the population. This relationship between the public and public health led to an expansion of the vaccination programme and provided the authority for its maintenance. But this relationship still needed tending. Uptake was not always optimal, and occasional bouts of apathy (either across the population or in specific localised examples) required the intervention of MOHs and the Ministry of Health. In some cases, the government reminded parents of their responsibilities and the very real dangers posed by diseases that might return. In others, such as smallpox, general disinterest among the population, coupled with expert analyses of the risks posed by the disease and the vaccine, meant that the United Kingdom's smallpox vaccination programme was dismantled in advance of those of many other European countries.

The two crises outlined in Part II of the book, somewhat paradoxically, provide the best example of how the British public believed in vaccination. For while specific vaccines could become the centre of controversy at certain times, the vaccination system *as a whole* stood firm. With both pertussis vaccination and MMR vaccine, immunisation rates recovered relatively quickly following initial scares. Furthermore, uptake of vaccines that were not directly associated to whole-cell pertussis vaccine or MMR was not dramatically affected. Similarly, there were reports in both cases of parents demanding separate vaccines in order to avoid the Urabe mumps strain within the trivalent vaccines that had been identified as potentially dangerous. Nevertheless, the public understood the relative risks of disease symptoms and vaccines, and the inconvenience of presenting children for vaccination, differently to epidemiologist advisers in the government. Faith in vaccination still relied upon the moral and political authority of the scientific and administrative communities that vouched for the safety and efficacy of both the vaccines themselves and the mass immunisation programmes that underpinned them. In the aftermath of the thalidomide or BSE crises, or during major political debates about the viability and future of the welfare state, such authority was dented. Experiences with these crises led to a reappraisal of how vaccinators communicated with the public, producing a greater academic and administrative emphasis on hesitancy and decision making about vaccination. The hope was that analysing and monitoring for signs of faltering confidence could predict and prevent such crises before they occurred.

The five themes explored in this book – apathy, nation, demand, risk and hesitancy – all help to answer the main question posed in the Introduction: how did routine vaccination become normalised in Britain after the Second World War? In drawing together these ideas, this conclusion makes some final observations on a thread that runs throughout the chapters. How did the public fit into British public health over the post-war period? How was the public identified; and what was public about public health? These are important questions, given the centrality of the relationship between British citizens and the British government across the vaccination programme. This relationship drove the development of the vaccination schedule. As we have seen, the government had expectations of the population and, in turn, the population made demands on its government. But these demands did not remain unchanged. The same is true of the public.

Janet Newman and John Clarke have argued that publicness – that is, representations of the concept of the public – is a useful lens for discussing historical change.[7] This form of analysis is designed to move away from solely talking about the public sphere. Partly this is because the public sphere is only one element of publicness; and partly it is because of the critique that many narratives surrounding the Habermasean public sphere often describe a decline from a "golden age".[8] Moreover, the limits of publicness have varied across time and according to what sort of public is under discussion. Newman and Clarke thus draw attention to three 'discursive chains', of which the public sphere is only one. First, there is the belief that the public is embodied by citizens, or the people, which in turn represents the nation. Second, one can argue that the public is manifested in the public sector, which represents the actions of the state. Third, the public are created through legal and democratic value systems, best expressed through the aforementioned concept of the public sphere.[9] This is the public space (physical or metaphorical) in which debates about the people and the state can be articulated. Each of these may have been considered more important relative to the others at different times or circumstances. This book has largely focused on how debates about publicness played out in the public sphere. Evidence of public activity is inferred and identified through official statistics, utterances in the press and the actions of voluntary organisations and representative bodies claiming to operate in the interests of the public. The two themes left to explore are what this public sphere activity says about the people and what this in turn says about the role of the state.

To tackle the first discursive chain, the public were discussed in public health discourse as "the population". The way that the government constructed apathy in Chapter 1 exemplifies this. Defining the public through statistical returns – and then inferring public behaviours through changes in these statistics – was a common practice in the vaccination programme throughout this book. Rises and falls in uptake and morbidity (either over time or in comparison to other national and local authorities) were used to measure the success of vaccination efforts. Thus, the drop in the number of immunisations between 1949 and 1950 was considered troublesome in its own right. The solution, building on pre-existing ideas and conventions surrounding the dissemination of public health information and local MOHs led the Ministry of Health to focus its attempts on an advertising campaign. Resource constraints meant that it targeted its interventions on specific publics: those living in local authorities with low response rates relative to their peers. Over time, these statistical measures became more detailed, as did the means to analyse them. As Chapter 3 showed, the growth of the medical civil service both created and interpreted data for directing policy.[10] The foundation, first, of the JCPV (1955) and, later, of the JCVI (1962) provided the basis for this. In later years, health researchers paid greater attention not just to immunisation figures but to public attitudes through surveys. These had been performed as one-off studies in the 1940s for diphtheria but became routine from the late 1980s onwards through the Public Health Laboratory Service's COVER and regular studies of mothers' attitudes to immunisation.[11] These not only allowed for the identification of problematic behaviour within the public but also provided baseline measures to evaluate any intervention into such behaviour. This approach – which would form the basis of discussions around hesitancy in Chapter 5 – showed how conceptions of the public had evolved. Instead of semi-arbitrary target figures like 75 per cent for diphtheria or smallpox vaccination in the 1950s, epidemiologically and politically derived goals came from within the Department of Health and from internationally agreed standards with the WHO. Increasingly, outbreaks of manageable diseases became an embarrassment to the British authorities and the British public. During the MMR crisis, part of the education and risk communication campaign emphasised how other nations used immunisation. Advanced nations were supposed to avoid outbreaks of vaccine-preventable diseases; less-developed nations experienced them regularly.

Statistics were also used to sell the narrative that vaccination was not just for the good of the individual, but a sign of modernity, technological advancement and national pride. The national scope and character of the vaccination programme were therefore significant. Even where programmes were administered at the local level, they required national direction, financing and oversight. The national government's priorities and actions had been important in the inter-war period too. Experiences in other countries with diphtheria immunisation and BCG for tuberculosis had influenced the ways in which those vaccines were introduced in Britain.[12] Similarly, constant comparisons with the United States' IPV drove the course of the IPV campaign in Britain during the 1950s and early 1960s. While these discussions mainly concerned vaccines and the science surrounding them, they also reflected deeper ideas about who the "British public" were in "British public health". The nation (as highlighted in Chapter 2) came across strongly through the smallpox campaigns. Here, the British public was a body that needed to be protected from outside infection. Sometimes this was from foreign people, as seen with the reaction to Pakistani immigrants in the 1961/62 outbreak. At other times, foreign places were seen as the contagion, with people merely the mules, such as Australasian tourists in the 1950 outbreak. Even today, visitors to "exotic" countries are often obliged to receive vaccines against diseases such as yellow fever. Campaigns to control infectious disease also worked on a national level. This was true in their administration – decisions about national policy were taken jointly between the four home nations – and in their goals. Concerns over apathy towards the diphtheria programme were that a disease that was on the verge of elimination within Britain might return. The demand for polio vaccine in the 1950s reflected the British public's call to be protected from the disease, with vaccination and eventual eradication considered to be the most sensible way of achieving this. The management of risks, as discussed in Chapter 4, was also constructed at a national level. Immunisation was offered to all children in Britain to protect the entire population living there. At the same time, risks could be localised. This localisation could be geographic, such as with concentrated attempts to improve diphtheria or poliomyelitis vaccination in certain local authority areas; or demographic, such as with targeted rubella vaccination campaigns in the 1970s for girls and young women, or foreign-language adverts in South Asian newspapers. As discussed, internationally agreed targets would become increasingly important from the 1970s through the WHO and the rise of global public health initiatives.

While the state clearly defined the public in these administrative terms, the public also spoke back. Through this we can see that the government's definitions and treatment of the public did not always accord with the public's demands and expectations. Indeed, while it is clear that the British public demanded protection by the government against threats to the British public's health, it did not at all times agree that mass routine vaccination was the only or preferred solution. With smallpox, parents were more likely to avoid routine childhood vaccination than to present their children, but the immediate threat of disease could change behaviours. Fear was a motivating factor. In areas where there were outbreaks of smallpox, thousands would queue for hours outside the MOH's clinic for emergency vaccination. There appeared to be "soft" support for the polio vaccine among the general public, but it was only when a prominent footballer died that young adults presented themselves for vaccination in large numbers. Even with the success of the diphtheria programme in the 1940s, interest was revived in the 1950s by leveraging the greater demand for protection against whooping cough and creating multi-dose vaccines. The Ministry of

Health had hoped to revive demand for diphtheria immunisation as a good in its own right, but had to be pragmatic in order to achieve its public health goals. The pertussis and MMR crises also emphasised that the public weighed risks very differently to the government in some circumstances. For not only were people worried about infectious disease, but they were also anxious about the risks of the vaccines themselves. Voluntary and consumer organisations weighed in on the debate in this period, reflecting and creating a greater demand for choice and transparency in health-care decision making.[13] While the government demanded that the public continue to use the government-approved vaccine, many parents sought alternative forms of protection (such as separate vaccines or abstention from the process entirely until safety could be guaranteed). The government did retain a degree of authority throughout the period, as did the narrative that modern states and scientific methods could protect people through vaccination. Uptake recovered within a few years of both crises, reflecting a deeper long-term confidence in vaccination and the belief that it could protect the public from dangerous diseases. But in periods where the credibility of administrative, scientific and political establishments was under strain, the conditions were ripe for crises of confidence in vaccines and vaccination programmes.

If the government played a key role in defining and responding to the public as a population, it is also vital to interrogate the role of the public sector, or the second of Newman and Clarke's discursive chains. The government's use of bureaucratic and statistical tools was by no means restricted to public health policy. It reflected a wider shift in governance in Britain and other liberal democracies from the mid-twentieth century onwards.[14] Vaccination grew in importance during a period in which technocratic, state-led solutions to complex social problems were considered both viable and desirable. Newman and Clarke argue that the post-war period and the foundation of the welfare state mark a point where the public sector became a much more visible and important aspect of publicness.[15] This builds on T. H. Marshall's idea of the post-war period as an era of social rights, one in which health care and the wider welfare state became integral to the function of modern government.[16] Martin Moore has shown how public health and general practice increasingly routinised health care, a process that accelerated after the fiscal crisis of the 1970s. A greater emphasis on preventative medicine meant that the control of chronic conditions (or, in the case of vaccination policy, the risk of infectious disease outbreaks) became politically necessary, in line with the government's financial priorities. At the same time, developments in bureaucratic technologies for identifying and managing such risks had been harnessed and promoted by health professionals and co-opted by the state.[17] As Virginia Berridge has argued, post-war public health is characterised by the use of mass media, evidence-based medicine and a focus on individual behaviour.[18] The chapters of this volume also emphasise these changes. But what does this activity say about how the state constructed the public? Moreover, what does this say about what responsibilities the government felt that it had towards the public's health, and about what the public demanded from its government?

Government approaches to risk, as highlighted in Chapter 4, help to explain the relationship between the public sector and citizens during this period. Primarily, the state intended to reduce the burden of infectious disease through vaccination. In the 1950s, apathy was problematic because it risked the return of diphtheria as a common and widespread disease. Intervention through education and pressure on local authorities was considered a necessary health response because a deterioration in this element of public health was unacceptable to both the government and the general public. Similarly, the demand for IPV in the 1950s stemmed from the public's desire for protection from infectious disease and the belief that the British state had a duty to provide such protection. At the same time, collective responsibility for vaccination was re-emphasised through campaign literature and posters. While the private choice of parents remained, and compulsion was never re-introduced, citizens were expected to vaccinate both for the good of their own children and for the collective health of the nation as a whole. Such concepts of health citizenship were internalised as well as being imposed by government campaigning.[19] However, the risks to be managed through such behaviour changed over time. Once the state had succeeded in reducing the burden of infectious disease, it then sought to ensure that those infectious did not return. Complete eradication and its preservation required different forms of communication. The public had contradictory expectations with regard to disease management. On the one hand, parents had ceased to be overly concerned about diseases that were now so rare that few had direct experience of severe complications or death. To some extent this was evident in the diphtheria programme in the 1950s, but was considered especially prominent with pertussis in the 1970s and measles in the 1990s. On the other hand, reports of the increased morbidity of vaccine-preventable diseases reflected poorly on the government and the nation as a whole. These contradictions flared up in the pertussis crisis when the risks of both a whooping cough epidemic and a potentially dangerous vaccine had to be weighed against each other. In part, this led the government to strengthen its public health measures, such as incentivising general practitioners to vaccinate the entire child population, and the increased use of multi-dose vaccines like MMR.

This relationship between the public and the public sector was ever changing. This can be shown through the way in which hesitancy evolved as an analytical tool in the 2010s, as detailed in Chapter 5. Apathy was construed as a passive state by public health authorities in the 1950s with regard to diphtheria. In the twenty-first century, they were much more likely to talk about decision-making processes, hoping to influence these through effective risk communication. British governance structures had become more concerned with risk management and harm prevention in the post-war period.[20] Vaccination was no different – but the risks identified by public health authorities and the public changed over time. As in other arenas, risk became increasingly identified with financial cost. In the 1950s, apathy presented the possibility that diphtheria morbidity would cease to decline, perhaps even returning. Outbreaks of diphtheria remained the major cause of concern. As the vaccination programme established itself, however, these immediate threats dissipated. Many vaccine-preventable diseases became rare, meaning that any outbreak was damaging to the government's reputation. By the 1980s, disease rates were not framed as human tragedies so much as financial ones. Thus, the vaccination system became a front-line tool in reducing unnecessary public expenditure, and an investment whose benefits far outweighed the potential costs. These could be more accurately measured due to increased statistical monitoring both within Britain and by bodies such as the WHO.

The public, too, expressed risk in different ways. The general swell of approval for poliomyelitis vaccines showed a demand for protection from the disease. In the 1970s, such demands for protection were framed by voluntary organisations, consumer groups and advisory bodies. Moreover, while the public clearly felt that it was the job of the public sector to protect it from disease, it also expected protection from other dangers – which could include the vaccine itself. It would be simplistic to say that the public became less compliant with government advice over the post-war period. This was not some great rebellion as a result of the 1960s. Publics were non-compliant in the 1950s, as seen both in the decreasing uptake of smallpox and diphtheria vaccines among some populations and in the demands for improvements to the polio vaccination programme. Similarly, the acceptance rate of MMR in the mid-1990s – exceeding 90 per cent – suggests that in some ways there was greater compliance from the public in the later period. Rather, when there was a breakdown in trust between the public and the government, for reasons not always directly related to the science of vaccines or vaccination, the break was more dramatic and more vocal.

The public in 2018

From the autumn of 2017, hepatitis B was added to the British childhood vaccination schedule.[21] The clamour over extending meningitis vaccine to all children also shows that parents continue to demand that the government protects them from infectious disease.[22] In 2017–18, uptake of MMR remains well above 90 per cent in all home nations of the United Kingdom. By the standards of the 1960s, this is a remarkable achievement. The vast majority of people appear to accept the general narrative that vaccinations work, they are safe and they are an integral part of a modern functioning state.[23]

The challenges facing public health authorities today are different than they were some eighty years ago when nation-wide diphtheria immunisation was introduced. Throughout this volume, the government's attempts to improve uptake were based mainly on increasing national vaccination rates. At times, this meant focusing on particular local authorities and specific vaccines. But, broadly, successes or failures have been measured by increases or decreases in national statistics relative to various targets. Today, mature vaccination programmes are having to deal with different threats. There are geographically and socially concentrated communities whose children are under-vaccinated for a variety of reasons. Some of those have been convinced that certain vaccines do not work – such as through the influence of anti-vaccination campaigners on the Somali-American community in Minnesota.[24] Others, particularly middle-class parents, doubt the need for or safety of vaccines produced by pharmaceutical companies and governments whose motives they find suspicious.[25]

There is a narrative among some in the public health community that this is inevitable. Public health is a victim of its own success.[26] Robert Chen and Beth Hibbs offer a model of the evolution of an immunisation programme. As vaccine coverage increases, the disease declines; but through increased usage, the number of adverse events also climbs. At a certain point, this results in a loss in confidence. Because the disease is rare, the adverse events get more media coverage. As vaccination rates dip, an outbreak of the disease occurs – which is also rare, and therefore newsworthy. This restores faith in the vaccine until, eventually, the disease is fully eradicated.[27] Of course, this is an overly simplified model for explaining vaccine crises. Chen and Hibbs were writing after several pertussis scares in different countries, but before the MMR crisis started to bite. It neatly encapsulates, however, why apathy may set in and how this can lead to a drop in confidence in a particular vaccine. It also shows that public health researchers and practitioners are aware that progress towards disease eradication is rarely linear.

There is a clear issue here. These debates have been refracted through the politics of public health. Health authorities believe that vaccination is a universal good, that highly vaccinated populations are healthier and, therefore, that people ought to present themselves and their children for vaccination when required. This is a political view for which many have sympathy. But it means that explanations of the public's behaviour have centred on why people do not vaccinate and what can be done to get them to change their minds. Since the early 2010s work on vaccine confidence has begun to focus on the factors that affect parents' choices, but much of this work is also used to assess hesitancy.[28] Since parents' decisions are known to be affected by their communities, local and national circumstances, and attitudes towards medical science, culture plays a key role. And if parents behave differently according to culture and space, they also behave differently across time. This is where history can offer insights for vaccination debates. The demand for IPV in the 1950s might inform debates about vaccine confidence;

the apathy around diphtheria might say something about complacency. Perhaps more pertinently, the debates around vaccination policy in Britain since the Second World War show us that the ways in which the public's behaviour has been described have also been historically specific. Vaccine confidence and hesitancy happen to be the latest in a global context. Through approaching these issues historically, we can explore these other constructions of public behaviour and see how publics have responded to authorities in different ways.

To end, it is worth taking another historical perspective – that of scale. Public health authorities believe that we are heading into another period of crisis. The return of measles in North America and several European countries has left governments puzzled and worried in equal measure. In Italy, there have been violent clashes with doctors over the introduction of stricter compulsion laws.[29] Protests in California have followed the decision to end conscientious objection to vaccination for parents wishing to enrol their children in public schools.[30] Even in Britain, where the spectre of compulsory smallpox vaccination loomed over the twentieth century, there is serious consideration about whether forcing parents to vaccinate their children might improve public health outcomes.[31] Opponents appear to be emboldened by online communities, protests and legal cases. A 2017 ruling in the European Court of Justice appears to pave the way for circumstantial evidence to be accepted as proof of vaccine injury in compensation cases, rather than the use of scientific evidence "beyond reasonable doubt". The consequences for vaccine manufacturers could be devastating – and, given the already-rising costs of vaccines and the declining number of companies producing them, this could threaten the stability of vaccination programmes that have taken decades to evolve.[32]

In a world where the risk of measles and other infectious diseases can be managed through vaccination, it is not surprising that governments and publics have sought to ensure that protection is universally available. But, as Mark Drakeford and Ian Butler demonstrate in their work on scandals, crises have to be manufactured. They do not emerge value-free from scientific facts.[33] If there is a crisis today, it is a historically specific one. The 1950s IPV supply crisis was rooted in post-war anxieties about Britain's place in the world and the unfulfilled promises of technological progress. The 1970s pertussis crisis emerged alongside deep concerns about the role and function of the British welfare state.

The 2000s MMR crisis flourished in an age of mass media, the internet and mistrust of political and medical authority following a host of scandals. So what of today's crises? They are portrayed as a result of a declining faith in science, the rampant individualism of certain types of parents and a sense that we have forgotten just how deadly measles, polio and diphtheria really were. This is not just a crisis about declining vaccination rates – it reflects a wider moral panic about globalisation, "post-truth politics" and the lack of faith in traditional forms of expertise.

Uptake of key vaccinations has stalled or even declined among certain populations. Nevertheless, uptake remains historically high. Given that well over 90 per cent of children in the United Kingdom receive the recommended vaccines, it would suggest that the vaccine narrative has survived among the vast majority of the public. The events and processes described in this book do not deny that there is a crisis brewing today. But they suggest that this too shall pass. Public health authorities are in the unenviable position of seeking a perfection which they may never obtain. The public may elude precise measurement and may not completely comply with official advice. For the most part, however, they want and demand vaccination – for (and of) themselves and others.

Notes

1 Diphtheria, tetanus, pertussis, polio, haemophilus influenza type b (Hib), pneumococcal infection, rotavirus, meningitis B, meningitis C, measles, mumps, rubella, human papilloma virus (for girls only), meningitis, influenza and hepatitis B. National Health Service, 'Childhood vaccines timeline' (16 July 2016) www.nhs.uk/Conditions/Vaccinations/Pages/Childhood-vaccination-schedule.aspx (accessed 12 January 2018).

2 Health and Social Care Information Centre, 'NHS immunisation statistics: England, 2014–15' (23 September 2015) http://digital.nhs.uk/catalogue/PUB18472/nhs-immu-stat-eng-2014–15-rep.pdf (accessed 23 August 2017).

3 Public Health England, 'Notifiable diseases: Historic annual totals' (28 November 2016) www.gov.uk/government/publications/notifiable-diseases-historic-annual-totals (accessed 5 May 2017).

4 Jacob Heller, *The Vaccine Narrative* (Nashville, TN: Vanderbilt University Press, 2008).

5 See Public Health Wales, 'Measles outbreak: Data' (19 February 2015) http://www.wales.nhs.uk/sitesplus/888/page/66389 (accessed 27 July 2018); and for minor outbreaks of measles in England in 2018 see Public Health England, 'Measles outbreaks across England' (25 July 2018) https://www.gov.uk/government/news/measles-outbreaks-across-england (accessed 27 July 2018).
6 Dorothy Porter, *Health Citizenship: Essays in Social Medicine and Biomedical Politics* (Berkeley: University of California Press, 2011); Frank Huisman and Harry Oosterhuis, 'The politics of health and citizenship: Historical and contemporary perspectives', in Frank Huisman and Harry Oosterhuis (eds), *Heath and Citizenship: Political Cultures of Health in Modern Europe* (London: Pickering and Chatto, 2014), pp. 1–40.
7 Janet Newman and John Clarke, *Publics, Politics and Power: Remaking the Public in Public Services* (London: Sage, 2009).
8 Jürgen Habermas, *The Structural Transformation of the Public Sphere: An Inquiry into a Category of Bourgeois Society* (Cambridge, MA: MIT Press, 1989); Richard Sennett, *The Fall of Public Man* (Cambridge: Cambridge University Press, 1977).
9 Newman and Clarke, *Publics, Politics and Power*.
10 Sally Sheard, 'Quacks and clerks: Historical and contemporary perspectives on the structure and function of the British medical civil service', *Social Policy & Administration*, 44:2 (2010), 193–207.
11 See Norman T. Begg, O. N. Gill and Joanne M. White, 'COVER (cover of vaccination evaluated rapidly): Description of the England and Wales scheme', *Public Health*, 103:2 (1989), 81–9; Joanne Yarwood, Karen Noakes, Dorian Kennedy, Helen Campbell and David Salisbury, 'Tracking mothers' attitudes to childhood immunisation 1991–2001', *Vaccine*, 23:48–49 (2005), 5670–87.
12 Jane Lewis, 'The prevention of diphtheria in Canada and Britain 1914–1945', *Journal of Social History*, 20:1 (1986), 163–76; Linda Bryder, ' "We shall not find salvation in inoculation": BCG vaccination in Scandinavia, Britain and the USA, 1921–1960', *Social Science & Medicine*, 49:9 (1999), 1157–67.
13 Alex Mold, *Making the Patient-Consumer: Patient Organisations and Health Consumerism in Britain* (Manchester: Manchester University Press, 2015).
14 Alan R. Petersen and Deborah Lupton, *The New Public Health: Health and Self in the Age of Risk* (London: Sage Publications, 2000); Michel Foucault, *The Birth of the Clinic: An Archaeology of Medical Perception* (London: Tavistock, 1973); David Armstrong, *Political Anatomy of the Body: Medical Knowledge in Britain in the Twentieth Century* (Cambridge: Cambridge University Press, 1983).

15 Newman and Clarke, *Publics, Politics and Power*.
16 T. H. Marshall, *Citizenship and Social Class, and Other Essays*. (Cambridge: Cambridge University Press, 1950).
17 Martin D. Moore, *Managing Diabetes, Managing Medicine: Chronic Disease and Clinical Bureaucracy in Post-War Britain* (Manchester: Manchester University Press, 2019).
18 Virginia Berridge, *Marketing Health* (Oxford: Oxford University Press, 2007).
19 Porter, *Health Citizenship*; Huisman and Oosterhuis, 'The politics of health and citizenship'.
20 See, for example, the history of health and safety and changing notions of "risk" for the British state in this period. Christopher Sirrs, 'Accidents and apathy: The construction of the "Robens philosophy" of occupational safety and health regulation in Britain, 1961–1974', *Social History of Medicine*, 29:1 (2016), 66–88.
21 Ingrid Torjesen, 'UK adds hepatitis B to infant vaccination schedule', *British Medical Journal*, 358 (2017), j3357.
22 UK Government and Parliament Petitions, 'Petition: Give the meningitis B vaccine to ALL children, not just newborn babies' (15 September 2015) https://petition.parliament.uk/petitions/108072 (accessed 23 August 2017).
23 Heller, *The Vaccine Narrative*.
24 Owen Dyer, 'Measles outbreak in Somali American community follows anti-vaccine talks', *British Medical Journal*, 357 (2017), j2378.
25 Philip J. Smith, Susan Y. Chu and Lawrence E. Barker, 'Children who have received no vaccines: who are they and where do they live?', *Pediatrics*, 114:1 (2004), 187–95; Laura Donnelly, 'Private school measles alert', *Daily Telegraph* (27 April 2013), p. 1; Ian Steadman, 'Anti-vaxxers have revived measles in the US, but what about the UK?', *New Statesman* (6 February 2015) www.newstatesman.com/lifestyle/2015/02/anti-vaxxers-have-revived-measles-us-what-about-uk (accessed 9 August 2017).
26 This phrase appears in numerous places. Some include: Matthew Janko, 'Vaccination: A victim of its own success', *Virtual Mentor*, 14:1 (2012), 3; David Edwards, 'Vaccination: a victim of its own success?', *Journal of Small Animal Practices*, 45:11 (2004), 535; Ricki Lewis, 'Vaccines: Victims of their own success?', *The Scientist* (19 July 2004) www.thescientist.com/?articles.view/articleNo/15802/title/Vaccines–Victims-of-Their-Own-Success-/ (accessed 9 August 2017); James Best, 'Vaccination a victim of its own success', *Sydney Morning Herald* (21 September 2011) www.smh.com.au/lifestyle/life/vaccination-a-victim-of-its-own-success-20110920-1kixy.html (accessed 9 August 2017).

27 Robert T. Chen and Beth Hibbs, 'Vaccine safety: Current and future challenges', *Pediatric Annals*, 27:7 (1998), 445–55.
28 For example, although Heidi Larson's work at the London School of Hygiene and Tropical Medicine has focused on "confidence", the impetus for using this work with Gavi has been to help states to explain and counter vaccine scares and drops in uptake. See SAGE Working Group on Vaccine Hesitancy, *Report of the SAGE Working Group on Vaccine Hesitancy* (Geneva: World Health Organization, October 2014); Caitlin Jarrett, Rose Wilson, Maureen O'Leary, Elisabeth Eckersberger, Heidi J. Larson and SAGE Working Group on Vaccine Hesitancy, 'Strategies for addressing vaccine hesitancy – a systematic review', *Vaccine*, 33:34 (2015), 4180–90; Heidi J. Larson, William S. Schulz, Joseph D. Tucker and David M. D. Smith, 'Measuring vaccine confidence: Introducing a global vaccine confidence index', *PLOS Currents Outbreaks* (2015), doi: 10.1371/currents.outbreaks.ce0f6177bc97332602a8e3fe7d7f7cc4.
29 Michael Day, 'Doctor and MPs in Italy are assaulted after vaccination law is passed', *British Medical Journal*, 358 (2017), j3721.
30 Michael McCarthy, 'California ends vaccine exemptions on grounds of belief – will other states follow?', *British Medical Journal*, 351 (2015), h3635.
31 Denes Stefler and Raj Bhopal, 'Lessons to be learnt from other countries about mandatory child vaccination', *British Medical Journal*, 344 (2012), e4036; David Elliman and Helen Bedford, 'Should the UK introduce compulsory vaccination?', *The Lancet*, 381:9876 (2013), 1434–6; Tom Moberly, 'UK doctors re-examine case for mandatory vaccination', *British Medical Journal*, 358 (2017), j3414. On other countries, see Sophie Arie, 'Compulsory vaccination and growing measles threat', *British Medical Journal*, 358 (2017), j3429.
32 Clare Dyer, 'Courts can decide that vaccine has caused harm despite lack of evidence', *British Medical Journal*, 357 (2017), j3081. On the financial pressures on vaccine companies, see: Paul A. Offit, 'The Cutter Incident, 50 years later', *New England Journal of Medicine*, 352:14 (2005), 178–84.
33 Mark Drakeford and Ian Butler, *Scandal, Social Policy and Social Welfare*, 2nd edn (Bristol: Policy Press, 2006).

Select bibliography

Archival sources

The National Archives, Kew, London
BD 25/104, Smallpox outbreak in South Wales: Reports and correspondence
BN 10/229, Leaflets, posters and press advertisements: diphtheria immunisation
BN 13/360, Vaccine Damage Payments Act 1979
BN 35/57, Immunisation and vaccination statistics
BN 124/10, Vaccine Damage Payments Scheme: Ministerial discussions
BS 14/28, Rubella vaccination campaign
CAB 128/61/18, Cabinet minutes 5 May 1977
CAB 129/195/14, Cabinet memoranda 29 April 1977
CAB 129/195/16, Cabinet memoranda 2 May 1977
EF 7/2998, Advisory committees on dangerous pathogens and genetic manipulation: Smallpox vaccination for laboratory workers
FD 1/8290, First report on BCG and vole bacillus vaccines in the prevention of TB in adolescents
FD 4/272, A study of diphtheria in two areas of Great Britain
FD 23/1028, Continuation of vaccine trials during 1957
FD 23/1031, Press conference on polio vaccine held on 27th February 1957
FD 23/1058, Polio vaccine crisis 1957 to January 1960: Papers produced in 1957
FD 23/1059, Polio vaccine crisis 1957 to January 1960: Papers produced in 1958
FD 23/1060, Polio vaccine crisis 1957 to January 1960: Papers produced in 1959
HO 45/10768/273078, Anti-inoculation propaganda among the troops issued by the British Union for the Abolition of Vivisection
INF 12/238, Ministry of Health: Diphtheria immunisation 1953–1954
LCO 20/1293, The National Association for Deaf Blind and Rubella Children
MH 55/293, National Anti-Vaccination League: Anti-vaccination inoculation and immunisation propaganda

Select bibliography 237

MH 55/902, Smallpox vaccination: Publicity
MH 55/936, Diphtheria immunisation campaign
MH 55/1720, Vaccination and innoculation: objections to anti-vaccination propaganda
MH 55/1828, Outbreak on board SS Mooltan: Minutes
MH 55/1829, Outbreak on board SS Mooltan: Correspondence
MH 55/1830, Outbreak on board SS Mooltan: Quarantine control procedure
MH 55/1836, Memorandum on smallpox control
MH 55/2191, Diphtheria prophylaxis: Publicity campaign
MH 55/2458, Poliomyelitis policy 1953–56
MH 55/2460, Poliomyelitis policy 1956–57
MH 55/2461, Poliomyelitis policy 1957
MH 55/2464, Poliomyelitis policy 1958–59
MH 55/2469, Poliomyelitis policy 1960–61
MH 55/2472, Poliomyelitis policy 1961
MH 55/2473, Policy: Introduction of live oral vaccine for routine vaccination
MH 55/2510, Vaccination and control: Representations by British Medical Association
MH 134/151, Diphtheria and whooping cough: Combined prophylactic
MH 134/156, Inoculation campaign: Statistical results
MH 148/364, Vaccination policy after declaration of eradication
MH 154/61, Smallpox vaccination sub-committee 1963–65
MH 154/62, Smallpox vaccination sub-committee 1962–63
MH 154/268, Withdrawal of recommendation for vaccination in early childhood
MH 154/270, Cessation of commercial supplies by Lister Institute pending world wide eradication of smallpox
MH 154/404, Importations of smallpox into England and Wales 1936–1970
MH 154/1053, Compensation for victims of immunisation and accidents
MH 154/1057, European Commission of Human Rights application number 7154/75 by the Association of Parents of Vaccine Damaged Children
MH 154/1464, Joint Committee on Vaccination and Immunisation: Rubella vaccination sub-committee 1976–78
MH 154/1465, Joint Committee on Vaccination and Immunisation: Rubella vaccination sub-committee 1978
MH 154/1466, Joint Committee on Vaccination and Immunisation: Rubella vaccination sub-committee 1978
MH 154/1471, Joint Committee on Vaccination and Immunisation: Rubella vaccination sub-committee 1979
PIN 35/549, Association of Parents of Vaccine Damaged Children

Legislation

Education (Administrative Provisions) Act 1907.
National Health Service Act 1946.
National Health Service (Scotland) Act 1947.
Vaccination Act 1840.
Vaccination Act 1853.
Vaccination Act 1898.
Vaccination Act 1907.
Vaccine Damage Payments Act 1979.

Newspapers

Coventry Evening Telegraph
Coventry Standard
Daily Express
Daily Mail
Daily Mirror
Daily Post [Liverpool]
Daily Telegraph
Guardian
Herald
Independent
Manchester Guardian
New Statesman
Scotsman
Sunday Pictorial
Sunday Times
The Times

Secondary sources

Abbasi, Kamran, 'Man, mission, rumpus', *British Medical Journal*, 322:7281 (2001), 306.
Abel-Smith, Brian and Peter Townsend, *The Poor and the Poorest: A New Analysis of the Ministry of Labour's Family Expenditure Surveys of 1953–54 and 1960* (London: Bell, 1965).
Action Medical Research, 'History' (undated) www.action.org.uk/about-us/history (accessed 24 August 2017).
Agerholm, Margaret, 'Importation of poliomyelitis vaccine', *The Lancet*, 2:6986 (1957), 270.

Select bibliography

Agnew, R. A. L., 'Vaccination against smallpox', *British Medical Journal*, 1:5276 (1962), 482.
Alaszewski, Andy and Tom Horlick-Jones, 'How can doctors communicate information about risk more effectively?', *British Medical Journal*, 327:7417 (2003), 728–31.
Alcock, Sharon, 'How parents decide on MMR', *British Medical Journal*, 324:7335 (2002), 492.
Allen, Arthur, *Vaccine: The Controversial Story of Medicine's Greatest Lifesaver* (New York: W. W. Norton, 2007).
Anon, 'A measles vaccine withdrawn', *British Medical Journal*, 1:5647 (1969), 794–5.
———, 'American polio vaccine', *British Medical Journal*, 1:5029 (1957), 1229–30.
———, 'Annual Meeting, Belfast: Scientific proceedings: Symposium: Virus diseases', *British Medical Journal*, 2:5300 (1962), 318–20.
———, 'British poliomyelitis vaccine', *British Medical Journal*, 1:5030 (1957), 1291–2.
———, 'Epidemiology section', *British Medical Journal*, 1:4658 (1950), 914–15.
———, 'For further debate', *British Medical Journal*, 3:5767 (1971), 129.
———, 'Help for victims of immunizations', *British Medical Journal*, 1:5856 (1973), 758–9.
———, 'Immunization ups and downs', *British Medical Journal*, 2:5299 (1962), 250.
———, 'Polio fantasies', *British Medical Journal*, 1:5018 (1957), 571–2.
———, 'Poliomyelitis vaccine', *British Medical Journal*, 2:5041 (1957), 405–6.
———, 'Prevention of whooping-cough by vaccination', *British Medical Journal*, 1:4721 (1951), 1463–71.
———, 'Smallpox in England', *British Medical Journal*, 1:5272 (1962), 164–5.
———, 'Social survey of diphtheria immunization', *British Medical Journal*, 2:4461 (1946), 21.
———, 'Vaccination against smallpox', *British Medical Journal*, 2:5300 (1962), 311–12.
———, 'Whooping-cough immunisation', *British Medical Journal*, 2:6078 (1977), 5–6.
AP Archive, 'Polio inoculations' (original video clip dated 13 April 1959) www.aparchive.com/metadata/youtube/4bdf81b34ff4492ea60082787a 97e807 (accessed 24 August 2017).
Arie, Sophie, 'Compulsory vaccination and growing measles threat', *British Medical Journal*, 358 (2017), j3429.
Armstrong, David, 'Origins of the problem of health-related behaviours: A genealogical study', *Social Studies of Science*, 39:6 (2009), 909–26.

———, *Political Anatomy of the Body : Medical Knowledge in Britain in the Twentieth Century* (Cambridge: Cambridge University Press, 1983).
Arnold, David, *Colonizing the Body: State Medicine and Epidemic Disease in Nineteenth-century India* (Berkeley: University of California Press, 1993).
Arnoldi, Jakob, *Risk: An Introduction* (Cambridge: Polity, 2009).
Artenstein, Andrew W., 'Smallpox', in Andrew W. Artenstein (ed.), *Vaccines: A Biography* (New York: Springer, 2010), pp. 61–9.
———, ed. *Vaccines: A Biography* (New York: Springer, 2010).
Artenstein, Nicholas C. and Andrew W. Artenstein, 'The discovery of viruses and the evolution of vaccinology', in Andrew W. Artenstein (ed.), *Vaccines: A Biography* (New York: Springer, 2010), pp. 141–58.
Ashley, Jack, *Acts of Defiance* (London: Reinhardt, 1992).
Ashraf, Haroon, 'US expert group rejects link between MMR and autism', *The Lancet* 357:9265 (2001), 1341.
Ashtiyani, S. C. and A. Amoozandeh, 'Rhazes diagnostic differentiation of smallpox and measles', *Iranian Red Crescent Medical Journal*, 12:4 (2010), 480–3.
Axelsson, Per, 'The Cutter Incident and the development of a Swedish polio vaccine, 1952–1957', *Dynamis* 32:2 (2012), 311–28.
Ayo, Nike, 'Understanding health promotion in a neoliberal climate and the making of health conscious citizens', *Critical Public Health*, 22:1 (2012), 99–105.
Badenoch, J., 'Big bang for vaccination', *British Medical Journal*, 297:6651 (1988), 750–1.
Baggott, Rob, *Public Health: Policy and Politics*, 2nd edn (Basingstoke: Palgrave Macmillan, 2012).
Baker, Jeffrey P., 'The pertussis vaccine controversy in Great Britain, 1974–1986', *Vaccine*, 21:25–26 (2003), 4003–10.
Barnes, Diana, 'The public life of a woman of wit and quality: Lady Mary Wortley Montagu and the vogue for smallpox inoculation', *Feminist Studies*, 38:2 (2012), 330–62.
Barratt, Helen, 'MMR vaccine row raises questions of clinical freedom', *British Medical Journal*, 323:7308 (2001), 300.
———, 'Scottish GPs to be sent discussion packs on MMR vaccine', *British Medical Journal*, 323:7312 (2001), 532.
Barrowcliffe, D. G., 'Vaccination against smallpox', *British Medical Journal*, 2:5306 (1962), 734.
Barry, Norman, 'Neoclassicism, the New Right and British social welfare', in Robert M. Pages and Richard Silburn (eds), *British Social Welfare in the Twentieth Century* (London: Macmillan, 1999), pp. 55–79.
Baxby, Derrick, 'The end of smallpox', *History Today*, 49:3 (1999), 14–16.

BBC, 'The Richard Dimbleby Lecture' (original broadcast 23 November 1978) www.bbc.co.uk/programmes/p00fr9fs (accessed 19 June 2017).
BBC News, 'Meningitis B petition becomes UK's most signed', *BBC News* (19 February 2016) www.bbc.co.uk/news/uk-england-kent-35614846 (accessed 20 August 2016).
Beaumont, Catriona, *Housewives and Citizens: Domesticity and the Women's Movement in England, 1928–64* (Manchester: Manchester University Press, 2013).
Beck, Ulrich, *Risk Society: Towards a New Modernity* (London: Sage, 1992).
———, *World at Risk* (Cambridge: Polity, 2009).
Bedford, Helen and David Elliman, 'Concerns about immunisation', *British Medical Journal*, 320:7229 (2000), 240–3.
Begg, N. T. and N. D. Noah, 'Immunisation targets in Europe and Britain', *British Medical Journal (Clinical Research Edition)* 291:6506 (1985), 1370–1.
Begg, Norman T., O. N. Gill and Joanne M. White, 'COVER (Cover of Vaccination Evaluated Rapidly): Description of the England and Wales scheme', *Public Health*, 103:2 (1989), 81–9.
Begg, Norman, Mary Ramsay, Joanne White and Zoltan Bozoky, 'Media dents confidence in MMR vaccine', *British Medical Journal*, 316:7130 (1998), 561.
Bellaby, Paul, 'Communication and miscommunication of risk: Understanding UK parents' attitudes to combined MMR vaccination', *British Medical Journal*, 327:7417 (2003), 725–8.
Bennett, Michael, 'Jenner's ladies: Women and vaccination against smallpox in early nineteenth-century Britain', *History*, 93:312 (2008), 497–513.
Berridge, Virginia, '"Hidden from history"? Oral history and the history of health policy', *Oral History*, 38 (2010), 99–100.
———, *Marketing Health* (Oxford: Oxford University Press, 2007).
———, 'Thinking in time: Does health policy need history as evidence?', *The Lancet*, 375:9717 (2010), 798–9.
———, 'Using history in policy and practice', in Virginia Berridge, Martin Gorsky and Alex Mold (eds), *Public Health in History* (Maidenhead: Open University Press, 2011), pp. 221–24.
Berridge, Virginia and Alex Mold, 'Professionalisation, new social movements and voluntary action in the 1960s and 1970s', in Matthew Hilton and James McKay (eds), *The Ages of Voluntarism: How We Got to the Big Society* (Oxford: Oxford University Press, 2011), pp. 114–34.
Beveridge, William H., *Social Insurance and Allied Services* (Cmd 6404) (London: HMSO, 1942).
Bhattacharya, Sanjoy, *Expunging Variola: The Control and Eradication of Smallpox in India, 1947–1977* (New Delhi: Orient Longman, 2006).

Birks, P. H., 'Vaccination against smallpox', *British Medical Journal*, 2:5300 (1962), 340.
Bivins, Roberta, *Alternative Medicine? A History* (Oxford: Oxford University Press, 2007).
———, '"The people have no more love left for the Commonwealth": Media, migration and identity in the 1961–62 British smallpox outbreak', *Immigrants & Minorities*, 25:3 (2007), 263–89.
———, *Contagious Communities: Medicine, Migration, and the NHS in Post-War Britain* (Oxford: Oxford University Press, 2015).
Blaxill, Luke and Jane K. Seymour, 'Adventures in text mining with the London MOH Annual Reports: Towards an alternative history of interwar public health', Conference paper (London Health Histories, Wellcome Trust, London, 26 May 2016).
Blume, Stuart, 'Anti-vaccination movements and their interpretations', *Social Science & Medicine*, 62:3 (2006), 628–42.
———, *Immunization: How Vaccines Became Controversial* (London: Reaktion, 2017).
Blyth Brooke, C. O. S., *Annual Report on the Public Health of Finsbury for the Year 1959* (Finsbury: The Metropolitan Borough of Finsbury, 1960).
Boddice, Rob, 'Vaccination, fear and historical relevance', *History Compass*, 14:2 (2016), 71–8.
Bonnett, E. J. S., 'Vaccination against smallpox', *British Medical Journal*, 2:5305 (1962), 675.
Borysiewicz, Leszek K., 'Prevention is better than cure', *The Lancet*, 375:9713 (2010), 513–23.
Bousfield, Guy, 'Smallpox vaccination', *British Medical Journal*, 3:5769 (1971), 302.
Bowden, Sue and Alex Sadler, 'Getting it right? Lessons from the interwar years on pulmonary tuberculosis control in England and Wales', *Medical History*, 59:1 (2015), 101–35.
Bower, Hilary, 'MMR vaccine policy is backed', *British Medical Journal*, 316:7136 (1998), 955.
Box, Kathleen, *Diphtheria Immunisation: An Inquiry Made by the Social Survey for the Ministry of Health* (London: The Social Survey, 1945).
Box, Kathleen and Geoffrey Thomas, 'The Wartime Social Survey', *Journal of the Royal Statistical Society*, 107:3/4 (1944), 151–89.
Boyce, Tammy, *Health, Risk and News: The MMR Vaccine and the Media* (New York: Peter Lang, 2007).
Bradford Hill, A. and J. Knowelden, 'Inoculation and poliomyelitis', *British Medical Journal*, 2:4669 (1950), 1–6.

British Medical Association Board of Science and Education, *Childhood Immunisation: A Guide for Healthcare Professionals* (London: British Medical Association, 2003).

Brown, Katrina F., J. Simon Kroll, Michael J. Hudson, Mary Ramsay, John Green, Charles A. Vincent, Graham Fraser and Nick Sevdalis, 'Omission bias and vaccine rejection by parents of healthy children: Implications for the influenza A/H1N1 vaccination programme', *Vaccine*, 28:25 (2010), 4181–5.

Brown, Katrina F., J. Simon Kroll, Michael J. Hudson, Mary Ramsay, John Green, Susannah J. Long, Charles A. Vincent, Graham Fraser and Nick Sevdalis, 'Factors underlying parental decisions about combination childhood vaccinations including MMR: A systematic review', *Vaccine*, 28:26 (2010), 4235–48.

Brown, Theodore M., Elizabeth Fee and Victoria Stepanova, 'Halfdan Mahler: Architect and defender of the World Health Organization "Health for All by 2000" declaration of 1978', *American Journal of Public Health*, 106:1 (2016), 38–9.

Browne, S. E., 'Press reports on Belfast', *British Medical Journal*, 2:5300 (1962), 340.

Brunton, Deborah, *The Politics of Vaccination: Practice and Policy in England, Wales, Ireland, and Scotland, 1800–1874* (New York: University Rochester Press, 2008).

Bryder, Linda, 'The King Edward VII Welsh National Memorial Association and its policy towards tuberculosis, 1910–48', *Welsh History Review* 13:2 (1986), 194–216.

———, '"We shall not find salvation in inoculation": BCG vaccination in Scandinavia, Britain and the USA, 1921–1960', *Social Science & Medicine*, 49:9 (1999), 1157–67.

Burgess, David C., Margaret A. Burgess and Julie Leask, 'The MMR vaccination and autism controversy in United Kingdom 1998–2005: Inevitable community outrage or a failure of risk communication?', *Vaccine*, 24:18 (2006), 3921–8.

Burnton, Simon, 'The forgotten story of … Jeff Hall, the footballer whose death turned the tide against polio', *Guardian* (9 December 2016) www.theguardian.com/football/blog/2016/dec/09/fogotten-story-jeff-hall-death-polio-birmingham-city (accessed 24 August 2017).

Bush, Barbara, 'Colonial research and the social sciences at the end of empire: The West Indian Social Survey, 1944–57', *Journal of Imperial & Commonwealth History*, 41:3 (2013), 451–74.

Butler, Declan, Ewen Callaway and Erika Check Hayden, 'How Ebola-vaccine success could reshape clinical-trial policy', *Nature*, 524:7563 (2015), 13–14.

Calhoun, Craig, 'Introduction: Habermas and the public sphere', in Craig Calhoun (ed.), *Habermas and the Public Sphere* (Cambridge: MIT Press, 1992), pp. 1–48.

Callender, David, 'Vaccine hesitancy: More than a movement', *Human Vaccines & Immunotherapeutics*, 12:9 (2016), 2464–8.

Calman, Kenneth C., 'Communication of risk: Choice, consent, and trust', *The Lancet*, 360:9327 (2002), 166–8.

Camargo, Kenneth and Roy Grant, 'Public health, science, and policy debate: Being right is not enough', *American Journal of Public Health*, 105:2 (2014), 232–5.

Campos-Outcalt, Doug, 'Measles: Why it's still a threat', *The Journal of Family Practice*, 66:7 (2017), 446–9.

Cantor, David, 'Representing "the public": Medicine, charity and the public sphere in twentieth-century Britain', in Steve Sturdy (ed.), *Medicine, Health and the Public Sphere in Britain: 1600–2000* (London: Routledge, 2002), pp. 145–68.

Carroll, Linda and Samuel Sarmiento, '"Striking" results from early Zika vaccine trial', *NBC News* (4 August 2016) www.nbcnews.com/storyline/zika-virus-outbreak/striking-results-early-zika-vaccine-trial-n623016 (accessed 19 August 2016).

Carroll, Patrick E., 'Medical police and the history of public health', *Medical History*, 46:4 (2002), 461–94.

Carter, Tim and Stephen E. Roberts, 'Infectious disease mortality in British merchant seamen and Lascars since 1900: From causes to controls', *International Journal of Maritime History*, 29:4 (2017), 788–815.

Casiday, Rachel, 'Risk communication in the British pertussis and MMR vaccine controversies', in Peter Bennett, Kenneth Calman, Sarah Curtis and Denis Fischbacher (eds), *Risk Communication and Public Health*, 2nd edn (Oxford: Oxford University Press, 2010), pp. 129–46.

Casper, Monica J. and Laura M. Carpenter, 'Sex, drugs, and politics: The HPV vaccine for cervical cancer', *Sociology of Health & Illness*, 30:6 (2008), 886–99.

Cassier, Maurice, 'Producing, controlling, and stabilizing Pasteur's anthrax vaccine: Creating a new industry and a health market', *Science in Context*, 21:2 (2008), 253–78.

Castle, Barbara, *Fighting All the Way* (London: Pan Books, 1994).

Centers for Disease Control and Prevention, 'Pertussis (whooping cough)' (27 June 2016) www.cdc.gov/pertussis/about/index.html (accessed 6 June 2017).

Chalke, H. D., *Report of the Medical Officer of Health for the Year 1959* (Camberwell: Metropolitan Borough of Camberwell, 1960).

Chalmers, Iain and Andy Haines, 'Commentary: Skilled forensic capacity needed to investigate allegations of research misconduct', *British Medical Journal*, 342 (2011): d3977.

Chatterjee, Archana and Catherine O'Keefe, 'Current controversies in the USA regarding vaccine safety', *Expert Review of Vaccines*, 9:5 (2010), 497–502.

Chen, Robert T. and Frank DeStefano, 'Vaccine adverse events: Causal or coincidental?', *The Lancet*, 351:9103 (1998), 611–12.

Chen, Robert T. and Beth Hibbs, 'Vaccine safety: Current and future challenges', *Pediatric Annals*, 27:7 (1998), 445–55.

Church, M., 'Return of whooping cough', *British Medical Journal*, 1:6157 (1979), 195.

Clark, Peder, '"Problems of today and tomorrow": prevention and the National Health Service in the 1970s', *Social History of Medicine* (forthcoming).

Cohen, Jon, *Shots in the Dark: The Wayward Search for an AIDS Vaccine* (London: Norton, 2001).

Coker, Richard, 'Civil liberties and public good: Detention of tuberculous patients and the Public Health Act 1984', *Medical History*, 45:3 (2001), 341–58.

Colgrove, James, *State of Immunity: The Politics of Vaccination in Twentieth-Century America* (Berkeley: University of California Press, 2006).

———, 'The McKeown thesis: A historical controversy and its enduring influence', *American Journal of Public Health*, 92:5 (2002), 725–9.

Condie, Roy G., 'Smallpox vaccination', *British Medical Journal*, 3:5773 (1971), 534.

Cox, P. J., *Report of the Committee of Inquiry into the Smallpox Outbreak in London in March and April 1973* (Cmnd 5626) (London: HMSO, 1974).

Crawford, L. A., 'Rubella vaccination', *British Medical Journal*, 1:6125 (1978), 1485.

Cusick, James, 'Meningitis B: Petition calling for vaccine breaks government website record', *Independent* (19 February 2016) www.independent.co.uk/life-style/health-and-families/health-news/meningitis-b-petition-calling-for-vaccine-breaks-government-website-record-a6884946.html (accessed 20 August 2016).

Dale, Iain, *Conservative Party General Election Manifestos 1900–1997* (Abingdon: Routledge, 2000).

Daley, Allen, *Report of the County Medical Officer of Health and School Medical Officer for the Year 1949* (London: London County Council, 1950).

Daley, Allen, *Report of the County Medical Officer of Health and School Medical Officer for the Year 1950* (London: London County Council, 1951).

Daly, Ann, *Inventing Motherhood: The Consequences of an Ideal* (New York: Schocken, 1983).

Dane, D. S., G. W. A. Dick, J. H. Connolly, O. D. Fisher, Florence McKeown, Moya Briggs, Robert Nelson and Dermot Wilson, 'Vaccination against poliomyelitis with live virus vaccines', *British Medical Journal*, 1:5010 (1957), 59–74.

Davenport, Romola J., Jeremy Boulton and Leonard Schwarz, 'Urban inoculation and the decline of smallpox mortality in eighteenth-century cities – A reply to Razell', *Economic History Review*, 69:1 (2016), 188–214.

Davenport, Romola, Leonard Schwarz and Jeremy Boulton, 'The decline of adult smallpox in eighteenth-century London', *Economic History Review*, 64:4 (2011), 1289–314.

Davies, S. and W. H. Crichton, 'Smallpox vaccination', *British Medical Journal*, 3:5771 (1971), 430–1.

Davies, Sara E. and Belinda Bennett, 'A gendered human rights analysis of Ebola and Zika: Locating gender in global health emergencies', *International Affairs*, 92:5 (2016), 1041–60.

Davis, Angela, *Modern Motherhood: Women and Family in England, c. 1945–2000* (Manchester: Manchester University Press, 2012).

Day, Alison, '"An American tragedy". The Cutter Incident and its implications for the Salk polio vaccine in New Zealand 1955–1960', *Health & History: Journal of the Australian & New Zealand Society for the History of Medicine*, 11:2 (2009), 42–61.

——, '"The magical formula": Reactions and responses to diphtheria immunisation in New Zealand 1920–1960', *Health & History: Journal of the Australian & New Zealand Society for the History of Medicine*, 15:2 (2013), 53–71.

Day, Michael, 'Doctor and MPs in Italy are assaulted after vaccination law is passed', *British Medical Journal*, 358 (2017): j3721.

Deer, Brian, 'How the case against the MMR vaccine was fixed', *British Medical Journal*, 342 (2011), c5347.

——, 'Reflections on investigating Wakefield', *British Medical Journal*, 340 (2010), c672.

Dennison, F. Roy, *Annual Report on the Health Services for the Year 1955* (West Ham: County Borough of West Ham, 1956).

——, *Annual Report on the Health Services for the Year 1956* (West Ham: County Borough of West Ham, 1957).

Department of Health, *Building on the Best: Choice, Responsiveness and Equity in the NHS* (Cm 6079) (London: TSO, 2003).

——, *The Health of the Nation: A Strategy for Health in England* (Cm 1986) (London: HMSO, 1992).

Department of Health and Social Security, *Promoting Better Health: The Government's Programme for Improving Primary Health Care* (Cm 249) (London: HMSO, 1987).

———, *Public Health in England: The Report of the Committee of Inquiry into the Future Development of the Public Health Function* (Cm 289) (London: HMSO, 1988).
Department of Health and Social Security, Committee on Safety of Medicines and Joint Committee on Vaccination and Immunisation, *Whooping Cough: Reports from the Committee on Safety of Medicines and the Joint Committee on Vaccination and Immunisation* (London: HMSO, 1981).
Department of Health and Social Security, Department of Education and Science, Scottish Office and Welsh Office, *Prevention and Health* (Cmnd 7047) (London: HMSO, 1977).
Dick, G. W. A., 'Letter: Whooping-cough vaccine', *British Medical Journal*, 4:5989 (1975), 161.
———, 'Routine smallpox vaccination', *British Medical Journal*, 3:5767 (1971), 163–6.
———, 'Epidemiology of poliomyelitis', *British Medical Journal*, 1:5122 (1959), 618–19.
———, 'Prevention of virus diseases in the community', *British Medical Journal*, 2:5315 (1962), 1275–80.
Dick, G. W. A. and D. S. Dane, 'Live poliomyelitis vaccine', *British Medical Journal*, 1:5125 (1959), 853–4.
———, 'Vaccination against poliomyelitis with live virus vaccines', *British Medical Journal*, 2:5106 (1958), 1184–6.
Dick, George, 'Obituary: Duncan Guthrie', *Independent* (20 October 1994) www.independent.co.uk/news/people/obituary-duncan-guthrie-1444138.html (accessed 24 August 2017).
Dixon, C. W., 'Vaccination against smallpox', *British Medical Journal*, 1:5287 (1962), 1262–6.
———, *Smallpox* (London: J. & A. Churchill, 1962).
Dobson, Roger, 'Parents' champion or loose cannon?', *British Medical Journal*, 324:7334 (2002), 386.
Donoughue, Bernard, *Prime Minister: The Conduct of Policy under Harold Wilson and James Callaghan* (London: Cape, 1987).
Douglas, John and William Edgar, 'Smallpox in Bradford, 1962', *British Medical Journal*, 1:5278 (1962), 612–14.
Douglas, Mary and Aaron Wildavsky, *Risk and Culture* (Berkeley: University of California Press, 1983).
Downs, Julie S., Wändi Bruine de Bruin and Baruch Fischhoff, 'Parents' vaccination comprehension and decisions', *Vaccine*, 26:12 (2008), 1595–607.
Drakeford, Mark and Ian Butler, *Scandal, Social Policy and Social Welfare*, 2nd edn (Bristol: Policy Press, 2006).

Dredger, Alice, 'What if not all parents who question vaccines are foolish and anti-science?', *New Statesman* (4 June 2015) https://www.newstatesman.com/2015/05/heretic-academy (accessed 29 March 2018).

Dubé, Eve, Maryline Vivion and Noni E. MacDonald, 'Vaccine hesitancy, vaccine refusal and the anti-vaccine movement: Influence, impact and implications', *Expert Review of Vaccines*, 14:1 (2015), 99–117.

Duncan, Peter, 'Failing to professionalise, struggling to specialise: The rise and fall of health promotion as a putative specialism in England, 1980–2000', *Medical History*, 57:3 (2013), 377–96.

Durbach, Nadja, *Bodily Matters: The Anti-Vaccination Movement in England, 1853–1907* (Durham, NC: Duke University Press, 2005).

———, 'Class, gender, and the conscientious objector to vaccination, 1898–1907', *Journal of British Studies*, 41:1 (2002), 58–83.

Dyer, Clare, 'Co-author of Wakefield paper on MMR vaccine wins his appeal against decision by GMC to strike him off', *British Medical Journal*, 344 (2012), e1745.

———, 'Commission withdraws Legal Aid for parents suing over MMR vaccine', *British Medical Journal*, 327:7416 (2003), 640.

———, 'Courts can decide that vaccine has caused harm despite lack of evidence', *British Medical Journal*, 357 (2017), j3081.

———, 'NHS told to pay £10m to patients infected with hepatitis C', *British Medical Journal*, 322:7289 (2001), 751.

Dyer, Owen, 'Measles outbreak in Somali American community follows anti-vaccine talks', *British Medical Journal*, 357 (2017), j2378.

Edgerton, David, 'C. P. Snow as anti-historian of British science: Revisiting the technocratic moment, 1959–1964', *History of Science*, 43:2 (2005), 187–208.

Editors of The Lancet, 'Retraction – Ileal-lymphoid-nodular hyperplasia, non-specific colitis, and pervasive developmental disorder in children', *The Lancet*, 375:9713 (2010), 445.

Edwards, David, 'Vaccination: A victim of its own success?', *Journal of Small Animal Practice*, 45:11 (2004), 535.

Elliman, David and Helen Bedford, 'MMR vaccine: The continuing saga', *British Medical Journal*, 322:7280 (2001), 183–4.

———, 'Safety and efficacy of combination vaccines', *British Medical Journal*, 326:7397 (2003), 995–6.

———, 'Should the UK introduce compulsory vaccination?', *The Lancet*, 381:9876 (2013), 1434–6.

Engels, Eric A., Hormuzd A. Katki, Nete M. Nielsen, Jeanette F. Winther, Henrik Hjalgrim, Flemming Gjerris, Philip S. Rosenberg and Morten Frisch, 'Cancer incidence in Denmark following exposure to poliovirus vaccine contaminated with simian virus 40', *Journal of the National Cancer Institute*, 95:7 (2003), 532–9.

Engineer, Amanda, 'Illustrations from the Wellcome Library: The Society of Medical Officers of Health: Its history and its archive', *Medical History*, 45:1 (2001), 97–114.

Erichsen, Vibeke, 'The health of the school child?: An historical comparison of inspection schemes in Britain and Norway', *Dynamis*, 13 (1993), 29–53.

Eriksen, Anne, 'Advocating inoculation in the eighteenth century: Exemplarity and quantification', *Science in Context*, 29:2 (2016), 213–39.

———, 'Cure or protection? The meaning of smallpox inoculation, ca 1750–1775', *Medical History*, 57:4 (2013), 516–36.

Evans, M., H. Stoddart, L. Condon, E. Freeman, M. Grizzell and R. Mullen, 'Parents' perspectives on the MMR immunisation: A focus group study', *The British Journal of General Practice*, 51:472 (2001), 904–10.

Farrington, P., M. Rush, E. Miller, S. Pugh, A. Colville, A. Flower, J. Nash and P. Morgan-Capner, 'A new method for active surveillance of adverse events from diphtheria/tetanus/pertussis and measles/mumps/rubella vaccines', *The Lancet*, 345:8949 (1995), 567–9.

Federman, Ross S., 'Understanding vaccines: A public imperative', *The Yale Journal of Biology and Medicine*, 87:4 (2014), 417–22.

Fenner, Frank, Donald A. Henderson, Isao Arita, Jezek Zdenek, Ivan Danilovich Ladnyi and World Health Organization, *Smallpox and Its Eradication* (Geneva: World Health Organization, 1988).

Ferriman, Annabel, 'London Mayor attacked for doing "irreparable damage" on MMR', *British Medical Journal*, 325:7355 (2002), 66.

Fine, Paul, 'Stopping routine vaccination for tuberculosis in schools', *British Medical Journal*, 331:7518 (2005), 647–8.

Fischoff, Baruch and John Kadvany, *Risk: A Very Short Introduction* (Oxford: Oxford University Press, 2011).

Fisher, Tim, 'Fatherhood and the British fathercraft movement, 1919–39', *Gender & History*, 17:2 (2005), 441–62.

Fitzpatrick, Mike, 'Choice', *The Lancet*, 363:9409 (2004), 668.

Foucault, Michel, *Discipline and Punish: The Birth of the Prison* (New York: Pantheon Books, 1977).

———, *The Birth of the Clinic: An Archaeology of Medical Perception* (London: Tavistock, 1973).

Fox, Rosemary, *Helen's Story* (London: John Blake, 2006).

Francis, Thomas, *Evaluation of the 1954 Field Trial of Poliomyelitis Vaccine. Final Report* (Ann Arbor: University of Michigan, 1957).

Fraser, Nancy, 'Rethinking the public sphere: A contribution to the critique of actually existing democracy', *Social Text*, 25/26 (1990), 56–80.

Fraser, S. M., 'Leicester and smallpox: The Leicester Method', *Medical History*, 24:3 (1980), 315–32.
French, Henry, *Report of the Committee on the Cost of Home Information Services* (Cmnd 7836) (London: HMSO, 1949).
Fyfe, G. Matthew and J. B. Fleming, 'Encephalomyelitis after vaccination in Fife', *British Medical Journal*, 2:4325 (1943), 671–4.
Gachelin, Gabriel, 'The designing of anti-diphtheria serotherapy at the Institut Pasteur (1888–1900): The role of a supranational network of microbiologists', *Dynamis*, 27 (2007), 45–62.
Gangarosa, E. J., A. M. Galazka, C. R. Wolfe, L. M. Phillips, E. Miller, R. T. Chen and R. E. Gangarosa, 'Impact of anti-vaccine movements on pertussis control: The untold story', *The Lancet*, 351:9099 (1998), 356–61.
Geffen, D. H., 'The incidence of paralysis occurring in London children within four weeks after immunization', *The Medical Officer*, 83 (1950), 137–40.
General Medical Council, *Dr Andrew Jeremy Wakefield: Determination on Serious Professional Misconduct (SPM) and Sanction* (London: General Medical Council, 24 May 2010).
Gilbert, Pamela K., 'Producing the public, public medicine in private spaces', in Steve Sturdy (ed.), *Medicine, Health and the Public Sphere in Britain: 1600–2000* (London: Routledge, 2002), pp. 43–59.
Gillespie, James A., 'International Organizations and the Problem of Child Health, 1945–1960', *Dynamis* 23 (2003), 115–42.
Goldberg, David, 'MMR, autism, and Adam', *British Medical Journal*, 320:7231 (2000), 389.
Goldman, Stephen A., 'Limitations and strengths of spontaneous reports data', *Clinical Therapeutics*, 20 (1998), C40–4.
Goldstein, Diane E., *Once upon a Virus AIDS Legends and Vernacular Risk Perception* (Logan: Utah State University Press, 2004).
Gomi, Harumi and Hiroshi Takahashi, 'Why is measles still endemic in Japan?', *The Lancet*, 364:9431 (2004), 328–9.
Gorsky, Martin, 'Public health in interwar Britain: Did it fail?', *Dynamis*, 28 (2008), 175–98.
Gouyon, Jean-Baptiste, 'Making science at home: Visual displays of space science and nuclear physics at the Science Museum and on television in postwar Britain', *History & Technology*, 30:1/2 (2014), 37–60.
Global Polio Eradication Initiative, 'Global eradication of wild Poliovirus Type 2 declared' (20 September 2015) http://polioeradication.org/news-post/global-eradication-of-wild-poliovirus-type-2-declared/ (accessed 23 August 2017).
Grabenstein, John D., 'Toxoid vaccines', in Andrew W. Artenstein (ed.), *Vaccines: A Biography* (New York: Springer, 2010), pp. 105–24.

Grant, Mariel, 'Towards a Central Office of Information: Continuity and change in British government information policy, 1939–51', *Journal of Contemporary History*, 34:1 (1999), 49–67.

Gray, P. G. and Ann Cartwright, *Diphtheria Immunisation in 1951: An Inquiry Carried Out in May 1951 for the Ministry of Health* (London: The Social Survey, August 1951).

Greene, Jeremy A., 'Therapeutic infidelities: "Noncompliance" enters the medical literature, 1955–1975', *Social History of Medicine*, 3:1 (2004), 327–43.

Greenhalgh, Charlotte, 'The travelling social survey: Social research and its subjects in Britain, Australia and New Zealand, 1930s–1970s', *History Australia*, 13:1 (2016), 124–38.

Greenough, Paul, Stuart Blume and Christine Holmberg, 'Introduction', in Christine Holmberg, Stuart Blume, and Paul Greenough (eds), *The Politics of Vaccination: A Global History* (Manchester: Manchester University Press, 2017), pp. 1–16.

Griffiths, S., T. Jewell and P. Donnelly, 'Public health in practice: The three domains of public health', *Public Health*, 119:10 (2005), 907–13.

Habermas, Jürgen, *The Structural Transformation of the Public Sphere: An Inquiry into a Category of Bourgeois Society* (Cambridge, MA: MIT Press, 1989).

Hagan, Pat, 'Routine vaccination for tuberculosis ends in UK', *British Medical Journal*, 331:7509 (2005), 128.

Hall, Stuart, 'The great moving right show', in Stuart Hall and Martin Jacques (eds), *The Politics of Thatcherism* (London: Lawrence & Wishart, 1983) pp. 19–39.

Hamborsky, Jennifer, Andrew Kroger and Charles Wolfe (eds), *Epidemiology and Prevention of Vaccine-Preventable Diseases*, 13th edn (Washington, DC: Centre for Disease Control and Prevention, 2015).

Hamlin, Christopher, *Public Health and Social Justice in the Age of Chadwick: Britain, 1800–1854* (Cambridge: Cambridge University Press, 1998).

Hammond, Phil, 'The editor asks M.D. to peer review Private Eye's MMR coverage', *Dr Phil Hammond.com* (18 February 2010) www.drphilhammond.com/blog/2010/02/18/private-eye/dr-phil%E2%80%99s-private-eye-column-issue-1256-february-17-2010/ (accessed 11 July 2017).

Hampton, Jameel, *Disability and the Welfare State in Britain: Changes in Perception and Policy 1948–1979* (Bristol: Policy Press, 2016).

Hanley, Anne, *Medicine, Knowledge and Venereal Diseases in England, 1886–1916* (Basingstoke: Palgrave Macmillan, 2016).

Hanley, James G., 'The public's reaction to public health: Petitions submitted to Parliament, 1847–1848', *Social History of Medicine*, 15:3 (2002), 393–411.

Hardy, Anne, *The Epidemic Streets: Infectious Disease and the Rise of Preventive Medicine, 1856–1900* (Oxford; New York: Clarendon Press; Oxford University Press, 1993).

Hargreaves, Ian, Justin Lewis and Tammy Speers, *Towards a Better Map: Science, the Public and the Media* (London: Economic and Social Research Council, 2003).

Hartley, Percival Horton-Smith, *A Study of Diphtheria in Two Areas of Great Britain: With Special Reference to the Antitoxin Concentration of the Serum of Inoculated and Non-Inoculated Patients and Other Persons; and the Relation of This to the Incidence, Type and Severity of the Disease* (London: HMSO, 1950).

Hawker, Jeremy I., Babatunde Olowokure, Annette L. Wood, Richard C. Wilson and Richard Johnson, 'Widening inequalities in MMR vaccine uptake rates among ethnic groups in an urban area of the UK during a period of vaccine controversy (1994–2000)', *Vaccine*, 25:43 (2007), 7516–19.

Hay, Colin, 'Chronicles of a death foretold: The winter of discontent and construction of crisis of British Keynesianism', *Parliamentary Affairs*, 63 (2010), 446–70.

Hays, J. N., *Epidemics and Pandemics: Their Impact on Human History* (Santa Barbara: ABC-CLIO, 2005).

Health and Social Care Information Centre, 'NHS immunisation statistics: England, 2004–05' (22 September 2005) http://content.digital.nhs.uk/catalogue/PUB00176 (accessed 23 August 2017).

———, 'NHS immunisation statistics: England, 2014–15' (23 September 2015) http://digital.nhs.uk/catalogue/PUB18472/nhs-immu-stat-eng-2014-15-rep.pdf (accessed 23 August 2017).

Heller, Jacob, *The Vaccine Narrative* (Nashville, TN: Vanderbilt University Press, 2008).

Heller, Tom, Dick Heller, Stephen Pattison and Tom Heller, 'Vaccination against mumps, measles, and rubella: Is there a case for deepening the debate?', *British Medical Journal*, 323:7317 (2001), 838–40.

Hendriks, Jan and Stuart Blume, 'Measles vaccination: Before the measles-mumps-rubella vaccine', *American Journal of Public Health*, 103:8 (2013), 1393–401.

Hennock, E. P., 'Vaccination policy against smallpox, 1835–1914: A comparison of England with Prussia and Imperial Germany', *Social History of Medicine*, 11:1 (1998), 49–71.

Heyck, Hunter and David Kaiser, 'Introduction', *Isis*, 101:2 (2010), 362–66.

Hilton, Matthew, Nick Crowson, Jean-François Mouhot and James McKay, *The Politics of Expertise: How NGOs Shaped Modern Britain* (Oxford: Oxford University Press, 2013).

History and Policy, 'History and policy' (undated) www.historyandpolicy.org (accessed 30 September 2016).

Hobbins, Peter, '"Immunisation is as popular as a death adder": The Bundaberg Tragedy and the politics of medical science in interwar Australia', *Social History of Medicine* 24, no. 2 (August 2011): 426–44.

Hobson-West, Pru, '"Trusting blindly can be the biggest risk of all": Organised resistance to childhood vaccination in the UK', *Sociology of Health & Illness*, 29:2 (2007), 198–215.

Honigsbaum, Mark, 'Between securitisation and neglect: Managing Ebola at the borders of global health', *Medical History*, 61:2 (2017), 270–94.

Hooker, Claire, 'Diphtheria, immunisation and the Bundaberg Tragedy: A study of public health in Australia', *Health and History*, 2:1 (2000), 52–78.

Hooker, Claire and Alison Bashford, 'Diphtheria and Australian public health: Bacteriology and its complex applications, c. 1890–1930', *Medical History*, 46:1 (2002), 41–64.

Horkheimer, Max and Theodor W. Adorno, *Dialectic of Enlightenment* (London: Verso, 1997).

Horton, Richard, 'A statement by the editors of The Lancet', *The Lancet*, 363:9411 (2004), 820–1.

———, *MMR: Science and Fiction – Exploring a Vaccine Crisis* (London: Granta, 2004).

———, 'The lessons of MMR', *The Lancet*, 363:9411 (2004), 747–9.

Howard, Colin R., 'The impact on public health of the 19th century anti-vaccination movement', *Microbiology Today*, 30:1 (2003), 22–5.

Howell, Philip, 'A private Contagious Diseases Act: Prostitution and public space in Victorian Cambridge', *Journal of Historical Geography*, 26:3 (2000), 376–402.

Hoyt, Kendall, *Long Shot: Vaccines for National Defense* (Cambridge, MA: Harvard University Press, 2012).

Huisman, Frank and Harry Oosterhuis, 'The politics of health and citizenship: Historical and contemporary perspectives', in Frank Huisman and Harry Oosterhuis (eds), *Heath and Citizenship: Political Cultures of Health in Modern Europe* (London: Pickering and Chatto, 2014), pp. 1–40.

Hüntelmann, Axel C., 'Diphtheria serum and serotherapy. Development, production and regulation in "fin de siecle" Germany', *Dynamis*, 27 (2007), 107–31.

Huzair, Farah and Steve Sturdy, 'Biotechnology and the transformation of vaccine innovation: The case of the hepatitis B vaccines 1968–2000', *Studies in History & Philosophy of Biological & Biomedical Sciences*, 64 (2017), 11–21.

Information Services Division Scotland, 'Trends in immunisation uptake by quarter, calendar and financial year – Scotland' (Edinburgh, June 2016).

International Conference on Primary Health Care, *Declaration of Alma-Ata* (Alma-Ata: World Health Organization, 1978).

Jalabi, Raya, 'California declares Disneyland measles outbreak over as vaccine fight rages on', *Guardian* (17 April 2015) https://www.theguardian.com/society/2015/apr/17/california-declares-disneyland-measles-outbreak-over (accessed 12 January 2018).

Janko, Matthew, 'Vaccination: A victim of its own success', *Virtual Mentor*, 14:1 (2012), 3.

Jarrett, Caitlin, Rose Wilson, Maureen O'Leary, Elisabeth Eckersberger, Heidi J. Larson and SAGE Working Group on Vaccine Hesitancy, 'Strategies for addressing vaccine hesitancy – a systematic review', *Vaccine*, 33:34 (2015), 4180–90.

Jefferies, Sally, Sylvia McShane, Juliet Oerton, Christina R. Victor and Rosemary Beardow, 'Low immunization uptake rates in an inner-city health district: Fact or fiction?' *Journal of Public Health*, 13:4 (1991), 312–17.

Jenner, Edward, *An Inquiry into the Causes and Effects of the Variolæ Vaccinæ a Disease Discovered in Some of the Western Counties of England, Particularly Gloucestershire and Known by the Name of the Cow Pox* (London: Sampson Low, 1789).

Johnson, Norman, *The Welfare State in Transition: The Theory and Practice of Welfare Pluralism* (Amherst: University of Massachusetts Press, 1987).

Joint Committee on Vaccination and Immunisation, *Whooping Cough Vaccination: Review of the Evidence on Whooping Cough Vaccination* (London: HMSO, 1977).

Jones, Allan, 'Elite Science and the BBC: A 1950s Contest of Ownership', *British Journal for the History of Science*, 47:4 (2014), 701–23.

Jose, Jim and Kasey McLoughlin, 'John Stuart Mill and the Contagious Diseases Acts: Whose law? Whose liberty? Whose greater good?' *Law & History Review*, 34:2 (2016), 249–79.

Journal of Molecular Pathology, 'Pre-published Molecular Pathology paper', *Journal of Molecular Pathology* (3 February 2002) http://jcp.bmj.com/content/55/1/suppl/DC1 (accessed 5 January 2017).

Kaplan, Colin, 'Vaccination against smallpox', *British Medical Journal*, 2:5298 (1962), 189.

Keja, K., C. Chan, G. Hayden and R. H. Henderson, 'Expanded programme on immunization', *World Health Statistics Quarterly*, 41:2 (1988), 59–63.

Kennedy, Catriona, Carol Gray Brunton and Rhona Hogg, '"Just that little bit of doubt": Scottish parents', teenage girls' and health professionals' views of the MMR, H1N1 and HPV vaccines', *International Journal of Behavioral Medicine*, 21:1 (2014), 3–10.

Kennedy, Ian, *The Report of the Public Inquiry into Children's Heart Surgery at the Bristol Royal Infirmary 1984–1995: Learning from Bristol* (Cm 5207) (London: TSO, 2001).
Kickbusch, I., 'The development of international health policies – accountability intact?' *Social Science & Medicine* 51:6 (2000), 979–89.
Kimura, Mikio and Harumi Kuno-Sakai, 'Pertussis vaccines in Japan – a clue toward understanding of Japanese attitude to vaccines', *Journal of Tropical Pediatrics*, 37:1 (1991), 45–7.
Kinrade, Derek, *Alf Morris: People's Parliamentarian: Scenes from the Life of Lord Morris of Manchester* (London: National Information Forum, 2007).
Kirk, Dudley, 'Demographic transition theory', *Population Studies*, 50:3 (1996), 361–87.
Kitta, Andrea, *Vaccinations and Public Concern in History: Legend, Rumor, and Risk Perception* (New York: Routledge, 2012).
Klein, N., K. Morgan and M. H. Wansbrough-Jones, 'Parents' beliefs about vaccination: The continuing propagation of false contraindications', *British Medical Journal*, 298:6689 (1989), 1687.
Klein, Rudolf, *The New Politics of the NHS: From Creation to Reinvention*, 7th edn (Oxford: Radcliffe, 2013).
Kmietowicz, Zosia, 'Government launches intensive media campaign on MMR', *British Medical Journal*, 324:7334 (2002), 383.
———, 'Separate vaccines could endanger children', *British Medical Journal*, 323:7315 (2001), 711.
Kuehni, Claudia E., Adrian M. Brooke, Anthony Davis and Michael Silverman, 'Vaccinations as risk factors for wheezing disorders', *The Lancet*, 358:9288 (2001), 1186.
Kulenkampff, M., J. S. Schwartzman and J. Wilson, 'Neurological complications of pertussis inoculation', *Archives of Disease in Childhood*, 49:1 (1974), 46–9.
Lancet, The, 'Time to look beyond MMR in autism research', *The Lancet*, 359:9307 (2002), 637.
Larson, Heidi J., 'The world must accept that the HPV vaccine is safe', *Nature*, 528:7580 (2015), 9.
———, 'Vaccine trust and the limits of information', *Science*, 353:6305 (2016), 1207–8.
Larson, Heidi J., Louis Z. Cooper, Juhani Eskola, Samuel L. Katz and Scott Ratzan, 'Addressing the vaccine confidence gap', *The Lancet*, 378:9790 (2011), 526–35.
Larson, Heidi J., Alexandre de Figueiredo, Zhao Xiahong, William S. Schulz, Pierre Verger, Iain G. Johnston, Alex R. Cook and Nick S. Jones, 'The state

of vaccine confidence 2016: Global insights through a 67-country survey', *EBioMedicine*, 12 (2016), 295–301.

Larson, Heidi J., Caitlin Jarrett, Elisabeth Eckersberger, David M. D. Smith and Pauline Paterson, 'Understanding vaccine hesitancy around vaccines and vaccination from a global perspective: A systematic review of published literature, 2007–2012', *Vaccine*, 32:19 (2014), 2150–9.

Larson, Heidi J., William S. Schulz, Joseph D. Tucker and David M. D. Smith, 'Measuring vaccine confidence: Introducing a global vaccine confidence index', *PLOS Currents Outbreaks* (2015), doi: 10.1371/currents.outbreaks. ce0f6177bc97332602a8e3fe7d7f7cc4.

LeBas, Elizabeth, ' "When every street became a cinema": The film work of Bermondsey Borough Council's Public Health Department, 1923–1953', *History Workshop Journal*, 39 (1995), 42–66.

Lee, Catherine, 'Prostitution and Victorian society revisited: The Contagious Diseases Acts in Kent', *Women's History Review*, 21:2 (2012), 301–16.

Leveson, Lord, *An Inquiry into the Culture, Practices and Ethics of the Press. Report*, Volume II (HC 780-II, 2012–13) (London: TSO, 2012).

Lewis, Jane, 'The medical profession and the state: GPs and the GP contract in the 1960s and the 1990s', *Social Policy & Administration*, 32:2 (1998), 132–50.

———, *The Politics of Motherhood: Child and Maternal Welfare in England, 1900–1939* (London: Croom Helm, 1980).

———, 'The prevention of diphtheria in Canada and Britain 1914–1945', *Journal of Social History*, 20:1 (1986), 163–76.

———, *What Price Community Medicine? The Philosophy, Practice, and Politics of Public Health since 1919* (Brighton: Wheatsheaf Books, 1986).

Lindner, Ulrike and Stuart S. Blume, 'Vaccine innovation and adoption: Polio vaccines in the UK, the Netherlands and West Germany, 1955–1965', *Medical History*, 50:4 (2006), 425–46.

Lishman, F. J. G., 'Smallpox vaccination', *British Medical Journal*, 3:5773 (1971), 534.

Loughlin, Kelly, 'The history of health and medicine in contemporary Britain: Reflections on the role of audio-visual sources', *Social History of Medicine*, 13:1 (2000), 131–45.

Maartens, Brendan, 'From propaganda to "information": Reforming government communications in Britain', *Contemporary British History* (2016).

McCarthy, Michael, 'California ends vaccine exemptions on grounds of belief – will other states follow?', *British Medical Journal*, 351 (2015), h3635.

McCarthy, Nick, 'Polio campaigning widow of Blues legend Jeff Hall dies after cancer battle' (7 June 2016) www.birminghammail.co.uk/news/

midlands-news/polio-campaigning-widow-blues-legend-11437906 (accessed 24 August 2017).
McCloskey, Bertram P., 'The relation of prophylactic inoculations to the onset of poliomyelitis', *The Lancet*, 255:6606 (1950), 659–63.
MacFarlane, John T. and Michael Worboys, 'Showers, sweating and suing: Legionnaires' disease and "new" infections in Britain, 1977–90', *Medical History*, 56:1 (2012), 72–93.
McKeown, Thomas and R. G. Brown, 'Medical evidence related to English population changes in the eighteenth century', *Population Studies*, 9:2 (1955), 119–41.
Maglen, Kristen, ' "The first line of defence": British quarantine and the port sanitary authorities in the nineteenth century', *Social History of Medicine*, 15:3 (2002), 413–28.
Majeed, Azeem, 'Referral of Dr Peter Mansfield to the GMC', *British Medical Journal*, 323:7309 (2001), 356.
Manning, Nathan, 'The relational self and the political engagements of young adults', *Journal of Sociology*, 50:4 (2014), 486–500.
Marshall, T. H., *Citizenship and Social Class, and Other Essays*. (Cambridge: Cambridge University Press, 1950).
Martin, J. K., 'Local paralysis in children after injections', *Archives of Disease in Childhood*, 25:121 (1950), 1–14.
Marx, Karl, *The Eighteenth Brumaire of Louis Bonaparte* (London: FQ Publishing, 2007).
Mayor, Susan, 'Medical Research Council review sets research agenda for autism', *British Medical Journal*, 324:7328 (2002), 10.
———, 'Researcher from study alleging link between MMR and autism warns of measles epidemic', *British Medical Journal*, 327:7423 (2003), 1069.
Mazumdar, Tulip, 'Zika vaccine possible "within months" ', *BBC News* (4 March 2016) www.bbc.co.uk/news/health-35727047 (accessed 19 August 2016).
Medical Research Council, 'B.C.G. and vole bacillus vaccines in the prevention of tuberculosis in adolescents', *British Medical Journal*, 1:4964 (1956), 413–27.
———, 'B.C.G. and vole bacillus vaccines in the prevention of tuberculosis in adolescents', *British Medical Journal*, 2:5149 (1959), 379–96.
———, *Review of Autism Research: Epidemiology and Causes* (London: Medical Research Council, 2001).
———, 'Vaccination against whooping-cough; Relation between protection in children and results of laboratory tests; A report to the Whooping-Cough Immunization Committee of the Medical Research Council and to the Medical Officers of Health for Cardiff, Leeds, Leyton, Manchester,

Middlesex, Oxford, Poole, Tottenham, Walthamstow, and Wembley', *British Medical Journal*, 2:4990 (1956), 454–62.

Meldrum, Marcia, '"A calculated risk": The Salk polio vaccine field trials of 1954', *British Medical Journal*, 317:7167 (1998), 1233–6.

Melling, Joseph and Pamela Dale, 'Medical Officers of Health, gender and government responses to the problem of cancer in Britain, 1900–1940', *Medical History*, 53:4 (2009), 537–60.

Mercer, A. J., 'Smallpox and epidemiological-demographic change in Europe: The role of vaccination', *Population Studies*, 39:2 (1985), 287–307.

Meszaros, Jacqueline R., David A. Asch, Jonathan Baron, John C. Hershey, Howard Kunreuther and Joanne Schwartz-Buzaglo, 'Cognitive processes and the decisions of some parents to forego pertussis vaccination for their children', *Journal of Clinical Epidemiology*, 49:6 (1996), 697–703.

Mills, Heather, *Private Eye Special Report: MMR: The Story So Far* (London: Pressdam, 2002).

Millward, Gareth, 'A disability act? The Vaccine Damage Payments Act 1979 and the British government's response to the pertussis vaccine scare', *Social History of Medicine*, 30:2 (2016), 429–47.

———, '"A matter of commonsense": The Coventry poliomyelitis epidemic 1957 and the British public', *Contemporary British History*, 31:3 (2017), 384–406.

———, 'Social security policy and the early disability movement – expertise, disability and the government, 1965–1977', *Twentieth Century British History*, 26:2 (2015), 274–97.

Ministry of Health, *Annual Report of the Ministry of Health for the Year 1967* (Cmnd 3702) (London: HMSO, 1968).

———, *Report of the Ministry of Health Covering the Period from 1st April, 1950 to 31st December, 1951. Part II on the State of the Public Health, Being the Annual Report of the Chief Medical Officer for the Year 1950* (Cmd 8582) (London: HMSO, 1952).

———, *Report of the Ministry of Health Covering the Period from 1st April, 1950 to 31st December, 1951. Part III on the State of the Public Health* (Cmd 8787) (London: HMSO, 1953).

———, *Report of the Ministry of Health for the Year 1957. Part II on the State of the Public Health Being the Annual Report of the Chief Medical Officer* (Cmnd 559) (London: HMSO, 1958).

———, *Report of the Ministry of Health for the Year 1958. Part II on the State of the Public Health Being the Annual Report of the Chief Medical Officer* (Cmnd 871) (London: HMSO, 1959).

———, *Report of the Ministry of Health for the Year 1960. Part II. On the State of the Public Health. Being the Annual Report of the Chief Medical Officer* (Cmnd 1550) (London: HMSO, 1961).

———, *Report of the Ministry of Health for the Year Ended 31st December, 1953 Part II on the State of the Public Health* (Cmd 9307) (London: HMSO, 1954).
———, *Report of the Ministry of Health for the Year Ended 31st December, 1954 Part II on the State of the Public Health Being the Report of the Chief Medical Officer for the Year 1954* (Cmd 9627) (London: HMSO, 1955).
———, *Report of the Ministry of Health for the Year Ended 31st December, 1955 Part II on the State of the Public Health* (Cmnd 16) (London: HMSO, 1956).
———, *Report of the Ministry of Health for the Year Ended 31st December, 1956. Part II on the State of the Public Health Being the Annual Report of the Chief Medical Officer for the Year 1956* (Cmnd 325) (London: HMSO, 1957).
———, *Summary Report by the Ministry of Health for the Period from 1st April, 1939 to 31st March 1941* (Cmd 6340) (London: HMSO, 1942).
———, *Summary Report of the Ministry of Health for the Year Ended 31st March, 1943* (Cmd 6468) (London: HMSO, 1943).
MMR Expert Group, 'Report of the MMR Expert Group', *Scottish Government* (April 2002) www.gov.scot/Publications/2002/04/14619/3779 (accessed 24 August 2017).
Moberly, Tom, 'UK doctors re-examine case for mandatory vaccination', *British Medical Journal*, 358 (2017), j3414.
Mold, Alex, *Making the Patient-Consumer: Patient Organisations and Health Consumerism in Britain* (Manchester: Manchester University Press, 2015).
Mooney, Graham, *Intrusive Interventions: Public Health, Domestic Space, and Infectious Disease Surveillance in England, 1840–1914* (Rochester: University of Rochester Press, 2015).
Mooney, Helen, 'More "responsible" science reporting is needed, Leveson Inquiry hears', *British Medical Journal*, 343 (2011), d8051.
Moore, Martin D., *Managing Diabetes, Managing Medicine: Chronic Disease and Clinical Bureaucracy in Post-War Britain* (Manchester: Manchester University Press, 2019).
Morgan, Montagu Travers, *Annual Report of the Medical Officer of Health to 31st December, 1949* (London: Port of London Health Authority, 1950).
Morris, A. and D. Aldulaimi, 'New evidence for a viral pathogenic mechanism for new variant inflammatory bowel disease and development disorder?', *Molecular Pathology*, 55:2 (2002), 83.
Moulin, Anne Marie, 'La metaphore vaccine: de l'inoculation a la vaccinologie', *History and Philosophy of the Life Sciences*, 14:2 (1992), 271–97.
Moxon, E. Richard and Claire-Anne Siegrist, 'The next decade of vaccines: Societal and scientific challenges', *The Lancet*, 378:9788 (2011), 348–59.
Mukherjee, Siddhartha, 'The race for a Zika vaccine', *New Yorker* (22 August 2016) www.newyorker.com/magazine/2016/08/22/the-race-for-a-zika-vaccine (accessed 19 August 2016).

Murch, Simon, Mike Thomson and John Walker-Smith, 'Autism, inflammatory bowel disease, and MMR vaccine', *The Lancet*, 351:9106 (1998), 908.

Murch, Simon H., Andrew Anthony, David H. Casson, Mohsin Malik, Mark Berelowitz, Amar P. Dhillon, Michael A. Thomson, Alan Valentine, Susan E. Davies and John A. Walker-Smith, 'Retraction of an interpretation', *The Lancet*, 363:9411 (2004), 750.

Naqvi, Nasim Hasan, 'A medical classic: Al-Razi's treatise on smallpox and measles', *Muslim Heritage* (2009) www.muslimheritage.com/article/medical-classic-al-razi%E2%80%99s-treatise-smallpox-and-measles (accessed 19 September 2016).

Nathanson, Neal and Alexander D. Langmuir, 'The Cutter Incident. Poliomyelitis following formaldehyde-inactivated poliovirus vaccination in the United States during the spring of 1955', *American Journal of Epidemiology*, 78:1 (1963), 29–60.

National Health Service, 'Childhood vaccines timeline' (16 July 2016) www.nhs.uk/Conditions/Vaccinations/Pages/Childhood-vaccination-schedule.aspx (accessed 12 January 2018).

National Health Services Scotland, 'Childhood immunisation statistics Scotland: Quarter and year ending 31 December 2015' (22 March 2016) www.isdscotland.org/Health-Topics/Child-Health/Publications/2016-03-22/2016-03-22-Immunisation-Report.pdf (accessed 23 August 2017).

Newlands, Emma, *Civilians into Soldiers: War, the Body and British Army Recruits, 1939–45* (Manchester: Manchester University Press, 2014).

Newman, Janet and John Clarke, *Publics, Politics and Power: Remaking the Public in Public Services* (London: Sage, 2009).

NHS Digital, 'Childhood vaccination coverage statistics, England, 2016–17' (20 September 2017) https://digital.nhs.uk/catalogue/PUB30085 (accessed 12 January 2018).

NHS Digital, 'NHS Immunisation Statistics: England, 2015–16', (London, September 2016).

Nicoll, A. and D. Jenkinson, 'Decision making for routine measles/MMR and whooping cough immunisation', *British Medical Journal*, 297:6645 (1988), 405–7.

Nicoll, Angus, David Elliman and Euan Ross, 'MMR vaccination and autism 1998', *British Medical Journal*, 316:7133 (1998), 715–16.

Nigam, Aruna, Pikee Saxena, Anita S. Acharya, Archana Mishra and Swaraj Batra, 'HPV vaccination in India: Critical appraisal', *ISRN Obstetrics and Gynecology*, 2014 (2014), http://dx.doi.org/10.1155/2014/394595.

O'Brien, Sarah J., Ian G. Jones and Peter Christie, 'Autism, inflammatory bowel disease, and MMR vaccine', *The Lancet*, 351:9106 (1998), 906–7.

Ocaña, Esteban Rodríguez, 'The social production of novelty: Diphtheria sero-therapy, "herald of the new medicine"', *Dynamis*, 27 (2007), 21–31.
Offit, Paul A., 'The anti-vaccination epidemic: Whooping cough, mumps and measles are making an alarming comeback, thanks to seriously misguided parents', *Wall Street Journal (Online)* (24 September 2014) www.wsj.com/articles/paul-a-offit-the-anti-vaccination-epidemic-1411598408 (accessed 19 August 2016).
———, 'The Cutter Incident, 50 years later', *New England Journal of Medicine*, 352:14 (2005), 1411–12.
———, *The Cutter Incident: How America's First Polio Vaccine Led to the Growing Vaccine Crisis* (New Haven, CT: Yale University Press, 2005).
———, *Vaccinated: One Man's Quest to Defeat the World's Deadliest Diseases* (New York: Smithsonian Books, 2007).
O'Hara, Glen, 'Towards a new Bradshaw? Economic statistics and the British state in the 1950s and 1960s', *Economic History Review* 60:1 (2007), 1–34.
Oliver, Michael, *The Politics of Disablement* (London: Macmillan Education, 1990).
Opal, Steven M., 'A brief history of microbiology and immunology', in Andrew W. Artenstein (ed.), *Vaccines: A Biography* (New York: Springer, 2010), pp. 31–56.
Oshinsky, David M., *Polio: An American Story* (Oxford: Oxford University Press, 2005).
Pareek, M. and H. M. Pattison, 'The two-dose measles, mumps, and rubella (MMR) immunisation schedule: Factors affecting maternal intention to vaccinate', *The British Journal of General Practice*, 50:461 (2000), 969–71.
Parish, H. J., *A History of Immunization* (Edinburgh: Livingstone, 1965).
Parrish, David, 'A party contagion: Party politics and the inoculation controversy in the British Atlantic world, c.1721–1723', *Journal for Eighteenth-Century Studies*, 39:1 (2016), 41–58.
Paul, John Rodman, *A History of Poliomyelitis* (New Haven, CT: Yale University Press, 1971).
Payling, Daisy, '"The people who write to us are the people who don't like us": Public responses to the Government Social Survey's Survey of Sickness, 1943–1952', *Journal of British Studies* (forthcoming, 2018).
Pearson, Colin, *Royal Commission on Civil Liability and Compensation for Personal Injury Vol.1* (Cmnd 7054-I) (London: HMSO, 1978).
Pearson, Jessica, 'French colonialism and the battle against the WHO Regional Office for Africa', *Hygiea Internationalis: An Interdisciplinary Journal for the History of Public Health*, 13:1 (2016), 65–80.
Peckham, C. A., 'Action Research for the Crippled Child, British Postgraduate Medical Federation, Institute of Child Health and Department of Paediatric

Epidemiology', *The Peckham Report: National Immunisation Study: Factors Influencing Immunisation Uptake in Childhood* (London: Department of Paediatric Epidemiology, Institute of Child Health; Horsham, West Sussex: Action Research for the Crippled Child, 1989).

Petersen, Alan R. and Deborah Lupton, *The New Public Health: Health and Self in the Age of Risk* (London: Sage, 2000).

Petrovic, Marko, Richard Roberts and Mary Ramsay, 'Second dose of measles, mumps, and rubella vaccine: Questionnaire survey of health professionals', *British Medical Journal*, 322:7278 (2001), 82–5.

Pickstone, John, 'Production, community and consumption: The political economy of twentieth-century medicine', in Roger Cooter and John Pickstone (eds), *Medicine in the Twentieth Century* (Abingdon: Routledge, 2003), 1–20.

Poliomyelitis Vaccines Committee (Medical Research Council), 'Assessment of the British vaccine against poliomyelitis', *British Medical Journal*, 1:5030 (1957), 1271–77.

Porras, María Isabel and María Victoria Cabellero, 'Vaccines and vaccination against smallpox and poliomyelitis: Economies and values', Conference paper (European Association for the History of Medicine and Health Conference, University of Cologne, September 2015).

Porter, Dorothy, *Health Citizenship: Essays in Social Medicine and Biomedical Politics* (Berkeley: University of California Press, 2011).

———, *Health, Civilization and the State: A History of Public Health from Ancient to Modern Times* (London: Routledge, 1999).

Porter, Dorothy and Roy Porter, 'The politics of prevention: Anti-vaccinationism and public health in nineteenth-century England', *Medical History*, 32:3 (1988), 231–52.

Price-Smith, Andrew, 'The plagues of affluence: Human ecology and the case of the SARS epidemic', *Environmental History*, 20:4 (2015), 765–78.

Public Health Agency [Northern Ireland], 'Vaccination coverage: COVER' (March 2017) www.publichealthagency.org/sites/default/files/directorates/files/24%20months%20of%20age_20.pdf (accessed 23 August 2017).

Public Health England, 'Measles notifications and deaths in England and Wales: 1940 to 2016', www.gov.uk/government/publications/measles-deaths-by-age-group-from-1980-to-2013-ons-data/measles-notifications-and-deaths-in-england-and-wales-1940-to-2013 (accessed 2 August 2017).

———, 'Measles outbreaks across England' (25 July 2018) https://www.gov.uk/government/news/measles-outbreaks-across-england (accessed 27 July 2018).

———, 'Notifiable diseases: historic annual totals' (28 November 2016) www.gov.uk/government/publications/notifiable-diseases-historic-annual-totals (accessed 5 May 2017).

———, 'Table 6: Pertussis notifications and deaths, England and Wales: 1940–2014' (5 May 2016) www.gov.uk/government/uploads/system/uploads/attachment_data/file/521438/Table_6_Pertussis_notifications_and_deaths__E_W__1940_-_2015.pdf (accessed 6 June 2017).

Public Health England and Department of Health, *Immunisation against Infectious Disease*, 2nd edn (London: Public Health England, 2013).

Parliamentary Commissioner for Administration, *Sixth Report for Session 1976–77: Whooping Cough Vaccination* (HC571) (London: HMSO, 1977).

Public Health Wales, 'Measles outbreak: Data' (19 February 2015) http://www.wales.nhs.uk/sitesplus/888/page/66389 (accessed 27 July 2018).

Rafferty, Sarah, Matthew R. Smallman-Raynor and Andrew D. Cliff, 'Variola minor in England and Wales: The geographical course of a smallpox epidemic and the impediments to effective disease control, 1920–1935', *Journal of Historical Geography*, 59 (2018), 2–14.

Ramsay, Mary E., J. Yarwood, D. Lewis, H. Campbell and J. M. White, 'Parental confidence in measles, mumps and rubella vaccine: Evidence from vaccine coverage and attitudinal surveys', *British Journal of General Practice*, 52:484 (2002), 912–16.

Ramsay, Sarah, 'UK government tries to control MMR panic', *The Lancet*, 359:9306 (2002), 590.

———, 'UK starts campaign to reassure parents about MMR-vaccine safety', *The Lancet*, 357:9252 (2001), 290.

Rāzī, Abū Bakr Muḥammad ibn Zakarīyā, William Alexander Greenhill and Naval Medical School (U.S.). *A Treatise on the Small-pox and Measles* (London: Sydenham Society, 1848).

Razzell, Peter, *The Conquest of Smallpox: The Impact of Inoculation on Smallpox Mortality in Eighteenth Century Britain* (Firle: Caliban Books, 1977).

———, 'The decline of adult smallpox in eighteenth-century London: A commentary', *Economic History Review*, 64:4 (2011), 1315–35.

Redden, Candace Johnson, 'Health as citizenship narrative', *Polity*, 34:3 (2002), 355–70.

Redfern, Michael, *The Royal Liverpool Children's Inquiry Report* (HC 12-II, 2000–01) (London: TSO, 2001).

Reinhardt, Bob H., *The End of a Global Pox: America and the Eradication of Smallpox in the Cold War Era* (Chapel Hill: University of North Carolina Press, 2015).

Riolo, Maria A., Aaron A. King and Pejman Rohani, 'Can vaccine legacy explain the British pertussis resurgence?', *Vaccine*, 31 (2013), 5903–8.
Roberts, Karen A., Mary Dixon-Woods, Ray Fitzpatrick, Keith R. Abrams and David R. Jones, 'Factors affecting uptake of childhood immunisation: A Bayesian synthesis of qualitative and quantitative evidence', *The Lancet*, 360:9345 (2002), 1596–9.
Roberts, Richard J., Quentin D. Sandifer, Merion R. Evans, Maria Z. Nolan-Farrell and Paul M. Davis, 'Reasons for non-uptake of measles, mumps, and rubella catch up immunisation in a measles epidemic and side effects of the vaccine', *British Medical Journal*, 310:6995 (1995), 1629–39.
Roemer-Mahler, Anne and Stefan Elbe, 'The race for Ebola drugs: Pharmaceuticals, security and global health governance', *Third World Quarterly*, 37:3 (2016), 487–506.
Rogers, Chris, 'The politics of economic policy making in Britain: A reassessment of the 1976 IMF crisis', *Politics & Policy*, 37:5 (2009), 971–94.
Rogers, Naomi, *Dirt and Disease: Polio before FDR* (New Brunswick: Rutgers University Press, 1992).
———, *Polio Wars: Sister Elizabeth Kenny and the Golden Age of American Medicine* (Oxford: Oxford University Press, 2014).
Rosen, George, *A History of Public Health* (New York: MD Publications, 1958).
Rouse, A., 'Autism, inflammatory bowel disease, and MMR Vaccine', *The Lancet*, 351:9112 (1998), 1356.
RTS,S Clinical Trials Partnership, 'Efficacy and safety of RTS,S/AS01 malaria vaccine with or without a booster dose in infants and children in Africa: Final results of a phase 3, individually randomised, controlled trial', *The Lancet*, 386:9988 (2015), 31–45.
Ruane, Kevin and James Ellison, 'Managing the Americans: Anthony Eden, Harold Macmillan and the pursuit of "power-by-proxy" in the 1950s', *Contemporary British History*, 18:3 (2004), 147–67.
Runciman, W. G., 'Review of Strukturwandel der Öffentlichkeit, Jürgen Habermas', *British Journal of Sociology*, 15:4 (1964), 366.
Rusnock, Andrea, 'Medical statistics and hospital medicine: The case of the smallpox vaccination', *Centaurus*, 49:4 (2007), 337–59.
———, *Vital Accounts: Quantifying Health and Population in Eighteenth-Century England and France* (Cambridge: Cambridge University Press, 2002).
Russell, Patrick and James Piers Taylor (eds), *Shadows of Progress: Documentary Film in Post-war Britain* (London: British Film Institute, 2010).
SAGE Working Group on Vaccine Hesitancy, *Report of the SAGE Working Group on Vaccine Hesitancy* (Geneva: World Health Organization, 2014).
Salmon, R. L., 'Science in the face of disaster', *The Lancet*, 363:9414 (2004), 1084–5.

Savage, Mike, *Identities and Social Change in Britain since 1940: The Politics of Method* (Oxford: Oxford University Press, 2010).

———, 'Affluence and social change in the making of technocratic middle-class identities: Britain, 1939–55', *Contemporary British History*, 22:4 (2008): 457–76.

Schar, M., 'Vaccination against smallpox', *British Medical Journal*, 1:5275 (1962), 403.

Schmalstieg, Frank C. and Armond S. Goldman, 'Birth of the science of immunology', *Journal of Medical Biography*, 18:2 (2010), 88–98.

Schmidt, James, 'Publicity and the public sphere – reading Habermas as a historian of concepts', *Persistent Enlightenment* (31 March 2013) https://persistentenlightenment.wordpress.com/2013/03/31/publicity-publicsphere-habermas/ (accessed 25 August 2016).

Scott, J. A., *Report of the County Medical Officer of Health and Principal School Medical Officer for the Year 1957* (London: London County Council, 1958).

———, *Report of the County Medical Officer of Health and School Medical Officer for the Year 1951* (London: London County Council, 1952).

———, *Report of the County Medical Officer of Health and School Medical Officer for the Year 1952* (London: London County Council, 1953).

———, *Report of the County Medical Officer of Health and School Medical Officer for the Year 1953* (London: London County Council, 1954).

———, *Report of the County Medical Officer of Health and School Medical Officer for the Year 1954* (London: London County Council, 1955).

———, *Report of the County Medical Officer of Health and School Medical Officer for the Year 1955* (London: London County Council, 1956).

———, *Report of the County Medical Officer of Health and School Medical Officer for the Year 1956* (London: London County Council, 1957).

———, *Report of the County Medical Officer of Health and School Medical Officer for the Year 1957* (London: London County Council, 1958).

Sennett, Richard, *The Fall of Public Man* (Cambridge: Cambridge University Press, 1977).

Sewell, Claire, ' "If one member of the family is disabled the family as a whole is disabled": Thalidomide children and the emergence of the family carer in Britain, c. 1957–1978', *Family & Community History*, 18:1 (2015), 37–52.

Seymour, Jane K., Martin Gorsky and Shakoor Hajat, 'Health, wealth and party in inter-war London', *Urban History*, 44:3 (2017), 464–91.

Shaw, Alison, 'Gordon Stewart, expert in public health and colleague of Fleming who helped pioneer the use of penicillin', *Herald* (15 November 2016) www.heraldscotland.com/opinion/obituaries/14904952.Obituary___Gordon_Stewart___expert_in_public_health_and_colleague_of_Fleming_who_helped_pioneer_the_use_of_penicillin/ (accessed 19 June 2017).

Sheard, Sally, 'Quacks and clerks: Historical and contemporary perspectives on the structure and function of the British medical civil service', *Social Policy & Administration*, 44:2 (2010), 193–207.

———, *The Passionate Economist: How Brian-Abel Smith Shaped Global Health and Social Welfare* (Bristol: Policy Press, 2013).

Shooter, R. A., *Report of the Investigation into the Cause of the 1978 Birmingham Smallpox Occurrence* (HC 668, 1979–80) (London: HMSO, 1980).

Sibbald, Bonnie, Ian Enzer, Cary Cooper, Usha Rout and Valerie Sutherland, 'GP job satisfaction in 1987, 1990 and 1998: Lessons for the future?', *Family Practice*, 17:5 (2000), 364–71.

Simon, Jonathan, 'The origin of the production of diphtheria antitoxin in France, between philanthropy and commerce', *Dynamis*, 27 (2007), 63–82.

Sirrs, Christopher, 'Accidents and apathy: The construction of the "Robens philosophy" of occupational safety and health regulation in Britain, 1961–1974', *Social History of Medicine*, 29:1 (2016), 66–88.

Smallman-Raynor, Matthew and Andrew D. Cliff, 'The geographical spread of the 1947 poliomyelitis epidemic in England and Wales: Spatial wave propagation of an enigmatic epidemiological event', *Journal of Historical Geography*, 40 (2013), 36–51.

Smith, F. B., 'Ethics and disease in the later nineteenth century: The Contagious Diseases Acts', *Historical Studies*, 15:57 (1971), 118–35.

Smith, Jennifer, 'Illustrations from the Wellcome Institute Library: The Archive of the Health Visitors' Association in the Contemporary Medical Archives Centre', *Medical History*, 39:3 (1995), 358–67.

Smith, Kendall A., 'Louis Pasteur, the father of immunology?', *Frontiers in Immunology*, 3:68 (2012).

Smith, Philip J., Susan Y. Chu and Lawrence E. Barker, 'Children who have received no vaccines: Who are they and where do they live?', *Pediatrics*, 114:1 (2004), 187–95.

Smith, Richard, 'Do patients need to read research?', *British Medical Journal*, 326:7402 (2003), 1307.

Smith, T., 'Measles and the government', *British Medical Journal (Clinical Research Edition)*, 294:6578 (1987), 989–90.

South, Mary, 'Smallpox inoculation campaigns in eighteenth-century Southampton, Salisbury and Winchester', *The Local Historian*, 43:2 (2013), 122–37.

Speers, Tammy and Justin Lewis, 'Journalists and jabs: Media coverage of the MMR vaccine', *Communication & Medicine*, 1:2 (2004), 171–81.

Spier, R. E., 'Perception of risk of vaccine adverse events: A historical perspective', *Vaccine*, 20: Supplement 1 (2001), S78–84.

Stanton, Jennifer, 'What shapes vaccine policy? The case of hepatitis B in the UK', *Social History of Medicine*, 7:3 (1994), 427–46.
Starkey, Pat, 'The feckless mother: Women, poverty and social workers in wartime and post-war England', *Women's History Review*, 9:3 (2000), 539–57.
Stefanoff, Pawel, Svenn-Erik Mamelund, Mary Robinson, Eva Netterlid, Jose Tuells, Marianne A. Riise Bergsaker, Harald Heijbel and Joanne Yarwood, 'Tracking parental attitudes on vaccination across European countries: The Vaccine Safety, Attitudes, Training and Communication Project (VACSATC)', *Vaccine*, 28:35 (2010), 5731–7.
Stefler, Denes and Raj Bhopal, 'Lessons to be learnt from other countries about mandatory child vaccination', *British Medical Journal*, 344 (2012), e4036.
Stephen, Wendy E., 'Re: UK doctors re-examine case for mandatory vaccination', *British Medical Journal*, 358 (2017), j3414.
Stewart, A. B., *Report of the County Medical Officer of Health and Principal School Medical Officer for the Year 1964* (London: London County Council, 1966).
Stewart, G. T., 'The law tries to decide whether whooping cough vaccine causes brain damage: Professor Gordon Stewart gives evidence', *British Medical Journal (Clinical Research Edition)* 293:6540 (1986), 203–4.
———, 'Vaccination against whooping-cough', *The Lancet*, 1:8005 (1977), 234–7.
Stewart, James, 'Smallpox1962 – An online archive of the outbreaks in Wales and England' (2012) www.smallpox1962.org.uk (accessed 5 April 2017).
Straus, Eugene and Alex Straus, *Medical Marvels: The 100 Greatest Advances in Medicine* (Amherst: Prometheus Books, 2006).
Sturdy, Steve, 'Introduction: Medicine, health and the public sphere', in Steve Sturdy (ed.), *Medicine, Health and the Public Sphere in Britain: 1600–2000* (London: Routledge, 2002), pp. 1–24.
Styles, W. M., 'Rubella immunisation', *British Medical Journal*, 2:6140 (1978), 834.
Sunday Times, *Suffer the Children: The Story of Thalidomide* (New York: Viking Press, 1979).
Sutcliffe-Braithwaite, Florence, 'Discourses of "class" in Britain in "New Times"', *Contemporary British History*, 31:2 (2017), 294–317.
Swansea Research Unit of the Royal College of General Practitioners, 'Effect of a low pertussis vaccination uptake on a large community', *British Medical Journal (Clinical Research Edition)*, 282:6257 (1981), 23–6.
Szreter, Simon, 'The importance of social intervention in Britain's mortality decline c.1850–1914: A re-interpretation of the role of public health', *Social History of Medicine*, 1:1 (1988), 1–38.

Telegraph, 'Boys should get HPV vaccine to protect them from throat cancers, experts say', *Telegraph* (10 July 2016) www.telegraph.co.uk/news/2016/07/09/boys-should-get-hpv-vaccine-to-protect-them-from-throat-cancers/ (accessed 19 August 2016).

Thane, Pat, Melanie Oppenheimer and Nicholas Deakin (eds), *Voluntary Action in Britain since Beveridge* (Manchester: Manchester University Press, 2011).

Thomas, Patricia, *Big Shot: Passion, Politics, and the Struggle for an AIDS Vaccine* (New York: Public Affairs, 2001).

Topley, W. W. C. and G. S. Wilson, 'The spread of bacterial infection. The problem of herd-immunity', *The Journal of Hygiene*, 21:3 (1923), 243–9.

Torjesen, Ingrid, 'UK adds hepatitis B to infant vaccination schedule', *British Medical Journal*, 358 (2017), j3357.

Towghi, Fouzieyha, 'The biopolitics of reproductive technologies beyond the clinic: Localizing HPV vaccines in India', *Medical Anthropology*, 32:4 (2013), 325–42.

Ueda, Kohji, Chiaki Miyazaki, Yasufumi Hidaka, Kenji Okada, Koichi Kusuhara and Ryo Kadoya, 'Aseptic meningitis caused by measles-mumps-rubella vaccine in Japan', *The Lancet*, 346:8976 (1995), 701–2.

Uhlmann, V., C. M. Martin, O. Sheils, L. Pilkington, I. Silva, A. Killalea, S. B. Murch, J. Walker-Smith, M. Thomson, A. J. Wakefield and J. J. O'Leary, 'Potential viral pathogenic mechanism for new variant inflammatory bowel disease', *Molecular Pathology*, 55:2 (2002), 84–90.

UK Government and Parliament Petitions, 'Petition: Give the meningitis B vaccine to ALL children, not just newborn babies' (15 September 2015) https://petition.parliament.uk/petitions/108072 (accessed 23 August 2017).

UNdata, 'Internet users (per 100 people)'. http://data.un.org/Data.aspx?d=WDI&f=Indicator_Code%3AIT.NET.USER.P2 (accessed 22 June 2017).

Vara, Vauhini, 'The race for an Ebola vaccine', *New Yorker* (25 November 2014) www.newyorker.com/business/currency/race-ebola-vaccine (accessed 19 August 2016).

Vargha, Dora, 'Between East and West: Polio vaccination across the Iron Curtain in Cold War Hungary', *Bulletin of the History of Medicine*, 88:2 (2014), 319–42.

Various, 'Health professionals' attitudes to MMR vaccine', *British Medical Journal*, 322:7294 (2001), 1120.

Various, 'MMR vaccination and autism 1998', *British Medical Journal*, 316:7147 (1998), 1824.

Various, 'MMR vaccine debate', *British Medical Journal*, 324:7339 (2002), 733.

Verweij, M. F. and Angus Dawson, 'The meaning of "public" in "public health"', in M. F. Verweij and Angus Dawson (eds), *Ethics, Prevention, and Public Health* (Oxford: Clarendon Press, 2007), pp. 13–29.

Vyse, A. J., N. J. Gay, J. M. White, M. E. Ramsay, D. W. G. Brown, B. J. Cohen, L. M. Hesketh, P. Morgan-Capner and E. Miller, 'Evolution of surveillance of measles, mumps, and rubella in England and Wales: Providing the platform for evidence-based vaccination policy', *Epidemiologic Reviews*, 24:2 (2002), 125–36.
Wakefield, A. J. and S. M. Montgomery, 'Measles, mumps, rubella vaccine: Through a glass, darkly', *Adverse Drug Reactions and Toxicological Reviews*, 19:4 (2000), 265–83; discussion 284–92.
Wakefield, A. J., S. H. Murch, A. Anthony, J. Linnell, D. M. Casson, M. Malik, M. Berelowitz, A. P. Dhillon, M. A. Thomson, P. Harvey, A. Valentine, S. E. Davies and J. A. Walker-Smith, 'RETRACTED: Ileal-lymphoid-nodular hyperplasia, non-specific colitis, and pervasive developmental disorder in children', *The Lancet*, 351:9103 (1998), 637–41.
Walker-Smith, John, 'Autism, bowel inflammation, and measles', *The Lancet*, 359:9307 (2002), 705–6.
Walkowitz, Judith R., *Prostitution and Victorian Society: Women, Class, and the State* (Cambridge: Cambridge University Press, 1980).
Warner, Michael, *Publics and Counterpublics* (Cambridge: Zone Books, 2002).
Wartime Social Survey, *Diphtheria Immunisation Enquiry: A Survey of 2,026 Parents Made in July–August 1942, for the Ministry of Health* (London: Wartime Social Survey, 1942).
Webster, Charles, 'Healthy or hungry thirties?', *History Workshop*, 13 (1982), 110–29.
Weisz, George, *Chronic Disease in the Twentieth Century* (Baltimore: Johns Hopkins University Press, 2014).
Welshman, John, '"Bringing beauty and brightness to the back streets": Health education and public health in England and Wales, 1890–1940', *Health Education Journal*, 56:2 (1997), 199–209.
———, 'Compulsion, localism, and pragmatism: The micro-politics of tuberculosis screening in the United Kingdom, 1950–1965', *Social History of Medicine*, 19:2 (2006), 295–312.
———, 'In search of the "problem family": Public health and social work in England and Wales 1940–70', *Social History of Medicine*, 9:3 (1996), 447–65.
———, *Municipal Medicine: Public Health in Twentieth-Century Britain* (Bern: Peter Lang, 2000).
———, 'The Medical Officer of Health in England and Wales, 1900–1974: Watchdog or lapdog?', *Journal of Public Health*, 19:4 (1997), 443–50.
Whiteley, Paul and Steve Winyard, *Pressure for the Poor: The Poverty Lobby and Policy Making* (London: Methuen, 1987).
Williams, Gareth and Ray Loadman, *Paralysed with Fear: The Story of Polio* (Basingstoke: Palgrave Macmillan, 2013).

Williamson, Stanley, *The Vaccination Controversy: The Rise, Reign and Fall of Compulsory Vaccination for Smallpox* (Liverpool: Liverpool University Press, 2007).
Wilson, G. S., 'B.C.G. vaccination in control of tuberculosis', *British Medical Journal*, 2:4534 (1947), 855–9.
Wise, Jacqui, 'Finnish study confirms safety of MMR vaccine', *British Medical Journal*, 322:7279 (2001), 130.
Wolfe, Robert M. and Lisa K. Sharp, 'Anti-vaccinationists past and present', *British Medical Journal*, 325:7361 (2002), 430–2.
Worboys, Michael, *Spreading Germs: Disease Theories and Medical Practice in Britain, 1865–1900* (Cambridge: Cambridge University Press, 2000).
World Health Organization, *Global Vaccine Action Plan* (Geneva: World Health Organization, 2013).
World Health Organization, 'Measles continues to spread and take lives in Europe' (11 July 2017) www.euro.who.int/en/media-centre/sections/press-releases/2017/measles-continues-to-spread-and-take-lives-in-europe (accessed 12 January 2018).
———, 'Statement on the 1st meeting of the IHR Emergency Committee on the 2014 Ebola outbreak in West Africa', (2014) www.who.int/mediacentre/news/statements/2014/ebola-20140808/en/ (accessed 19 August 2016).
———, 'Weekly epidemiological record' (7 January 2011) www.who.int/wer/2011/wer8601_02.pdf (accessed 24 August 2017).
———, 'Weekly epidemiological record' (29 January 2016) www.who.int/wer/2016/wer9104.pdf?ua=1 (accessed 24 August 2017).
———, 'WHO Director-General summarizes the outcome of the Emergency Committee regarding clusters of microcephaly and Guillain-Barré syndrome' (2016) www.who.int/mediacentre/news/statements/2016/emergency-committee-zika-microcephaly/en/ (accessed 19 August 2016).
World Health Organization, Rotary International, Centers for Disease Control and Prevention and UNICEF, *Global Polio Eradication Initiative Status Report 29 April 2013* (Geneva: Global Polio Eradication Initiative, 2013).
Wroe, Abigail L., Angela Bhan, Paul Salkovskis and Helen Bedford, 'Feeling bad about immunising our children', *Vaccine*, 23:12 (2005), 1428–33.
Yarwood, Joanne, 'Communicating vaccine benefit and risk – lessons from the medical field', *Veterinary Microbiology*, 117:1 (2006), 71–4.
Yarwood, Joanne, Karen Noakes, Dorian Kennedy, Helen Campbell and David Salisbury, 'Tracking mothers attitudes to childhood immunisation 1991–2001', *Vaccine*, 23:48–49 (2005), 5670–87.
Yuille, Duncan and Rowland Rogerson, 'Vaccination against smallpox', *British Medical Journal*, 1:5275 (1962), 402.

Zweiniger-Bargielowska, Ina, 'Raising a nation of "good animals": The New Health Society and health education campaigns in interwar Britain', *Social History of Medicine*, 20:1 (2007), 73–89.

Archived internet sources

Department of Health, 'Measles, mumps and rubella vaccine (MMR)'. http://web.archive.org/web/20021213092753/ http://www.doh.gov.uk/mmr/. Captured 13 December 2002, 09:27:53; accessed 11 July 2017.

———, 'MMR: myths and truths'. https://web.archive.org/web/20021019073221/ http://www.mmrthefacts.nhs.uk:80/basics/truths.php. Captured 19 October 2002, 07:32:21; accessed 11 July 2017.

———, 'MMR the facts'. https://web.archive.org/web/20020908120649/ http://www.mmrthefacts.nhs.uk:80/. Captured 8 September 2002, 12:06:49; accessed 11 July 2017.

———, 'MMR world map'. https://web.archive.org/web/20021214014604/ http://www.mmrthefacts.nhs.uk:80/worldmap/. Captured 14 December 2002, 01:46:04; accessed 11 July 2017.

———, 'Your questions answered'. https://web.archive.org/web/20021203001027/ http://www.mmrthefacts.nhs.uk:80/questions/. Captured 3 December 2002, 00:10:27; accessed 11 July 2017.

JABS, 'Fair warning'. http://web.archive.org/web/20011025144125/ http://www.jabs.org.uk:80/jabsinformation.htm. Captured 25 October 2001, 14:41:25; accessed 1 July 2017.

———, 'Welcome to JABS on the internet'. http://web.archive.org/web/20010405035243/ http://www.jabs.org.uk. Captured 5 April 2001, 03:52:43; accessed 1 July 2017.

Legal Services Commission, 'Decision to remove funding for MMR litigation upheld on appeal'. https://web.archive.org/web/20031010112531/ http://www.legalservices.gov.uk/misl/news/press/press-13-03.htm. Captured 10 October 2003, 11:25:31; accessed 5 January 2017.

Society for the Autistically Handicapped, 'Vaccines fact sheet'. http://web.archive.org/web/20000902060843/ http://www.autismuk.com:80/index1sub4.htm. Captured 2 September 2000, 06:08:43; accessed 1 July 2017.

Film

Ministry of Health, *Surprise Attack* (1951).

Index

advertisement (advert) 49, 52, 56–7, 130, 162, 165–6, 225
  see also advertising
advertising 12, 34, 46, 50–3, 85, 89, 115, 129, 150, 165–6, 195, 199, 220, 223
  see also advertisement; publicity
AIDS *see* HIV/AIDS
anti-vaccination 1, 11, 13, 33, 86, 204, 230
Anti-Vaccination League 86
apathy 14–17, 31–2, 34, 36, 38–9, 41–6, 48–50, 52–61, 72, 87, 95, 97, 102, 116, 136, 149, 182, 188, 205, 221–3, 225, 227–9, 230–1
Australia 34, 80–3
autism 180–1, 183, 189–95, 198, 201–2

Bacillus Calmette-Guérin (BCG) *see* tuberculosis
Belfast 95–6, 133
Bevan, Aneurin (Nye), Minister of Health 35, 54, 82
Blair, Leo, son of Prime Minister Tony 191, 198
bovine spongiform-encephalopathy (BSE) 183, 192, 194–5, 222

boys
  human papillomavirus (HPV) vaccine and 1
  mumps and 187
  rubella and 187
Bradford 91–6, 102
Bristol 50, 95
  heart scandal 195
Burroughs Wellcome *see* Wellcome
Burton-on-Trent 121–2

campaign *see* advertising; publicity
Canada
  polio vaccine and 133
  smallpox and 101
  see also North America
Cardiff 91–2, 95
Castle, Barbara, Secretary of State for Social Services 159
Central Office of Information (COI) 1, 38, 44, 49, 60, 74, 84, 88
Charles, John, Chief Medical Officer 87–9
children
  differentiation by age and 36–7, 50, 55–6, 75, 99, 114, 122
  parental attitudes and 37–8, 43–5, 49, 53–4, 58, 74, 86–7, 95, 123,

Index

133, 160, 163, 186, 189, 195, 201, 203–4
representation in health education 88–9
as target population 1–3, 31–2, 36–7, 47, 50–2, 74–5, 80, 92, 96, 120, 189, 225
vaccine damage and 33, 119–20, 154–8, 188, 190–1, 194–5
voluntary organisations and 115, 156–8, 164–5, 193–4
citizens 1
consumerism and 189
health citizenship and 6, 34–9, 45, 55, 101, 152, 184, 227
interactions with health authorities and 44, 54–5, 60, 80, 82, 93
nationality and 74
relationship with the state 3, 5–6, 9, 73, 150, 222
citizenship *see* citizens
civil service 73–4, 97, 124, 149, 223
Clarke, Kenneth, Secretary of State for Health 185
clinic 15, 37, 43, 47, 50, 54, 57–60, 84, 89, 122, 126, 151, 186, 197, 225
see also surgery
Cold War 4, 102, 116, 124
Committee on the Safety of Medicines (CSM) 160–3
Commonwealth 73–4, 90–1, 124
see also empire
compensation 151, 155–60, 163–4, 185, 196, 231
compulsion 1, 12, 77–8, 82, 85–8, 94, 221, 227, 231
see also compulsory vaccination

compulsory vaccination 11, 33, 75, 82, 87, 101, 231
see also compulsion
confidence
in vaccination 3–4, 16, 86, 100, 122, 127, 137, 150, 155, 159–60, 167, 170, 180–3, 188–9, 192, 195, 197, 204–6, 222, 226, 230–1
see also trust
Congenital Rubella Syndrome (CRS) 164–5, 167–9, 187
see also rubella
Connaught 134
conscientious objection 75, 77–8, 231
Consumers' Association 158
Coseley 53–4
Coventry 116, 125–7, 131
crisis 16, 83, 92, 159, 169, 226, 231
BSE 194
Ebola 2
HIV/AIDS 5
MMR 8, 17, 137, 149, 155, 170, 180–3, 188–9, 191–4, 196–7, 200, 202–5, 224, 230, 232
pertussis vaccine 16–17, 137, 150–6, 161, 165, 168–9, 180, 187, 193–4, 197, 204–5, 228, 231
rubella and lack of 164, 168
smallpox 92
vaccine supply 95, 134
see also scandal
CRS *see* Congenital Rubella Syndrome (CRS)
CSM *see* Committee on the Safety of Medicines (CSM)
Cutter Laboratories 119–20, 122, 126

damage
  from disease 88, 160, 164, 166
  to tourism 85
  to trade 91
  to vaccination programmes 16, 55, 149, 162, 182, 189
  vaccine 150–64, 168–9, 187–8, 193, 221
death
  from disease 1, 33, 36, 39–41, 75, 81, 84–5, 90, 116–17, 130, 132, 153–4, 156, 186, 228
  from vaccine 78
Deer, Brian, investigative journalist 189, 191, 202
demand
  for compensation 150–1, 156, 158
  for protection of health 35, 39, 45, 80, 82, 91–3, 114, 150–1, 182, 189
  for vaccination 2, 15–17, 78, 80, 82–5, 91–3, 99, 102–3, 114–16, 121–31, 133–6, 149–51, 162, 166–8, 182, 185–6, 188, 220–2, 225–32
Department of Health 185–202
  see also Department of Health and Social Security; Ministry of Health
Department of Health and Social Security 100, 149, 152–3, 158, 160–9, 182, 185, 224
  see also Department of Health; Ministry of Health
Derby 58
Dick, (Professor) George, epidemiologist 95–103, 133, 157
disability 45, 117, 153, 155–6, 158–9, 163, 167–9

Donaldson, Liam, Chief Medical Officer 198–9

Ebola 2
economy 15, 91, 124
Edinburgh 84–5
education 4, 53
  compulsion, opposite of 12, 38, 78
  health 14, 17, 33, 38–9, 48, 53–4, 56–60, 84, 89, 165–6, 183, 198, 220, 224, 227
emergency
  health 2, 83
  vaccination 15, 73, 83, 87, 94, 101, 114, 225
empire 73, 83
  see also Commonwealth
England 2, 8, 53, 72–3, 83–4, 95, 97, 117, 126, 130–1, 136, 150, 181, 201–2, 220
  see also individual town names
Ennals, David, Secretary of State for Social Services 158, 161
epidemic
  control 10, 73–4, 77, 79–80, 83, 91–2, 94–5, 98–9, 102, 129, 133, 135–7, 151, 203–4
  diphtheria 12, 46, 53
  pertussis 16, 152–3, 156, 160–2, 228
  polio 41, 114, 116–19, 125–6, 128, 133–4
  rubella 163–5, 167
  smallpox 72–4, 77, 80–1, 84–5, 90, 92, 96
  see also outbreak
epidemiology 7, 94, 128, 134, 150
error of commission see error of omission
error of omission 152

faith
  in government 42, 90, 169, 183
  in medical authority 137, 183, 232
  in vaccination 16, 94, 149, 161, 169, 191, 203, 222, 230
fathers 48–9, 89
  see also mothers; parents
fear
  of bioterrorism 102
  of immigration 93
  as irrational behaviour 42, 203
  lack of 32, 44–5, 60
  as motivation 45, 49, 53, 225
  of reputational damage 13, 156
  of socialised medicine 5
  of specific diseases 16, 31–2, 36, 43, 45, 53, 114, 117, 128, 153
  of vaccines 42–3, 54
Fletcher, Jackie, campaigner 193
foreigner 83, 89, 91, 93
  see also immigrant; traveller
Fox, Rosemary, campaigner 156, 158, 160

general practitioner (GP) 37, 88, 97, 134, 149, 166, 185–8, 192, 195–7, 201, 205, 228
German measles *see* rubella
girls
  human papillomavirus (HPV) vaccine and 1
  mumps and 187, 225
  rubella and 164–7
Glasgow 8, 80, 83–5, 92, 94
Glaxo 120, 123–4
global public health 5, 103, 170, 184–5, 200, 225
Godber, George, Chief Medical Officer 92

H1N1 *see* swine flu
Halifax 93, 136
Hall, Jeff, professional footballer 116, 130–2, 162
Hamilton 83–4
hazard 78, 99, 150–2, 157, 159, 161, 193
  see also risk
Health Education Council 165, 168
  see also education
herd immunity *see* immunity
hesitancy 16–17, 170, 181, 183, 204–5, 222, 224, 228, 230–1
HIV/AIDS 5, 8, 180
Hornby-Smith, Patricia, Minister of Health 50
HPV *see* human papillomavirus
Hull, Kingston upon 135
human papillomavirus (HPV) 1, 8
hygiene thesis 118

immigrant 6, 90, 93, 99, 165, 224
  see also foreigner; traveller
immunity 10, 74, 82–3, 87, 92–3, 118–21, 126, 130, 132–3
  herd 11, 80, 96–8, 150, 157, 186, 201, 204
inactivated poliomyelitis vaccine (IPV) 119–36, 224, 227, 230–1
  see also oral poliomyelitis vaccine (OPV)
injury 100, 154–9, 164, 231
  see also damage
internet 1, 181, 189, 193, 199–202, 205
Ipswich 134
IPV *see* inactivated poliomyelitis vaccine (IPV)

Japan 170, 192, 194
Joint Committee on Poliomyelitis Vaccine (JCPV) 98, 120, 127, 129, 133, 223
Joint Committee on Vaccination and Immunisation (JCVI) 97–8, 100, 102, 149, 157, 160–1, 163, 165–7, 223
Joseph, (Sir) Keith, Secretary of State for Social Services 100
Justice Awareness and Basic Support (JABS) 193

Koprowski, Hilary, vaccinologist 132–3

laboratory accidents 72, 101, 116
Legal Services Commission 191
Lennon, Rene, campaigner 156
Liverpool 81, 134, 162
London 38–9, 41, 44, 47, 49–50, 52, 55–8, 80–2, 88, 90, 92, 101, 166, 191, 196, 202–3

Macleod, Iain, Minister of Health 119
mad cow disease *see* bovine spongiform–encephalopathy (BSE)
Manchester 52, 56
March of Dimes 119
media 1–2, 7, 10, 52, 94, 115–16, 119, 123, 125–6, 136, 154, 156–7, 162, 165, 180–1, 189–91, 193–4, 198, 227, 230, 232
Medical Officer of Health (MOH)
  autonomy of 37, 53, 79, 121
  clinics and 37, 84
  education and 38, 46, 50, 56, 78–9, 85, 88–90, 223
  epidemic control and 73, 81–5, 88, 93, 96, 125, 225
  priorities of 13, 57–8, 97
  public and 44, 50, 55–6, 58–60, 78–9, 82, 84, 93
  role of 10, 13, 37–8, 41, 43–4, 60, 73
Medical Research Council (MRC) 13, 119–20, 122–5, 127, 129, 133–4, 153
meningitis 2, 194, 229
Ministry of Health 8, 12, 14, 31–2, 36, 39, 42, 46, 48, 52, 60, 72–4, 78, 80, 82, 88, 90–1, 94, 96, 100, 115, 119–20, 123–5, 127, 130, 135, 149, 220–1, 223
  see also Department of Health; Department of Health and Social Security
monitoring 7, 17, 35–6, 42, 52, 182, 184, 188, 205, 222, 228
  see also surveillance
mothers
  activism and 155–6, 193
  apathy and 31, 43, 47, 50–5, 87
  as at-risk population 1, 165
  as decision makers 42–3, 48–9, 87, 99, 120, 224
  as targets of health education 47–9, 54
  see also women
mumps 17, 180–1, 187, 190, 193–4, 196–7, 221

National Association for Deaf/Blind and Rubella Children (NADBRC) 164, 167–8
National Baby Welfare Council 89

National Health Service (NHS) 5, 10, 14, 32, 35, 37–9, 44, 81, 84, 130, 149, 184–5, 195, 197, 200
staff 86, 91, 93–4, 100, 201
North America
measles and 231
polio vaccine and 150
smallpox and 83, 101
see also Canada; United States
Northern Ireland 97
see also Belfast

oral poliomyelitis vaccine (OPV) 95, 97, 115, 116, 132–6, 157, 205
outbreak 6, 8, 10, 224, 230
diphtheria 53, 55–60, 228
food poisoning 45
measles 1, 191, 203, 220
pertussis 150, 162–3
polio 41–2, 135, 159
smallpox 73–8, 80–8, 90–6, 99–100
Zika 1
see also epidemic

panic 56, 82, 92–3, 96, 232
parents
activism and 2, 121, 156–8, 191, 193, 231
apathy and 14, 16–17, 31–2, 41–6, 50, 54–8, 87, 116, 149, 188
choice and 36, 47, 54, 99, 128, 158, 163, 181, 184, 189, 195–201, 227, 230–2
decision making and 1–3, 14, 17, 32, 36–7, 39, 42–3, 47–8, 87, 99, 123, 127–8, 131, 152–4, 158, 160–3, 180–3, 186–9, 193, 195–6, 198–205, 230–1
demand and 2, 16, 34, 121–3, 128, 131, 133, 221, 229

education and 43–7, 50, 53–4, 78, 158, 180, 189, 195, 198–201
health citizenship and 2, 34, 45, 54–5, 152, 221
as target of public health 14–15, 32, 44–8, 52–8, 78–9, 86–9, 116, 121–3, 149–50, 162, 180–3, 188, 198–204
see also fathers; mothers
Parke-Davis 130
Pfizer 130, 132, 134
pharmaceutical
companies 15, 115, 119, 121, 127, 133, 185–6, 230
industry 3, 103, 124
see also individual firms
polio season 42, 114
Powell, Enoch, Minister of Health 92, 97, 134
publicity 2, 59, 89, 93, 119, 150, 160, 193, 198
campaign 31, 46, 56, 88, 90, 115, 130, 161, 165–6, 191, 197–9
see also advertising

randomised-control trials see trials
risk
communication and 17, 44, 47, 99, 121, 152, 162, 166, 168–9, 183, 197–202, 224
factors 5
infectious disease and 4, 7, 10, 16, 32, 36, 41, 52, 55, 57, 72, 74, 84, 87, 96, 100–1, 124, 152, 155, 162–5, 167–9, 184, 188, 194, 196, 200–1, 221, 226–8, 231
management and 6, 13, 15–16, 35, 38, 42, 57, 73, 91, 124, 152, 155, 162–3, 167–9, 182, 184, 225, 227–8

public understanding and 16–17, 45–6, 57, 80, 99, 121, 128, 131, 152, 155, 162–5, 168–9, 181, 193, 196, 199, 205, 221, 226, 228
  reputation of authorities and 15–16, 33, 73, 99, 102, 120, 127, 135, 152, 162, 165
  sociological definition 150–3, 181, 198–9, 202, 205
  specific populations and 80–1, 91, 94, 100, 163–4, 199, 204, 226
  vaccines and 39, 41, 54, 72, 74, 78, 80, 95–6, 99–101, 120, 128, 150, 152, 155–60, 162–3, 169, 196, 200–1, 221, 226
routine vaccination 1–2, 7, 11, 15–16, 72–102, 114, 126, 133, 150, 153, 164, 167, 185–6, 220–5
rubella 17, 137, 153, 163–9, 180–1, 187, 190, 193, 196–7, 225
  see also Congenital Rubella Syndrome (CRS)

Sabin, Albert, vaccinologist 132, 133
Salk (vaccine) 120, 124, 126–30, 134–6, 150, 221
  see also inactivated poliomyelitis vaccine (IPV)
Salk, Jonas, vaccinologist 119, 132, 221
scandal 6, 84, 90–1, 102, 190, 231–2
  Alder Hey 195
  Bristol Heart 195
  BSE 192, 194
  pertussis vaccine 4, 156–7, 189
  thalidomide 155
  see also crisis
schedule 3, 15, 36, 117, 153, 205, 220, 222, 229
Scope *see* Spastics Society

Scotland 2, 73, 75, 80–1, 84–7, 92, 97, 126, 130–1, 198, 201–2
  see also Scottish Office and individual town names
Scottish Office 73, 84–5, 97, 100, 120
  see also Scotland
screening 166, 184
Shipman, Harold, general practitioner/serial killer 197
shortage 2, 93–4, 115–16, 123–4, 127–8, 131, 134, 162
smallpox eradication programme 5, 74, 100
Social Survey 39, 42–4, 48–60
Soviet Union 124, 132
Spastics Society (renamed Scope) 164–8, 197
Standing Medical Advisory Committee (SMAC) 97–8
Stoke-on-Trent 55
surgery (doctor's) 37, 87, 125
  see also clinic
surveillance 32, 36–7, 61, 74, 149, 183–4, 188
  see also monitoring
swine flu (H1N1) 204

targets (statistical benchmarks) 7, 14, 37, 41, 44, 89, 95, 149, 182, 185–7, 224–5, 229
technology 3, 6, 78, 97, 114–16, 123–4, 126, 132, 134, 136, 160–1, 188, 202, 204
thalidomide 155, 158, 160–1, 164, 194, 222
traveller 7, 80, 83, 85–6, 90, 94, 102
  see also foreigner; immigrant

Index

trials 1, 36, 74, 86, 95, 115, 119–20, 132–3, 136, 188
   randomised-control 78, 119
trust 60, 194–6, 198–200, 205, 229
   see also confidence; faith
tuberculosis 6, 11, 117
   Bacillus Calmette-Guérin (BCG) and 5, 12–14, 33–4, 78, 100, 120, 161, 224
Turton, Robin, Minister of Health 120, 126

United States
   attitudes to vaccination and 2, 5, 101, 137, 170, 196
   internet usage and 199–200
   polio vaccine and 115, 119–27, 132–4, 224
   smallpox vaccination and 101
   see also North America
uptake 10, 15–16, 31–2, 37–8, 41–4, 50, 52, 79–80, 87, 90, 95–7, 101, 121, 129–31, 136, 149–50, 160, 167, 180–3, 185–8, 202, 204, 221, 223, 226, 229, 232

Vaccination Acts 11, 85
vaccine-sceptic 189, 200–1
Vaccine Damage Payments Act 1979 152
variant Creutzfeldt-Jackob disease see bovine spongiform-encephalopathy (BSE)
variolation 10
Vaughan-Morgan, John, acting Minister of Health 125–6

Wakefield (town, West Yorkshire) 121
Wakefield, Andrew, medical researcher 180, 189–94, 196–7, 201–2
Wales 8, 72, 75, 83, 91, 95, 117, 126, 130–1, 136, 150, 220
   see also individual town names
Walker-Smith, Derek, Minister of Health 129–31
welfare state 3, 34–5, 55, 150–1, 157, 160, 168–9, 222, 226, 231
Wellcome 120–1, 124, 127, 133
West Bromwich 134
women
   attitudes towards 61
   as caregivers 48, 86–7
   rubella and 163–7
   as targets of health education 49–50, 52, 164–7, 225
   voluntary organisations and 89–90, 165–7
   see also girls; mothers
Women's Voluntary Service 89
World Health Organization (WHO) 16, 74–5, 96, 100, 181–2, 185–8, 200, 202, 204, 224–5, 228
World Wide Web see internet

yellow fever 7, 225
Yellowlees, (Sir) Henry, Chief Medical Officer 166–7

Zika 1

EU authorised representative for GPSR:
Easy Access System Europe, Mustamäe tee 50,
10621 Tallinn, Estonia
gpsr.requests@easproject.com

www.ingramcontent.com/pod-product-compliance
Ingram Content Group UK Ltd.
Pitfield, Milton Keynes, MK11 3LW, UK
UKHW021824140426
5217IPUK00004B/75